Children's Phonetic Disorders
Theory and Treatment

Children's Phonetic Disorders
Theory and Treatment

Paul R. Hoffman, Ph.D.
Associate Professor of Communication Disorders, Louisiana State University, Baton Rouge, Louisiana

Gordon H. Schuckers, Ph.D.
Professor of Communication Disorders and Associate Dean, School of Allied Health Professions, Louisiana State University Medical Center, Shreveport, Louisiana

Raymond G. Daniloff, Ph.D.
Professor and Director of Communication Disorders, Louisiana State University, Baton Rouge, Louisiana

A College-Hill Publication
Little, Brown and Company
Boston/Toronto/London

College-Hill Press
A Division of
Little, Brown and Company (Inc.)
34 Beacon Street
Boston, Massachusetts 02108

Library of Congress Cataloging in Publication Data
Main entry under title:

Hoffman, Paul R.
Children's phonetic disorders / Paul R. Hoffman, Gordon H. Schuckers, Raymond G. Daniloff.
p. cm.
"A College-Hill publication."
Bibliography: p.
Includes index.
ISBN 0-316-36837-7
1. Articulation disorders in children—Treatment. 2. Speech therapy for children. 3. English language—Phonetics.
I. Schuckers, Gordon. II. Daniloff, Raymond. III. Title.
RJ496.S7H56 1989
618.92'855—dc19 89-2788
CIP

Printed in the United States of America
EB

This volume is dedicated to

Our students
for constantly asking "Why?"

The children we've met in therapy and in studies
for supplying the answers

Don and Peg, Jeff and Mary, James and Mary
for raising us so that childhood and children are dear

Zack, Jeff, and Brent
for reminding us to look at the world through children's eyes

Mary Ann, Rita, and Joanne
for reminding us to be adults, now and then

Contents

Preface

This text is intended for use in courses in articulation disorders. The title highlights our concern with *phonetic* processing (i.e., the way speech sounds are produced by the vocal tract and perceived by eye and ear) because children's speech is recognized as being outside the normal developmental sequence at this most peripheral level of analysis. Furthermore, clinicians measure and attempt to improve children's speech by asking them to observe, listen to, and produce speech.

These emphases differ from many currently available texts addressing disordered speech that use the label "phonological." This difference is not because we dismiss the importance of cognitive processing implicit in the phonological approach. Rather, we believe that cognitive processing is intimately related to phonetic level articulatory movements and auditory, visual, and somesthetic feedback characteristics of speech production.

To speak of a distinction between phonetic and phonological disorders implies that the two are somehow disconnected, that phonological disorders are "mentalistic" and therefore distinct from "physical" realities of speech production and perception. This view implies that phonological knowledge can be separated from language and targeted in speech production and perception exercises. Instead, we advocate the synergistic unity of cognition and sensation in phonetic behavior.

In particular, we think that cognitive processing involved in speech sound production and perception uses as its most basic units the sensory perceptions derived from the vocal tract, as well as auditory and visual systems. We are convinced that these basic perceptions are integrated in the nervous system, through learning, into phonemic, word, and higher-order *concepts* related to propositions. Thus, control of speech production is intimately related to propositions that a child interprets and produces in social interactions.

The result of this assumption is that treatment of disordered sound production must occur in a social interaction in which the child attempts to communicate with others. We advocate that the clinician assume the role of a "partner-in-communication" who expedites the child's interpretations and productions of speech acts, including the phonetic level detail of those speech acts.

Besides providing information specific to the nature of children's disordered speech production, its measurement, and its treatment, we want to instill the concept that clinicians are scientists. Clinicians must know how to ask questions about their clients, must find ways of measuring improved performance, and must realize that their own performance can be measured and varied when needed. We have attempted to exemplify this process throughout the text.

The topical organization of this text is designed to suit the needs of most majors in speech-language pathology. Such students typically take a course in articulation disorders as one of their first courses in disordered communication. Before taking this course, the student should have taken courses in phonetics, anatomy and physiology of speech production, introductory linguistics, and language acquisition. It has been our experience that students have a difficult time assimilating such information into a unified body of knowledge. They learn static descriptions of speech sounds using place-manner-voicing categories in articulatory phonetics. They learn the bones, cartilages, and muscles related to speech production in anatomy and physiology of speech. But they often don't discover that abstract categories of the phonetician are assumed to function as control parameters in the nervous system, directing the contraction of muscles to produce specific movements of articulators to approximate those speech sound categories. Often, none of these courses teaches students about acoustic attributes of speech or the kind of cognitive processing involved in speech perception. The student may learn a schedule of normal speech sound development but may not relate this information to concurrent development of language at other levels, or the relationship between speech sound development and the anatomical growth of the vocal tract.

We sought to rectify this situation by presenting in Chapter 1 a model of adult phonetic processing based on parallel distributed processing models of cognition being developed for a wide range of cognitive functions (Rumelhart and McClelland and others, 1986). The model contains levels of cognitive organization that are hierarchically embedded in one another. The model is said to be parallel because processing occurs at all levels simultaneously. A speaker is simultaneously aware of wanting to have an effect on a listener, the concepts that are most salient in a particular situation, the proposition to be expressed about those concepts, and, to a lesser degree, the English phrases and words that are part of the utterances produced. The speaker typically uses knowledge of syllables, phonemes, and features of those language units in a fairly automatic, nonconscious manner.

The student will have been introduced to higher levels of this model (i.e., meaning, concepts, propositions, and meaningful linguistic units) in introductory linguistics courses. The middle layers of the model, syllables and phonemes, are introduced to most students in a course in articulatory phonetics. The lowest level, features, discusses the anatomical system that controls speech production, a topic introduced in courses in anatomy and physiology of speech production.

This model is described as "distributed" because each level does not exist as discrete entities that pass inputs and outputs to one another. Rather, representations of conceptual knowledge are contained in learned connections among the most basic units or perceptible features. Each phoneme exists as an intersection of connections among the applicable vocal tract, auditory, and visual features at the lower level and the words in which they occur at higher levels. Connections that are formed represent patterns of language structure and use that are often characterized using rule statements in phonological models.

The main topics discussed in each chapter are listed at the beginning of the chapters to help students organize information. A perusal of these lists will show the instructor where topical emphasis has been placed. At the conclusion of each chapter a few class activities are suggested. The activities are intended to be incorporated into class discussions to help the student assimilate the more important aspects of that chapter. In general, these build toward being more directly applicable to the conduct of therapy for misarticulating children. For example, at the end of the first chapter students are asked to create a narrative about a picture using sentences that vary in propositional complexity from descriptive to inferential. In the second chapter, students are asked to elicit and describe the propositional complexity of stories of normally developing children at a variety of ages. In the third, they are asked to repeat this process with children whose speech is disordered. In the fourth, articulation errors of these children are analyzed. In the fifth, students are asked to use the basic procedures detailed to produce improvements in a child's articulation during the telling of a story. One or two students, typically those who have children or who are currently enrolled in practicum classes, can be recorded in these activities and the class can participate in analysis and discussion of the recording. Alternatively, the instructor can construct tapes that illustrate these various exercises.

Chapter 1 is divided into three major topics: cognitive aspects, sensory-motor aspects, and auditory-perceptual aspects. The section on cognitive aspects presents an overview of the higher levels of the model—meaning, propositions, and linguistic meaning units in overview. The syllable structure level is discussed in somewhat more detail. The phonemic level receives comprehensive coverage and presents a review of the articulatory phonetic description of speech sounds.

The section on sensory-motor aspects exemplifies use of syllabic shape and phonemic levels in control of speech production. Primary emphasis is provided in describing the articulatory gestures used to actually approximate vocal tract shapes described in an articulatory phonetic classification of speech sounds. Muscles that provide the motive power for these movements are also detailed at this point, and nervous system components involved in directing the muscular contractions are overviewed.

The section on auditory-perceptual aspects provides a description of the acoustic elements of sound sources and filters, acoustic characteristics of speech sound classes, and effects of dynamic movement patterns on a sound's representation in different contexts. A model of speech perception based on the overall parallel distributed model is then presented.

Chapter 2 reviews normal development of phonetic processing using the major divisions of the first chapter. We make the basic assumption that development of language is an additive learning process in which the child develops closer and closer approximations of adult-like organization of basic perceptible features into conceptual categories of phonemes, words, propositions, and so forth.

This view contrasts with current phonological descriptions of this process suggesting that the child uses cognitive strategies to either "suppress" innate knowledge or "test hypotheses" about the structure of adult language. Both of these notions appear to us to attribute too much abstract knowledge to the developing child. Conversely, we assume that development is driven by the child's need to effectively interact with others in a social setting. Children refine their concepts to more closely match those of adults as they experience communication failures based on faulty concepts. The child's apparent cognitive goal is not to propose hypotheses about the structure of English, or any other parent language, but rather to have a desired effect on a listener. The child improves this communicative function by matching concepts, including phonemes, syllable shapes, and words, used in the environment.

Each section of this chapter is organized according to Nelson's (1985) stages of development—prelexical, cognitive, and semantic. The child's prelexical communication is bound directly to the social situation. Individual children use physiologically possible speech sound productions to express intentions within social situations. Speech sounds have not been organized into adult-like conceptual categories. The organization of language symbols becomes more adult-like as the child perceives patterns of speech produced by adults. Each time a syllabic or phonemic pattern is heard by the child, appropriate connections are established. The infant enters into this process with the ability to discriminate basic auditory features and coordinate them with visual and motoric features. Phonemic, syllabic, and word patterns are established among these features as caretakers talk to the child and provide opportunities for child responses.

Speech production during the prelexical stage is described with respect to the changing anatomy of the infant vocal tract, which defines at any age what sounds the child can produce for communicative purposes. Motoric patterns for adult-like syllables and phonemes are established as the child's sound productions are consequented by the caretaker (i.e., treated as though they were meaningful).

Development during the cognitive stage involves progressive approximation of syllabic, phonemic, and feature level concepts similar to those of the adult community as described in the first chapter. Inasmuch as all children have approximately the same physiological capabilities and are trying to approximate similar speech inputs from the adult community, their speech approximations and failures will be similar during this stage. These similarities are attributed in the current literature to the use of phonological processes or the child's postulation of linguistic rules. We maintain that the processes or rules are not cognitive mechanisms but are the results, or products, of conceptual development. For example, during early development in this stage, children typically produce few consonant clusters. This has been described as the result of a rule called "cluster reduction." Rather than suggesting that a child has proposed a rule that deletes consonants from clusters, we propose that their conceptual development at the syllabic level is not yet fully realized. As the child needs to refine productions of words like *tree* to contrast them with words like *tea,* he will necessarily develop such syllable shapes. Thus, the apparent rule of cluster reduction will appear to be suppressed. However, we maintain that the "rule" was only apparent—that it was the *result* not the *cause* of the child's cognitive organization.

During the semantic phase, children learn to use language concepts to form more abstract concepts. The child learns to use basic language concepts developed in the cognitive phase to mentally represent things not immediately perceptible—for example, past events and predictions about future events. It is at this stage of development that the child learns to use language to talk about language as an abstract set of objects such as words and sentences. During the conceptual stage, children use language as a social communication tool; in the semantic phase they start to use language as a thinking tool. Speech production continues to be refined during this period as the child apparently refines the use and overlapping of gestures to more efficiently produce speech.

The third chapter reviews what is generally known about children's disordered phonetic processing. An overview of the development of theories of children's misarticulations is provided as well as basic information about the process underlying conduct of empirical studies. The three major sections review the study of children's misarticulation from three historically-ordered perspectives—sensory-motor, auditory-perceptual, and cognitive-linguistic. The review of studies in each section is intended to be illustrative rather than exhaustive.

The sensory-motor section discusses the search for organic causes for misarticulation in anatomical structure and neurological deficits. The research cited provides examples of descriptive studies of speech production in populations with known organic problems and the physiological capabilities of children with functional misarticulation. It includes discussion of descriptive and treatment studies that analyzed effects of syllable position and phonetic context factors.

The auditory-perceptual section describes studies of speech productions of the hearing impaired. It also discusses evidence linking misarticulation with speech perception problems.

The cognitive-linguistic section discusses the relationship between speech production and general intelligence. It also describes the relationship between speech production errors and higher levels of language organization. Finally, the view that functional misarticulation is caused by faulty phonological processing is discussed.

The fourth chapter describes the clinical process of assessing phonetic ability as being similar to an empirical investigation. The first section describes how the clinician-scientist uses a case history to ask questions about a child, uses articulation tests to provide data, summarizes those data, and makes treatment decisions. Each of these stages is described with reference to published articulation tests and examples of data from two children. The discussion is intended to be illustrative rather than exhaustive. Particular test instruments are used as examples of the process. The clinical examples were chosen to represent what we consider to be the two major types of misarticulating children—a preschool child exhibiting multiple phoneme misarticulations and an elementary school child with a single phoneme misarticulation.

The chapter describes how clinicians determine if a child's speech is disordered or normal and how to describe disordered speech. Descriptions of children's misarticulation are presented using a variety of analyses—word position analysis, syllable position analysis, and analysis of common error approximations. Commonly occurring error approximations are described with respect to the syllabic, phonemic, and feature levels of the model presented in Chapter 1.

The final chapter discusses the clinical process of articulation therapy. We first describe components of this process by referring to a variety of treatment approaches proposed over the years from traditional to phonological. Perhaps the most important component is the role taken by the clinician. We view the clinician as being a counselor who seeks to help the child communicate more effectively. At the conclusion of this chapter, two overlapping treatment programs are suggested. These are intended to be used with children at different stages of language development. For the child in the semantic phase, the clinician can more directly discuss with the child the nature of speech sound production, the child's errors, and the process of actively practicing and monitoring aspects of speech production. For the younger child in the conceptual phase, we suggest a holistic approach to language improvement based on the child's ability to communicate effectively.

It is our hope that students who use this text will learn enough from it to direct their first clinical sessions with a sense of positive anticipation instead of trepidation. They will learn much from the children they serve if only they take the time to listen. We look forward to learning from our colleagues-to-be who use this text. We thank our current colleagues for the time they spend questioning our theories and suggesting alternatives. In particular, we thank Dr. Jan Norris for her suggestions regarding parallel distributed processing models and her keen clinical insight into therapy processes. Our appreciation also goes to Dr. Colleen Wilcox for supplying her artwork and to Jim Wilson for his excellent work on graphs and illustrations. And finally we thank the students who wrote the stories used as examples in the appendix.

P.R.H.
G.H.S.
R.G.D.

Children's Phonetic Disorders
Theory and Treatment

CHAPTER 1

Adult Phonetic Processing

Topics in this chapter include

- Cognitive Aspects
  - Meaning
  - Concepts
  - Propositions
  - Linguistic Meaning Units
  - Syllable Structures
  - Phonemes
- Sensory-Motor Aspects
  - Syllabic Organization
  - Phonemic Organization
  - Gestural Organization
  - Muscular Organization
- Auditory-Perceptual Aspects
  - Acoustic Representation of Speech
  - Model of Speech Perception

Phonetic processing refers to the production and perception of speech sounds, the most palpable stages of the synergistic process of verbal communication. Verbal communication is synergistic inasmuch as a variety of physiological, sensory, and cognitive processes interact with one another, causing unique higher order processes to emerge from the interaction of lower order processes. Verbal communication involves the production and interpretation of speech acts. A speech act is an action that is performed by speaking to alter the listener's attitudes, beliefs, or actions (Searle, 1969).

Consider the following speech act. You are sitting in the back of a classroom, next to the light switch, waiting for a lecture to start. The professor walks to a film projector, looks at you and says "Hit the switch." You turn off the lights, and the professor starts a film. The professor uttered the words "Hit the switch" for the purpose of altering your behavior. If you turned the lights off, the utterance served as the professor's instrument because it accomplished some task.

As the listener in this situation, you sought to interpret the intention motivating the professor's speech act. You have learned from your social interactions with others that language is sometimes used to direct one's actions. You know that it is socially appropriate for a professor to ask a student to do certain things related to classroom activities. You would react quite differently if the professor asked you to slap the person in the next seat, because slapping would usually be considered inappropriate behavior in the classroom social context.

To interpret this speech act, you had to determine its underlying proposition and concepts. This speech act contained a proposition coordinating two concepts. We can roughly characterize these concepts as "turn off" and "the lights." The concepts were represented by English phrases. The professor could have chosen a number of different English expressions, including "Turn off the lights," "Hit the switch," or "Kill those" (accompanied by a gesture toward the lights) to accomplish the same end.

Your interpretation depended on your conceptual knowledge. The propositions expressed must be related to a conceptual knowledge of objects and actions in the real world. To execute the professor's request, you needed to know enough about film projection to understand that it requires a darkened room. You needed to understand enough about electrical circuits to know how electrical lights are turned off using switches. When listeners do not have enough background knowledge, they fail to receive the intended message. Most of us would fail to carry out a request by an electrical engineer to "change the resistance in the lighting circuit" because we do not understand electricity at that conceptual level, and thus we would not be able to interpret the English expressions used to refer to the concepts of "circuits" and "electrical resistance."

In this first chapter, we will explore a model of the psychological and physiological processing required for verbal communication. This chapter is presented with the hope that it will set a context for the understanding of phonetic processes used by normal adults. The adult form of phonetic processing is the final stage of normal development as described in Chapter 2. The model of adult verbal communication and its developmental stages will provide us with points of comparison when we study disordered articulation in Chapter 3. The model of adult performance also serves as the goal for the speech-language pathologist who measures and treats disordered articulation as described in Chapters 4 and 5.

The first section of this chapter, entitled "Cognitive Aspects," discusses a model of the abstract-meaning linguistic system involved in verbal communication. It is intended to show how speech sound production is an integral part of verbal communication, an important consideration in determining how to test and plan for remediation of a patient's phonetic processing. Speech errors occur as part of the overall process and may not be easily changed if treated in isolation from the rest of the communication system.

The second section of this chapter, "Sensory-Motor Aspects," details physiological mechanisms involved in speech production. One aspect of phonetic processing is articulation of speech sounds. The verb *articulate* literally means "to bring together." Speech articulation refers to the process of bringing together parts of the vocal tract to produce speech sounds. The professor probably chose to represent this speech act verbally because speech production is faster and less ambiguous than using hand gestures or writing on the chalk board.

Although swift and seemingly effortless, speech production is a demanding physiological activity. In uttering the words "Hit the switch," the professor was simultaneously controlling the activities of 7 articulators. (Articulators are anatomical structures that move toward one another to form speech sounds.) For example, the *t* sound in the word *hit* was produced by raising the front of the tongue toward the upper front teeth. The movement of the tongue tip was coordinated with movement of the jaw (i.e., the jaw was raised to assist in raising the front of the tongue).

Not only does each speech sound's production involve the coordination of many articulators, the movements involved in the production of a particular speech sound are adjusted to take into account the speech sounds that surround it. If you utter the phrase "hit Tom," the front of the tongue will touch the bony ridge behind the front teeth rather than the upper front teeth, as was the case in "Hit the switch." To demonstrate the difference in these two phrases, say each aloud and stop yourself during the *t* sound of *hit*. By anticipating the tongue position for the next sound, a speaker produces faster, smoother speech than if each sound were produced the same way in all contexts. Such anticipation allows us to produce conversational speech at rates of 8 to 10 sounds per second.

An individual speech gesture, such as raising the tongue tip to the upper teeth, is produced by the coordinated contractions of a group of muscles. Individual muscle contractions must be adjusted to blend with the simultaneous contractions of all the other muscles involved in the movement of the articulator. For example, a muscle called the *superior longitudinal* acts to raise the tongue tip whereas the *inferior longitudinal* and the anterior portion of the *genioglossus* muscle act to lower the tongue tip. If a speaker simultaneously contracted all of these muscles strongly, the movement of the tongue would be stiff and unpredictable. Rather, the speaker must relax the muscles that lower the tongue tip while contracting those that raise the tongue tip to cause a smooth movement toward the roof of the mouth.

As with other automatized motor activities such as walking or reaching, the cognitive and physiological control of speech articulation is virtually unconscious. The professor, saying "Hit the switch," was primarily aware of an intention and to a lesser degree a choice of words. It is highly unlikely that the professor was aware of how the articulators were moving.

The third section of this chapter, "Auditory-Perceptual Aspects," presents a model of the psychological processing involved in perception of speech sounds. The acoustic characteristics of a speech sound depend on the shape of the vocal tract at each instant of time. Sound waves such as speech represent a flow of energy that can be described physically in terms of time-varying patterns of air pressure. Physical descriptors of sound waves include (1) intensity, which is primarily interpreted by a human listener as loudness, (2) frequency, which is primarily interpreted as pitch, and (3) spectral shape, which is interpreted as quality or timbre.

By overlapping the movements of articulators, the speaker not only increases speed of production but also produces different acoustic representations of a particular speech sound in different contexts. For example, say the words *see* and *sue*. As you say each, extend the *s* sounds. When you produce the word *sue*, your lips will be rounded. When you produce the word *see* your lips will be spread. These two *s* sounds differ acoustically. The lip-rounded *s* will have lower spectral frequencies than the lip spread *s*. Listeners learn to interpret these differing acoustic events as representatives of a single English phoneme *s*.

It is important for the speech-language pathologist to understand the process of speech perception because children learn to articulate speech largely through hearing their own speech and that of others. Some children may fail to develop acceptable articulation skills because they do not perceive speech well. Furthermore, the clinician's primary tools in altering a child's articulation are based in the clinician's speech acts that must be heard and acted on by the child.

COGNITIVE ASPECTS

In this section, a model of verbal communication is presented that is similar to the parallel distributed models of cognition proposed by Rumelhart, McClelland, and the PDP Research Group (1986). In such models, knowledge is organized into overlapping processing levels. For example, a per-

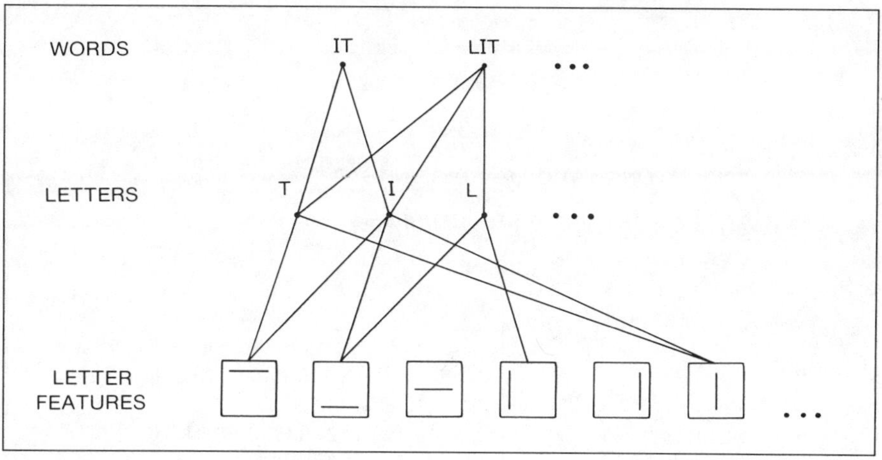

Fig. 1-1. Simplified parallel distributed model of reading.

son's knowledge of verbal communication no doubt involves a *word level* that contains processing units for each word known by that person. The processing units at each level exist as an organization of processing units present at lower and higher levels. For example, the processing units at the word level exist as connection strengths among more basic units such as speech sounds, visual characteristics of objects and actions, and auditory characteristics of objects and actions. The processing units at the word level are also associated with other word units via connections to propositions in which each has occurred in the individual's experience. For example, the words *man* and *woman* occur as "actors" in a variety of propositions and are thus related to one another inasmuch as both occur in propositions such as "The ______ is walking."

The organization of verbal knowledge in such models exists as connection strengths among units between levels and within a particular level. This organization is said to be *distributed* because information about a particular concept is not localized in a particular part of the nervous system. Except for the most basic units, which are sensory in nature, a unit does not exist as a discrete entity. Rather, a unit exists as a network of relationships among other units. Processing is said to be *parallel* because it occurs simultaneously at all levels. This parallel processing occurs because connection strengths cross all levels.

Consider the simplified model of reading shown in Fig. 1-1. This model has three processing levels: letter features, letters, and words. As a person reads a word, processing occurs at all three levels simultaneously. The elementary sensory-neural code generated by the eye activates appropriate *letter features.* Connections between the letter features and the letters activate certain letter units. Connections between the letter and word levels activate

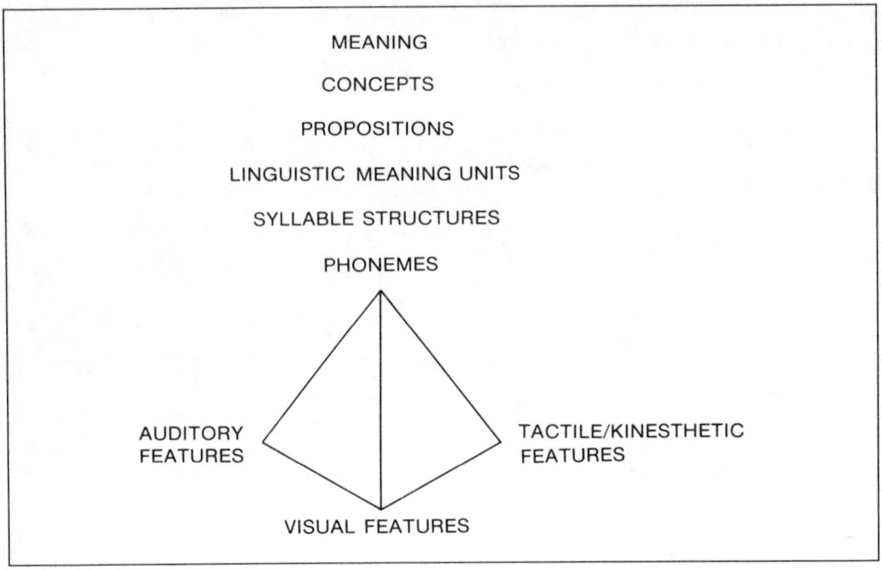

Fig. 1-2. Model of verbal communication.

certain word units. As a word is scanned from left to right, information at all levels is used to decide which word is present. This processing is bidirectional, moving up and down the levels of the model. The use of information at the word level makes recognition of the letter units faster if a word unit is known (i.e., connections already exist between the letter units at the word level). Thus, you will recognize the letter sequences *IT* and *LIT* faster than you will the sequence *ITI* because the former are also words that you have processed before and for which connection strengths already exist.

Each of the three levels contains units. The most basic units in this model are the six letter features: the high horizontal line, low horizontal line, central horizontal line, left-sided vertical line, right-sided vertical line, and central vertical line. The second highest level contains letter units. Each letter exists as connections among the various letter features. A *T* exists only as positive connections between a high horizontal line and a central vertical line. A *T* will also be related to other letters that share similar letter features (e.g., *T* is more strongly related to *I* than *L* because it shares two features with *I* and only one with *L*). When people misread letters they are more likely to make mistakes including letters that share more features because the perception of a particular feature activates all of the positively connected letters at the next level. The word units exist as connection strengths among the letter units. Connections among *L, I,* and *T* represent the spelling of the word *LIT*.

Figure 1-2 shows a model of the interconnected processing levels underlying verbal communication. It is divided into seven processing levels: meaning, concepts, propositions, linguistic meaning units, syllable structures, phonemes, and features. Each level is discussed in more detail below. As we move closer to the levels of production and perception of speech sounds, our discussion will become more detailed with respect to the nature of the units involved. The higher levels are briefly described to set a context for the production and perception of speech sounds.

MEANING

The *meaning level* represents the broadest level of cognitive organization. It contains all of the possible connections among the processing units within the person's cognitive system, including all of the subsequent levels: concepts, propositions, linguistic meaning units, and so forth. These connections have been established through an individual's social interactions, perceptions of sensory inputs, and patterns of action. This broad information base is available for creation of concepts with which a person can make inferences and denote attributes of objects, actions, and social interactions.

A person's development of meaning depends on the perceptual information available at the lowest level of the model. Consider the information base of a person who is blind from birth. This person's knowledge of objects and actions will be represented in connection strengths related to sensory inputs such as touch, taste, and sound. The lack of visual sensory experiences precludes a knowledge of "color" as experienced by the sighted person. Furthermore, the blind person's inability to track changes in the location of distant objects and their states makes it more difficult for the blind person to code these changes in a language system. Similarly, a hearing impaired person's knowledge of musical concepts will be different from that of a hearing person because many of the tonal qualities contained in music are not available for processing. The hearing impaired individual faces further problems coding experiences through verbally presented language forms.

CONCEPTS

Each individual organizes meaning into *concepts* by creating connection strengths between related perceptions and actions. For example, "color" and "music" are conceptual relationships among the possible perceptions that a person has actively organized. The person's social environment directs the individual's formation of concepts for those aspects of meaning that are considered important. In a mechanized society, certain mathematical skills are valued and actively taught to children. The degree of conceptual organization reached by an individual will depend on the person's participation in goal-directed sensory and motor experiences. The musician has actively organized the concepts of pitch, tone, and rhythm to a much higher degree than those of us who are "tone deaf." These concepts make the musician capable of finer analyses of music into discrete units than the untrained listener. The painter understands colors and their composition relative to the primary colors better than those of us who are content in the knowledge that "blue and yellow make green."

Consider some of the concepts associated with a simple coffee cup. At a basic level, coffee cups are expected to exist in a certain size range: A coffee cup should be smaller than a 40-gallon drum of oil. A coffee cup is expected to have a handle and is thus different from a bowl. Persons who have used coffee cups will also associate these concepts with their uses. A cup should hold drinkable liquids, unlike the oil drum. The handle is grasped by thumb and forefinger; therefore, part of your knowledge of coffee cups exists as connection strengths to appropriate hand and arm movements. The arm is used to lift the cup to the lips, and so on. A person who drinks coffee at home, at work, and at a coffee shop every day has probably organized concepts such as "coffee" and "coffee cups" differently and has created more connections than the child who has never had coffee and thinks that cups should hold milk.

PROPOSITIONS

In planning speech acts, or in processing the speech acts of others, an individual relates concepts to one another in *propositions.* Propositions are the basic underlying ideas expressed in a speech act. Propositions vary in complexity depending on the number of concepts that are related to one another and the degree to which these concepts must be supplied by the individual as opposed to being directly stimulated by the person's immediate surroundings. To illustrate different levels of propositions, we will present four types of propositions: *labels, descriptions, interpretations,* and *inferences.* Each of these levels is exemplified with reference to the first drawing in Appendix A. It is a typical summer street scene in which a woman is walking away from a vendor and his ice cream truck toward two boys who are playing catch with a baseball.

A proposition that *labels* a portion of the drawing represents the lowest level of propositionality. For example, the sentence "This is a boy" would provide a label for a portion of the visual perception of someone looking at this drawing. To apply this label, the speaker would have to relate the immediate perception of a portion of this scene to his or her concepts and language forms (i.e., the label *boy* and an appropriate sentence structure that points out this concept such as "This is a boy").

Description essentially adds another proposition to the original label that is readily apparent in the perceptual features of the scene. For example, "The boy is smiling" includes the label expressed in the first proposition and highlights some observable features of the boy's face (i.e., that his lips are spread). Both of these concepts are readily observable in the perceptual characteristics of the drawing. The act of adding information to a proposition in this fashion is called *predicating*.

In an *interpretation* the predication that is added to the original topic or label is displaced from the speaker's immediate perception. The predication may be about the internal states and motives underlying observable actions. For example, "The boy is happy to get the ice cream" assigns a quality (i.e., happiness) to something observable in the drawing (i.e., the smile and the ice cream). The quality itself is not directly observable but is attached to something that is observable. A number of language forms are used to express such relationships (e.g., "because," "if," "trying to," "sometimes," "when").

In an *inference* the speaker creates relationships among perceptual features from a knowledge of possible relationships. The speaker must infer actions that occurred before and after the depicted actions and changes in the spatial relationships among objects. For example, "The boy will eat the ice cream" predicts what will happen in this scene, even though the action of eating is not depicted in the picture. "The mother is rewarding the children for being good" infers the mother's motives and previous actions of the children.

LINGUISTIC MEANING UNITS

The concepts developed by an individual may be associated with linguistic symbols such as morphemes, words, and phrases. For example, in the sentence "The boy likes ice cream," "the boy" can be considered a phrase unit. The individual words of this unit are often associated with one another in English utterances so that a speaker of English senses that it is unnatural to say "Boy likes ice cream." The word *likes* involves two morpheme units, the word *like* and the *s* that relates this verb to an agent (the boy) who is singular and in the third person relative to the speaker of the utterance. Although these linguistic symbols are first used in conversations with others, they will eventually be usable in thought processes so that an individual can silently contemplate the world or even imagined worlds.

The basic units of meaning proposed here are words or morphemes, depending on the sophistication of the speaker/listener. A word is a combination of relationships among the perceptions and actions of the person that has been connected to a linguistic form. For example, the word *cow* is associated with a group of animals. Which group of animals this word refers to will depend on the person's conceptual knowledge. For children growing up in a city environment, *cow* may represent a relatively large, nonspecific group of animals. The child growing up on a farm will more quickly differentiate the animals labelled by *cow* from those labelled *bull* and will also learn to differentiate *dairy* from *beef* cows. The city dweller may not distinguish *cows* from *bulls* because the difference is unimportant to his or her day-to-day routine. However, the child of a farmer distinguishes between bulls and cows in part because of experiences with the two types of animals. A cow can be milked, and it is much less dangerous for the child to walk among the cows than it is to enter into the bull's area. Referring back to the electricity example used before, most of us understand something about the things that we can do with electricity (e.g., turn on lights and run dishwashers); however, most of us have difficulty distinguishing between "alternating current" and "direct current," labels that refer to much more specific concepts for the electrical engineer who uses these different types of electricity for different purposes.

Morphemes are units of meaning that may either stand alone as words (e.g., *cow, dog, run, his*), or are combined to make words (e.g., "re" "mark" "able"). Those morphemes that can stand alone as words are known as *free morphemes* (e.g., "mark"). Those that must be combined in words are called *bound morphemes* (e.g., "re"). Bound morphemes include common prefixes such as the "re" in *remarkable* and suffixes such as the "ish" in *bookish*. These morphemes may act to change the function of a word. For example, adding "ish" changes the function of the word *book* from being a label for a class of objects to being a description applied to a person. However, many people, including children at various stages of development, do not necessarily know that a word such as *bookish* is divisible into these smaller units. This knowledge may be something that is acquired when the person is taught how to read, write, and make reference to dictionaries that make use of morphemic units.

Perhaps a more basic type of bound morpheme consists of those morphemes that are used to express time relationships (e.g., *walk ing, walk s, walk ed*). These morphemes are learned by children as mechanisms for expressing differences in the time of occurrence of a particular action. Another morpheme that would appear to be learned regardless of a speaker's literacy is that which expresses plural number (e.g., *s* in *cats*).

As the person organizes more complex propositions, these basic meaningful units are related to one another using words that have meaning not because they refer to concepts but because they express relationships among propositions. For example, a number of propositions related to the first drawing in Appendix A might be as follows: "This is a boy," "This woman is the boy's mother," "The woman is giving the boy ice cream," "The boy likes ice cream," "The boy is happy." As a child develops the abilities to infer and interpret, these propositions could be expressed by combining them into a single sentence such as "The boy is happy because his mother is giving him the ice cream that she promised." Production of this utterance requires learning the use of a number of nonspecific words (i.e., words that refer to different persons, things, and actions depending on their linguistic

Table 1-1. COMMONLY OCCURRING ENGLISH SYLLABLE STRUCTURES

Syllable structure	*Word*
V	I
VC	it
VCC	ask
CV	pie
CCV	spy
CCCV	spry
CVC	pipe
CVCC	Max
CVCCC	lamps

context). This sentence employs pronouns such as "his" and "him," which refer to the boy, and "she," which refers to the mother. The meaning of these words changes with the context. The word *because* is used to express a relationship between otherwise unconnected propositions. This word does not have meaning outside of this relationship, which has been interpreted by the listener.

SYLLABLE STRUCTURES

Each meaningful unit is associated with a pattern of speech sounds that involves differing degrees of opening of the vocal tract. Speech sounds that are produced with very open vocal tracts allow more energy to escape to the listener who perceives these sounds as being louder. These louder sounds, typically vowels, are described as being *sonorant*. The sonorant sounds alternate with nonsonorant consonant sounds to form syllables. Each syllable has a vowel or a vowellike sound as its nucleus (or center) and may have consonants or combinations of consonants preceding or following the vowel. Table 1-1 shows some examples of words with a variety of syllable structures.

Some of the consonant sounds occur at the beginning and the end of syllables, whereas others occur only at the beginning or end. The sounds /w/, /j/, and /h/ all occur at the beginning of syllables but not at the end. These sounds are the first sounds in the words *wing, yes,* and *help,* but they do not occur as syllable-final sounds. The sound /ŋ/ does not occur at the beginning of syllables but does occur at the end of syllables (e.g., *wing*).

Only certain combinations of consonants cluster together in English at the beginning and end of words. Only /s/ begins a word-initial triple-consonant cluster. It must be followed by either /p/, /t/, or /k/, which must be followed by /l/ or /r/, as in the words — *spring, split, string,* and *scrap.*

Other sound combinations occur in two consonant clusters. In word-initial positions, the sound /s/ can be followed by /p, t, k, m, n, l, w/ as exemplified in the words *speak, steak, skate, smile, snake, slime,* and *swim.* The sounds /l, r/ can be preceded by a number of different consonants at the beginning of a syllable, as in the words *threat, flake, fry, play, pray, brake, blade, trade, drake, clown, crown, glow, grow.*

Other consonant clusters occur at the end of syllables. The sound /s/ is followed by /p, t, k/, as in *clasp, cast,* and *cask.* The sound /z/ is followed by /m/ as in *chasm.* The sound /n/ is followed by /t, d/ in *went* or *wind.* The sound /ŋ/ is followed by /k/ in *ink.* The sound /m/ is followed by /p/ in *camp;* /l/ is followed by /p, m, t, k/ in *help, helm, halt,* and *hulk,* and /t/ is preceded by /f, p, k/ in *aft, apt,* and *act.*

Morphemes or words may be multisyllabic as well as monosyllabic. When a word or morpheme contains more than one syllable, levels of syllable stress come into play. Such word-level stress patterns are generally predictable in English. However, stress is sometimes used in English to distinguish some aspects of word meaning. In a number of cases the difference between nouns and verbs is indicated by stress contour. For example, stress occurs on the first syllable of the nouns *conflict* and *insight* and on the second syllable of the verbs *conflict* and *incite.*

PHONEMES

The meaningful units are connected to particular sequences of distinctive speech sounds known as *phonemes.* Each phoneme is connected to a particular set of features. The features are all sensory in nature. Thus, the phoneme is a pattern of connections among auditory, visual, and tactile-kinesthetic sensations. These patterns guide the formulation of motoric plans for the production of sound segments and serve as sensory complexes used in the interpretation of another speaker's intended phonemes during speech perception.

The phonemic connections developed by an individual depend on the language the person learns. Learning phonemes involves finding out which sensory complexes are considered to be same and which are considered to be different. A child learns this by learning words that differ in phonemic structure. A phonemic contrast between two sounds will be established when the change from one feature complex to another is associated with changes in meaningful linguistic units. For example, a child learns that the distinction between the words *pea* and *bee* is associated with different feature patterns at the beginning of the word. Such words are called *minimal pairs.* For example, when we learned to produce and perceive the words *pea, bee, tea, Dee, key,* and *gee* as having different meanings, we were establishing phonemic differences among the sounds /p, t, k, b, d, ʤ/.

English speakers develop approximately 24 consonant phonemes and 16

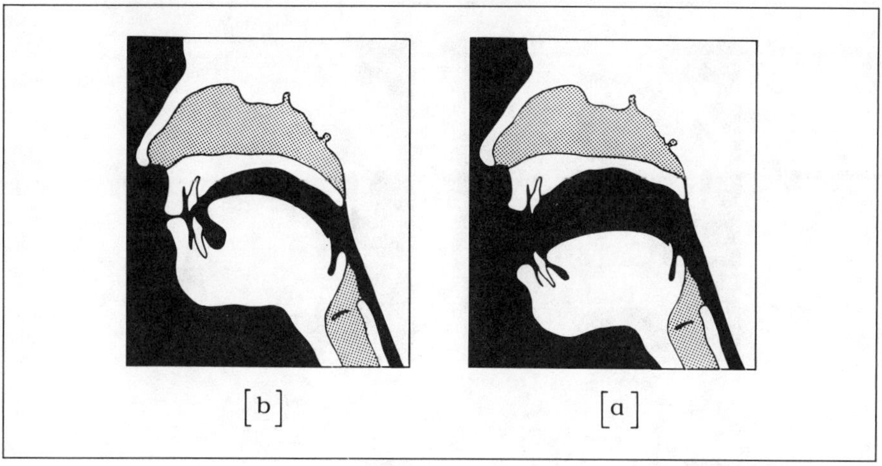

Fig. 1-3. Extremes of vocal tract opening illustrated by consonant [b] and vowel [a].

vowel phonemes, depending on the particular dialect encoded. These phonemes have been classified and described with respect to idealized versions of their articulation, which are related to the tactile-kinesthetic sensations organized by the language learner. The first major classification in an articulatory phonetic description of the phonemes of English is between the consonants and vowels. Vowels are produced with a relatively open vocal tract and may function as nuclei of syllables as described above. Consonants are produced with a relatively tight constriction in the vocal tract and serve as the onsets and offsets of syllables.

Figure 1-3 shows the polar extremes of vocal tract opening. The most extreme opening of the vocal tract occurs during production of the vowel /a/ as in the word *hot*. The most extreme closure of the vocal tract occurs when it is completely closed by the contact of two articulators as typified by the lip closure during production of /b/.

Vowels

The *vowels* of English are described along three dimensions. The first two, called *tongue horizontal position* and *tongue height* specify where in the vocal tract a constriction has been made. The third dimension, called *lip rounding,* refers to whether the lips are protruded or retracted.

Tongue Horizontal Position. The vowels are divided into front and back classes by the anterior-posterior positioning of the body of the tongue during their production. Figure 1-4 shows schematic drawings of the tongue positions in the four most extreme (point) vowels of English. The vowel /i/ as in the word *heat* is produced with the tongue body maximally forward in

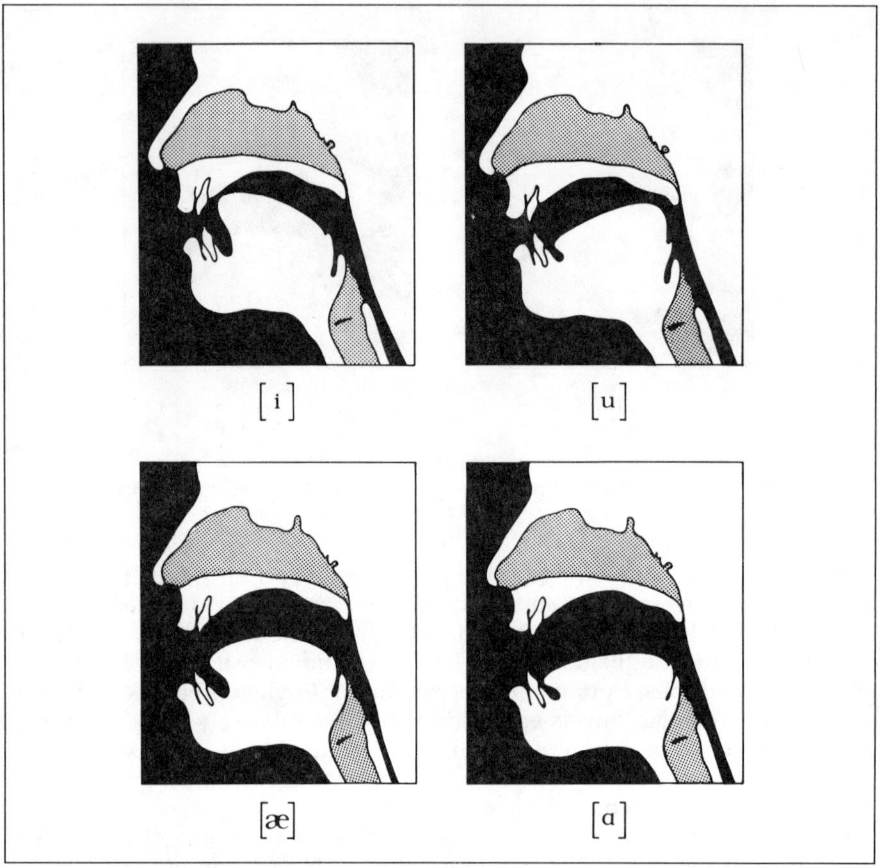

Fig. 1-4. Vocal tract configurations for the point vowels [i], [u], [æ], and [a].

the vocal tract. Thus, it is considered to be a front vowel. The vowel /i/ contrasts with the vowel /u/, as in the word *hoot*, inasmuch as /i/ is a front vowel and /u/ is a back vowel. Note the relative positions of the body of the tongue for these two vowels. You will note a similar difference in the front-back dimension between the vowels /æ/, as in *hat*, and /a/, as in *hot*. You can feel the differences in tongue position between these two sets of vowels by alternately saying a front vowel and a back vowel and feeling which teeth your tongue contacts.

Tongue Height. The second dimension of articulation used in describing vowels is *tongue height*, the degree to which the tongue is raised toward the roof of the mouth. The vowel /i/ differs from the other front vowel /æ/ in that the tongue dorsum is raised higher toward the palate for production of

Table 1-2. VOWELS OF AMERICAN ENGLISH DESCRIBED ACCORDING TO TONGUE BODY POSITION

Tongue height	*Tongue horizontal position*		
	Front	*Central*	*Back*
High	i (he) ɪ (hit)		u (who) ʊ (hook)
Mid	e (hay) ɛ (hem)	ɝ (her) ʌ (hut)	o (ho) ɔ (hawk)
Low	æ (hat)	ə (the)	a (hot)

/i/ than for /æ/. Similarly, the chief difference between /u/ and /a/ is also the position of the bulk of the tongue in a vertical dimension. You can demonstrate this dimension of articulation to yourself by prolonging the vowel /i/, as in the word *heat,* and slowly lowering your jaw. You should hear your vowel production change in quality from /i/ to something like the vowels in the words *hit* and *hate* before becoming the vowel /æ/ as in the word *hat.*

Table 1-2 lists the phonetic symbols used in transcription of the vowels of one dialect of English in the United States. These have been categorized according to the vertical and horizontal position of the tongue in the vocal tract, which is used in production of these sounds. The horizontal position of the constriction specifies whether a vowel is produced more toward the front of the mouth (e.g., /i/), or more toward the back (e.g., /u/). The vertical position specifies whether the tongue is raised high (e.g., /i/), causing a tight constriction, or is lowered (e.g., /æ/), causing a more open vocal tract.

Lip Rounding. There is another dimension of vowel production called *lip rounding,* which is not directly specified in Table 1-2. The most extremely lip-rounded vowel in English is /u/. At the other end of the lip-rounding continuum is the lip-spread vowel /i/. English does not contrast vowel sounds solely as a function of lip rounding. As you read the vowel chart from /i/ to /ɪ/ to /ɛ/ then around the bottom of the chart and back up toward /u/, each vowel becomes less spread and more rounded. One of the difficulties faced by the speaker of English who tries to learn French is to learn to produce front vowels that do contrast phonemically via lip rounding. For example, French contrasts the vowels /i/ and /y/. The vowel /y/ is produced with nearly the same tongue position as /i/ but is produced with rounded lips rather than spread lips.

Diphthongs

The vowels described above are referred to as *monophthongs* because they involve production of one vocal tract shape during their articulation. You can sustain the vocal tract shape and sound of an /i/ vowel indefinitely.

However, the *diphthongs* require that vocal tract shape be changed during their production. The symbols used for the diphthongs are combinations of the vowels that approximate the starting point and ending point of this vocal tract maneuver. For example, the diphthong /aɪ/ as in *sigh* starts near the vowel /a/ and ends near the vowel /ɪ/. Other diphthongs include /au/ as in *out* and /ɔɪ/ as in *boy*.

Consonants

As discussed earlier, the primary difference between consonants and vowels is that consonants are produced with a relatively tight constriction of the vocal tract. The classification of consonant phonemes describes the place of this constriction in the vocal tract and the tightness of constriction. These two dimensions are called *place of articulation* and *manner of articulation*. Two additional characteristics of consonants are related to the production of sound at the larynx during the consonant constriction (i.e., voicing) and whether sound is allowed to move through the nasal cavities during production (i.e., nasalization).

Place of Articulation. *Place of articulation* refers to where (and which) articulators are brought together to form a vocal tract constriction for a consonant sound. Figure 1-5 shows lateral views of the vocal tract, illustrating each of the places of articulation used to distinguish phonemes. *Bilabial* refers to the bringing together of the two lips as in the /b/ sound in *boy*. *Labiodental* constrictions occur between the lower lip and the upper front teeth, as in the /f/ in *fan*. *Dental* constrictions occur between the tip of the tongue and the upper front teeth, as in the /θ/ in *thumb*). *Alveolar* constrictions occur between the tip or blade of the tongue and the alveolar ridge (i.e., the portion of the hard palate just behind the teeth), as in /t/ in *tie*. *Palatal* sounds are produced between the oral dorsum of the tongue and the hard palate as in the /ʃ/ sound in the word *shoe*. *Retroflex* articulations involve complex tongue shapes that create two constrictions, one near the velum or oropharynx and one near the hard palate. They are used for production of /r/. *Velar* sounds are produced between the pharyngeal dorsum of the tongue and the velum, or soft palate (e.g., the /k/ sound in *cat*). *Glottal* sounds are produced with constrictions between the paired vocal folds within the larynx (e.g., /h/ in *Hi*).

Manner of Articulation. In most cases, *manner of articulation* refers to the degree of constriction (tightness) between the two articulators involved in the speech sound's production. *Obstruents* are those sounds with an oral constriction sufficiently tight to elevate the air pressure in the tract behind the constriction. These include the *stops*, *fricatives*, and *affricates*. Stops are produced with a complete articulatory closure that stops the flow of air through the vocal tract. The labial stops /p/ (*pie*) and /b/ (*buy*) stop the flow of air through the vocal tract at the lips, /t/ (*tie*) and /d/ (*die*) at the alveolar

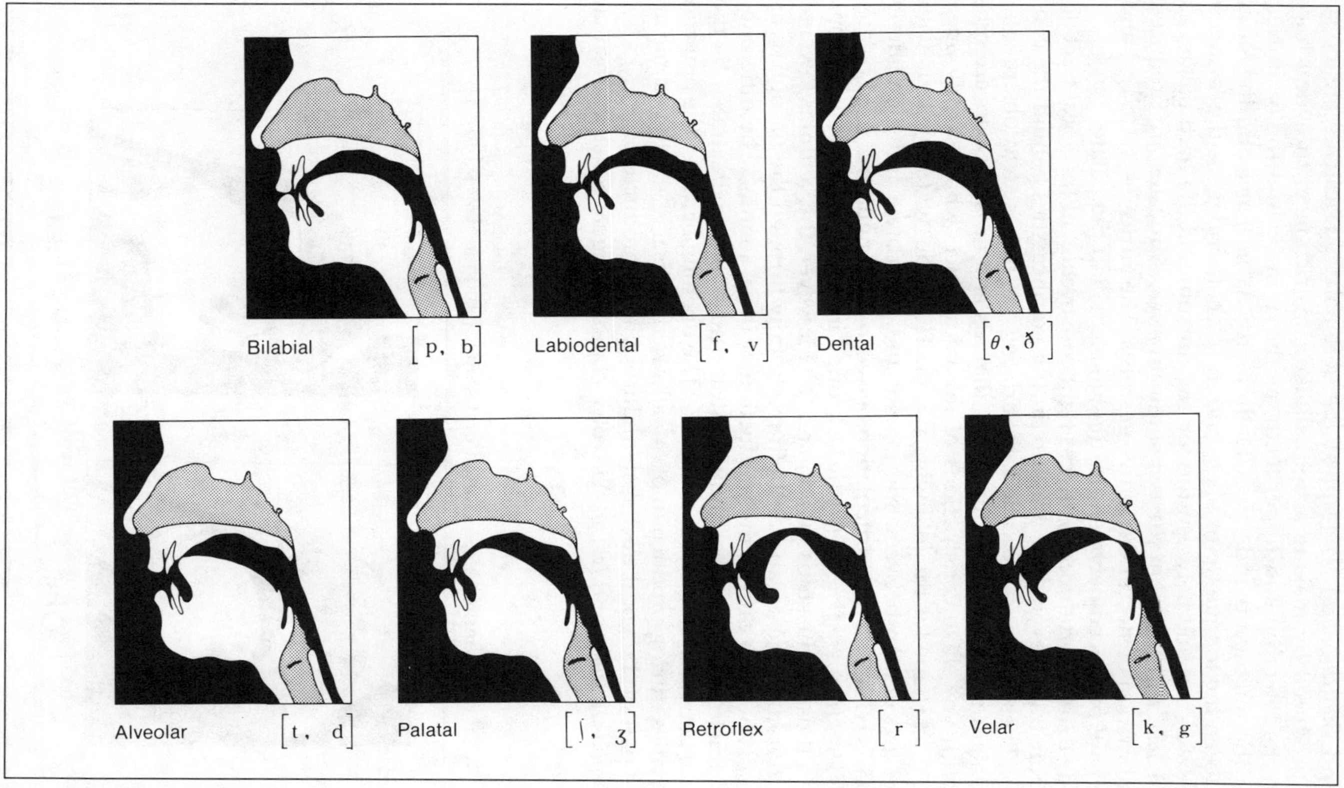

Fig. 1-5. Vocal tract configurations for bilabial, labiodental, dental, alveolar, palatal, retroflex, and velar consonant constrictions.

ridge, and /k/ (*cap*) and /g/ (*gap*) at the soft palate. Fricatives are noisy sounds produced by making a tight slitlike constriction of the vocal tract between the lower lip and upper teeth, as the /f/ in *fan* and the /v/ in *van;* between the tongue tip and upper teeth, as the /θ/ in *thumb* and the /ð/ in *this;* between the tongue tip or blade and the alveolar ridge, as the /s/ in *sue* and the /z/ in *zoo;* and between the tongue dorsum and the hard palate, as the /ʃ/ in *shoe* and the /ʒ/ in the last sound in *beige.* Affricates are produced as a combination of stop and fricative gestures. The affricates /tʃ/ (*cheap*) and /ʤ/ (*jeep*) are produced between the tongue blade and the palate.

Sounds that are produced with less tight constriction of the vocal tract do not demonstrate elevated air pressure in the vocal cavities behind the constriction. These sounds are called *approximants* as opposed to obstruents. Approximant sounds include the glides, liquids and nasals. *Glides* are produced with vowellike constrictions of the vocal tract, which swiftly open into the tract shape for the following vowel. The glide /w/ (*way*) starts with a /u/-like articulation between the tongue and soft palate and the glide /j/ (*yeah*) starts with an /i/-like articulation between the tongue and hard palate.

Nasals, /m/ (*me*), /n/ (*knee*), /ŋ/ (the last sound in *sing*), involve constrictions similar to those of the stops /b/, /d/, and /g/. However, the velum is lowered so that vibratory energy and air both freely flow through the nasopharynx and out of the nose during the production of these sounds. The difference in vocal tract shape for nasal and oral stop consonants is illustrated by the difference between /b/ and /m/ in Fig. 1-6. The opening between the oral and nasal cavities during production of /m/ allows the nasal cavity to become an effective part of the vocal tract system during nasal production.

The *liquids* /l/ (*lake*) and /r/ (*rake*) involve complex lingual constrictions that

Fig. 1-6. Vocal tract configurations for an oral stop [b] and nasal stop [m].

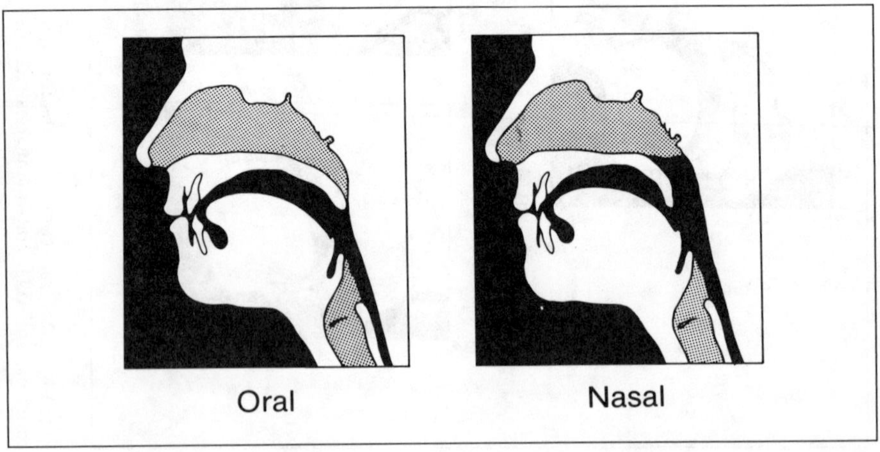

are not so tight that they usually produce friction noise in the vocal tract. The sound /r/ is produced with a retroflex constriction, whereas /l/ is produced with a central constriction flanked by lateral openings that allow sound energy and airflow to pass over both sides of the tongue laterally.

Voicing. Another dimension of consonant production is whether or not the vocal folds are vibrating during the interval of consonant production. Speech sounds in which the vocal fold vibrations are the only source of vibratory energy include the vowels and all of the approximants (i.e., the nasals, liquids, and glides). Obstruent consonants may be either voiced or voiceless. The fricatives can be divided into a group of *voiced* sounds that contain noise plus laryngeal voicing and *voiceless* sounds, which are noise only. The voiced fricatives are /v/, /ð/, /z/, and /ʒ/. Each of these has a voiceless counterpart or *cognate* (i.e., /f/, /θ/, /s/, and /ʃ/). The stop consonants also can be divided into voiced, /b, d, g/ and voiceless, /p, t, k/, cognates. However, the voicing of stop consonants is not related strongly to the presence or absence of voicing during the stop closure. Rather, the time lag between opening of the stop closure and the onset of laryngeal voicing for the following vowel (known as *voice onset time*) is the major cue for stop-consonant voicing.

Table 1-3 lists the phonetic symbols used for transcription of the consonant phonemes of English. Such descriptions of phonemes are necessarily abstract because place of articulation, manner of articulation, and voicing characteristics are rich in real physiological and acoustical details that cannot be captured by a symbol or two in a table. The process of changing phonemic target characteristics is discussed in the next section.

Features

Our model shows three interrelated feature types, all of which are based on physiological sensations (visual, auditory, tactile-kinesthetic) from the human vocal tract and the sensory systems of ear and eye. The *tactile-kinesthetic* (often termed somesthetic) features are related to the sensations of touch on the surfaces of the vocal tract (tactile sensations) and the spatial positions of the articulatory organs (kinesthetic sensations). Both forms of sensation arise as neurally encoded signals from sensory receptors in the vocal tract, which are transmitted up to the central nervous system. Tactile receptors discharge when the surface of an articulator is touched; kinesthetic receptors discharge when muscles tug on tendons and move bones at joints, while stretch receptors within muscles signal muscle length. *Auditory features* of speech are initially detected by receptor cells in the ear; *visual features* are initially detected by receptors in the eye.

These three classes of structurally interrelated perceptions are connected to one another, co-occurring during the act of articulation of a speech sound. Visual-auditory perceptions are gleaned from seeing and hearing

Table 1-3. CONSONANT PHONEMES OF ENGLISH

	Place of articulation							
Manner	*Labial*	*Labio dental*	*Dental*	*Alveolar*	*Palato-alveolar*	*Palatal*	*Velar*	*Glottal*
Stops	p b			t d			k g	
Nasals	m			n			ŋ	
Fricatives		f v	θ ð	s z	ʃ ʒ			h
Affricates					tʃ ʤ			
Liquids				l	r			
Glides	w					j	(w)	

another person's sound productions. Thus, phonemes are more "abstract" (a larger pattern of connections is made that includes the lower-level connections) in terms of neural organization than the initial sensory information, as words are more abstract than phonemes. For example, the word *dog* exists as connections to three phonemes and a larger number of auditory, visual, and tactile-kinesthetic feature patterns. The word also exists as connections to auditory, visual, and tactile-kinesthetic features of the interaction of that person with dogs, which is part of the conceptual meaning of *dogs* (i.e., the levels of the model that are higher and more general than the meaningful linguistic unit level).

An example of such neural organization is in order. The brain of the barn owl has been studied, revealing that certain areas of neural tissue respond to light energy whereas others respond to sound energy. These are the areas of brain tissue that are more directly associated with these particular sensory inputs. These areas are interconnected with one another and with the rest of the owl's nervous system in such a manner that other areas of the brain respond to either light or sound that comes from a particular position in space. This is useful to the owl because it must hunt for its food in the dark and uses both sight and sound to localize where a mouse might be moving. The pattern of excitation for a particular location in space is analogous to our phoneme level, which we suppose integrates sensations from the person's vocal tract with sensations of the auditory and visual system that are triggered by either the person's own or another person's production of that sound. Thus, we would say that the barn owl has developed a *localization level* that is similar to our *phonemic level* of organization.

SENSORY-MOTOR ASPECTS

In the preceding section, the cognitive organization underlying speech production and perception was described as having seven levels: meaning, concepts, propositions, meaningful linguistic units, syllable structure, phonemes, and features. This section will discuss how the perceptible features characteristic of a particular phoneme actually appear as physiological events during speech.

During speech production, all levels of the model cognitive system are simultaneously active. A potential speaker is constantly assessing the communicative situation by reference to the patterns in his or her conceptual system. The concepts stimulated are constantly being coordinated into propositions that are related to meaningful linguistic units, syllable structures, phonemes, and features. When the person decides to use speech for a purpose in a particular situation, the sensory features are used to guide the muscles of the vocal tract to produce speech sounds appropriate to the meaningful linguistic units.

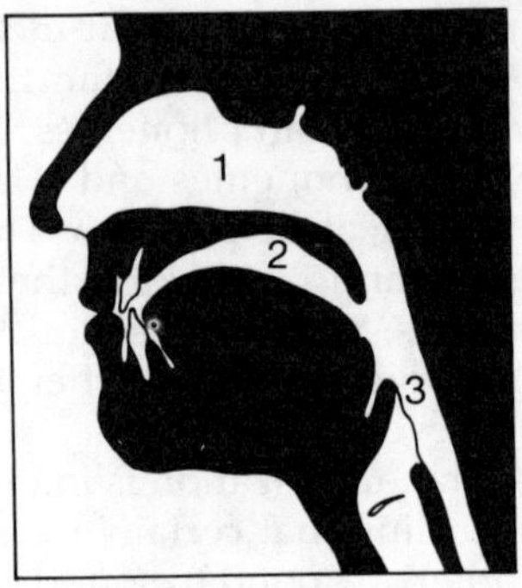

Fig. 1-7. Cavities of the vocal tract.

Tactile-kinesthetic sensory receptors allow speakers to monitor and control vocal tract shape and the resulting sound unique to each shape. Figure 1-7 presents a lateral profile of the cavities that form the vocal tract. The tract rises vertically in the neck from the larynx, passing through the pharynx (pharyngeal cavity), and splits at the level of the soft palate, branching forward into the oral cavity or coursing upward past the velum and then forward into the nasal cavity. The oral cavity begins at the lips and continues horizontally beneath the hard palate and above the tongue dorsum. It ends at the faucial pillars, the drapelike fleshy muscle bellies that you can see in a mirror inside your wide-open mouth. The pharyngeal cavity is complex, having oral, laryngeal, and nasal divisions. The oropharynx that joins the oral cavity at the faucial pillars courses backward and then downward into the neck to join the laryngopharynx at the level of the hyoid bone. The laryngopharynx continues downward, ending at the entrance to the larynx. The nasopharynx is ordinarily connected to the oropharynx by an open velopharyngeal port. The velum can be raised to close the velopharyngeal port, sealing off the nasopharynx. The nasopharynx runs superiorly and anteriorly from the velar opening, bending forward to join the twin nasal cavities.

It is important to understand that with the articulatory organs, the human speaker can dilate or constrict the width of the oral and pharyngeal cavities at many points. Constriction width can range from 2 to 3 cm down to zero when the cavity is fully constricted, and constriction length from a few millimeters to a few centimeters. These constrictions are created when an articulator is pulled, via muscular contraction, toward the vocal tract wall. The

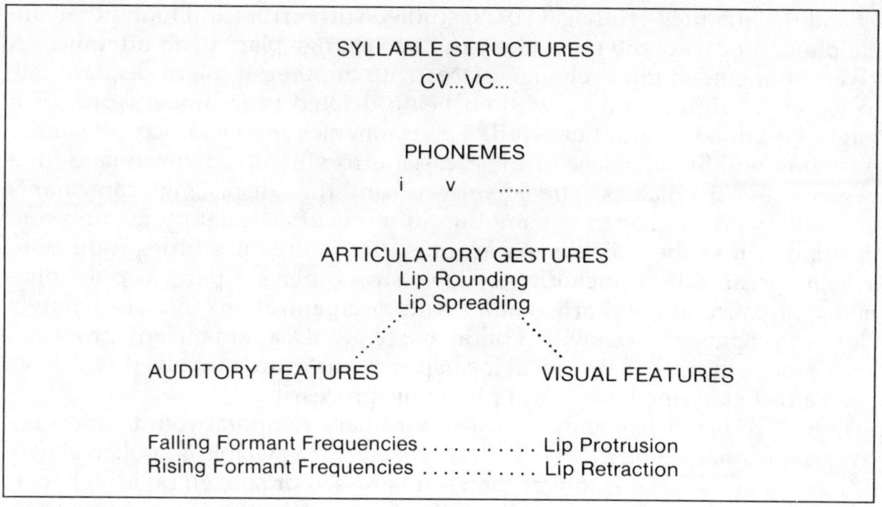

Fig. 1-8. Lower levels of the verbal communication model including example units.

following model describes how these constrictions might be controlled in the nervous system of the speaker.

Figure 1-8 presents an expanded version of the lower levels of the *verbal communication model* with examples of some of the basic units of the feature level. The tactile-kinesthetic features are used to generate and control articulatory gestures. For example, the lips can be spread or rounded. The speaker receives tactile-kinesthetic feedback that allows for sensation of the gestures produced. The effects of the lip-rounding or spreading gesture will be heard by both the speaker and listener as a lowering or raising of the frequencies of the sound produced. The listener will be able to see the visual characteristics of lip rounding or spreading.

SYLLABIC ORGANIZATION

As discussed earlier, English words are organized in syllable shapes that can be relatively simple (e.g., consonant & vowel [CV]), or relatively complex (e.g., CCCVCCC) in terms of their phonemic structure. Syllables within a word vary in degree of stress according to lexical stress and stress used by a speaker to emphasize a portion of an utterance.

The existence of a stage of syllabic organization during speech production has been demonstrated in studies of speech errors called "slips of the tongue." For example, the sentence "She sells sea shells" might be misproduced as "Sea shells she sells" by altering the positions of the phonemes

/s/ and /ʃ/. Shattuck-Hufnagel (1979) studied such errors and found that single phonemes were the most likely units to change place in an utterance. A given phoneme might exchange places with another; it might displace one to its left or right, with or without being deleted in its home word; or it might be added to another word. The phonemes involved occupy similar positions within syllables. In most cases errors involved consonants that began stressed syllables. The "displaced" and the "displacing" consonants generally were similar to one another in terms of articulatory features and position within the syllable. As an utterance is organized for production, syllabic organization, including syllabic stress, plays a part, as does phonemic organization and articulatory feature organization. In cases where a cluster exchanges places with a phoneme (e.g., "Dear old queen" produced as "Queer old dean") the syllabic shapes of the words involved will have been affected by the lower-level phonemic processing.

Recent research has shown an extraordinary temporal coordination between consonants and vowels within syllables. If a syllable is spoken slowly or heavily stressed, it is longer than if unstressed or spoken rapidly. Experiments have shown that regardless of rate or stress, the vowel begins at a point in time that is a constant fraction of the total syllable duration. (Kelso, Saltzman & Tuller, 1986). For example, in a particular CV syllable, the vowel might start one-third of the way through the syllable, however long or short it might be, depending on speed of utterance and syllable stress levels. Such relative invariance of consonant and vowel onsets has been observed for differing consonants, vowels, and articulatory organs. The temporal coordination of movements of articulatory organs within a syllable is quite precise under most conditions of speaking, suggesting that it is the smallest *autonomous* unit of cotiming and coordination of phonemes.

English speakers also tend to keep the length of syllables relatively constant. This requires that the lengths of the sounds within syllables be shortened if more complex syllable structures are employed. For example, the /s/ in the syllable /su/ will be longer than the /s/ in the syllable /stu/.

Figure 1-9 shows the organization of some of the units involved in an example utterance, "Sue saw Sally." At the syllabic organizational level, this utterance contains four syllables. The syllabic shapes associated with the words are CV (Sue), CV (saw), and CVCV (Sally). The name *Sally* contains two syllables. Each of the /s/s serves as the onset of a syllable, although the function of the /l/ is not quite as clear. As an "ambisyllabic" consonant it serves both to end the first syllable of *Sally* and to start the last syllable.

The speaker would choose to stress the syllable that is most important to his or her message. If answering the question "Who saw Sally?," the speaker would likely stress /su/. If answering the question "Did Sue hit Sally?," the speaker would likely stress /sɔ/. These syllables would be stressed by producing the consonants and vowels longer and more precisely and emphatically than usual. Thus, the /s/ contained in the stressed syllable will more closely approximate its ideal characteristics. The stressed syllable

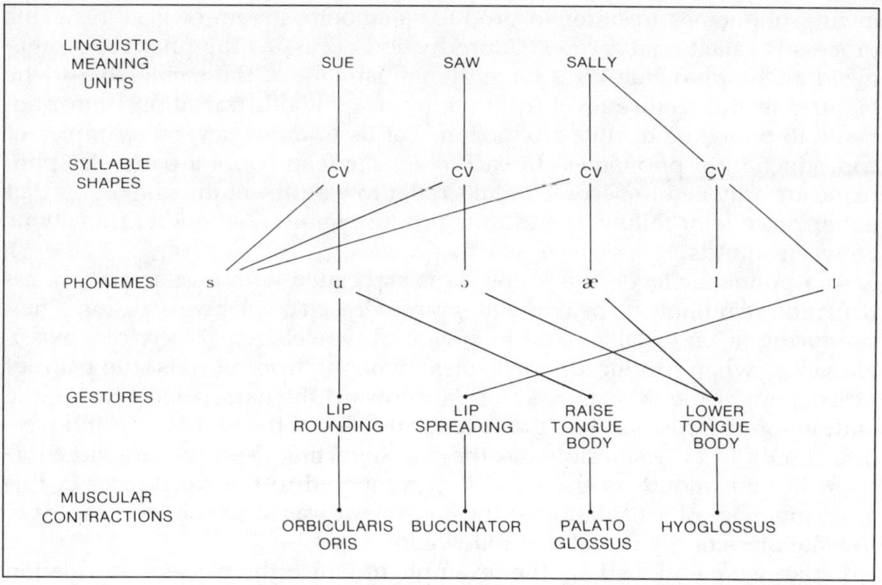

Fig. 1-9. Verbal communication model showing example units for the utterance "Sue saw Sally."

is generally longer, louder, and higher pitched. Reference to the lower levels of this figure is made in the following sections.

PHONEMIC ORGANIZATION

The syllable shapes and phonemes in an utterance are related to the meaningful units selected in the process of generating a proposition. Each phoneme of each word represents a unique set of place, manner, and voicing articulatory features. We suppose that the articulatory characteristics of a phoneme are learned as a target vocal tract configuration, as exemplified in the lateral views of the vocal tract used previously to illustrate different phonemes. Thus, organization of an utterance to express a proposition compels the organization of a string of vocal tract configurations through which the speech production system must navigate the articulatory organs. This syllabically organized series of articulatory configurations, each representative of a phoneme, in turn dictates the temporal sequence of articulatory gestures used in an utterance.

As the utterance is organized, the articulatory gestures for a given phoneme are adjusted and overlapped with the gestures for preceding and following phonemes in order to produce a smooth stream of gestures. This process is called *coproduction*. Coproduction occurs as the phonemes organized at the phoneme level force the adjustment of the tactile-kinesthetic features at the feature level to provide for a smooth transition from phoneme to phoneme during production. Let us examine several examples of coproduction of phonemes. In each case, the features of a particular phoneme are adjusted to become more similar to features of the phonemes that either precede or follow it, and thus produce shorter, smoother transitions between sounds.

At a phonemic level, the sound /k/ is associated with a velar place of articulation. An English speaker will typically reach a velar constriction when producing /k/ in syllables that involve back vowels (e.g., *coop, cop, coffee*). However, when produced in syllables involving front vowels, the place of articulation of the /k/ is moved forward toward the hard palate. Notice the shift in tongue position you produce for the /k/s in the words *coop* and *keep*. You should feel the sides of your tongue contacting teeth that are more forward in your mouth in the word *keep* compared to the word *coop*. In this case, the place of articulation of the consonant was altered to become more like the place of the vowel that followed it.

Earlier we mentioned another example in which the place of articulation of a consonant was adjusted to become more like that of consonants that followed it. Say the word *ten* and note where your tongue touches during the /n/ production. It should be making contact behind the upper front teeth, on the alveolar ridge. Now say the word *tenth* and note where the /n/ is produced. Your tongue is probably touching the upper front teeth. You have unconsciously anticipated the place of articulation of the /θ/ phoneme during the production of /n/. The alveolar place of articulation feature for /n/ has been adjusted to a dental place of articulation at the feature level. This adjustment is made even if the dental consonant is not in the same word. For example, you will dentalize /n/ in a phrase such as "Ban the bomb" because of the /ð/ that occurs in the following word. Our model accommodates this kind of effect because a whole proposition is being organized during speech production, not just the individual words or meaning units.

Adjustments in place of articulation are less likely to occur if the change in place of articulation would alter the identity of the phoneme being perceived. For example, you are less likely to dentalize the /s/ in "Pass the pepper" because /s/ and /θ/ contrast phonemically. Your listener might start to interpret your utterance as something like "Path the pepper." Dentalization of /t, d, n/ is unimportant to English speakers because these sounds do not contrast with dental stops at a phonemic level. However, sometimes articulatory adjustments are made that do alter phonemic contrasts. Say the phrase "I miss you" quickly. You probably produced the /s/ sound as a palatal /ʃ/ because you adjusted the place of articulation of the fricative sound to match that of the palatal /j/ in *you*.

Another common feature change that occurs in production of English involves nasalization of vowels. English speakers do not contrast oral and nasal vowels at a phonemic level, so when they produce vowels before or after nasal consonants, they tend to nasalize the vowel. Pinch your nose and listen to the difference in quality of the vowels in the words *pad* and *Pam*. You will find that you are already lowering your velum (causing nasalization of the vowel) in *Pam*, but not in *pad*.

The student should be aware that while coproduction causes many changes in a phoneme's gesture each time its neighboring sounds change within a syllable, certain portions of the gestures are unchanged, "frozen" into fixed movement patterns. These frozen snippets of movement, or "icebergs" as Fujimura (1986) called them, are found in consonant to vowel transitions. These invariant movements are joined by freely varying, coproduced movements. In the verbal communication model, these unchanging movements may be derived from the most basic, innate gestures captured in the tactile-kinesthetic features.

The articulatory features associated with a phoneme compose a mental "plan for action." This plan consists of a hierarchical network of neuronal circuits. Such plans have also been called *coordinative structures* or complex pattern generators, which control the coordinated movements for a given phonemic segment. Excitation of the mutually cooperating, coordinated motor control circuits associated with a phoneme will lead to its spoken production.

Following Perkell (1980), we speculate that the information needed to train and control speech motor movements is derived from a sensory feedback network. This is the basic feature network seen at the center of the cognitive model presented earlier. Because of their sensory nature, these learned feature networks for each phoneme provide a way of checking to see if the motor plans have been executed properly. The speaker can compare the sensory characteristics of the production plan with the sensory feedback that actually occurs during production. As feedback from the lower levels is compared with the plan of the utterance being produced, the plan may be altered to accommodate inconsistencies. This level of organization for a particular utterance will interact with the next level, the articulatory gestures, to account for coproduction and other phenomena discussed below.

The spatial goals for the three /s/s in the example utterance "Sue saw Sally" are coproduced with the other sounds in the utterance. The /s/ in *Sue* would be adjusted for the following /u/ vowel. The back of the tongue would be pulled back and up in anticipation of the high back vowel /u/. The lips would be rounded during production of the /s/ in anticipation of the lip rounding of /u/.

The second /s/ would be affected both by the /u/ that preceded it and the /ɔ/ that follows. Both of these are back vowels so the articulatory position for /s/ will be somewhat retracted. Both involve some degree of lip rounding, so the lips will remain rounded during the /s/. Both are voiced, so there will be some overlap of voicing into the /s/.

The third /s/ will involve a more forward tongue constriction as the body of the tongue advances to reach the target for /æ/. Again, because of its intervocalic position, this /s/ is likely to be partially voiced.

GESTURAL ORGANIZATION

The articulators are those *moveable* muscular or bony structures that form the walls of the vocal tract. In its relaxed state, an articulator sits at a resting, or neutral, position. When muscles attached to the articulator contract, they shorten in length and pull the articulator in one direction, producing one articulatory gesture. While one muscle (the agonist) is responsible for moving an articulator in one direction, antagonistic muscles reverse that motion to pull the organ in the opposite direction, producing the opposite articulatory gesture. You can observe opposing muscle systems in action by bending your elbow. The bicep flexes the elbow while the antagonistic tricep straightens the elbow. Thus, the "gesture" involved is *flexion-extension*. Similarly for speech, the lips can be pushed out from the face (rounded, protruded) or pulled back in toward the face (retracted, spread).

There are three fleshy, muscular articulators (lips, tongue, and velum) and one bony (mandible) articulator. In addition, the vocal folds of the larynx can form articulatorily useful constrictions (in addition to buzzing or being open and motionless) and can be considered an articulator. The articulators and their principal articulatory gestures are listed in Table 1-4. Notice

Table 1-4. INDEPENDENTLY CONTROLLED ARTICULATIONS

Articulatory gesture	*Muscles*
Lip rounding	Orbicularis oris Mentalis
Lip spreading	Buccinator Zygomaticus Risorius
Lip opening	(Raise upper lip) Zygomatic Levator labii superior Levator labii alaeque nasi (Lower lower lip) Depressor labii inferior
Lip closing	Orbicularis oris
Mandible raising	Internal pterygoid (mostly) Masseter Temporalis

Table 1-4. (continued)

Articulatory gesture	*Muscles*
Mandible lowering	External pterygoid Geniohyoid Digastricus—anterior belly Mylohyoid Genioglossus
Velum raising	Levator palatine
Velum lowering	Palatoglossus Palatopharyngeus
Tongue body forward	Genioglossus (posterior)
Tongue body backward	Styloglossus
Tongue body upward	Styloglossus Palatoglossus Genioglossus (posterior) Mylohyoid Geniohyoid
Tongue body downward	Hyoglossus
Tongue body concave	Styloglossus Palatoglossus Transverse
Tongue body convex	Hyoglossus Inferior longitudinal
Tongue tip forward	Transverse Genioglossus (posterior)
Tongue tip backward	Superior longitudinal Inferior longitudinal
Tongue tip upward	Superior longitudinal
Tongue tip downward	Inferior longitudinal Genioglossus (anterior)
Tongue tip groove	Vertical Transverse Inferior longitudinal
Tongue tip spread	Vertical
Tongue tip taper	Transverse
Pharyngeal wall constriction	Superior pharyngeal constrictor Middle pharyngeal constrictor Inferior pharyngeal constrictor
Pharyngeal wall expansion	Salpingopharyngeal
Vocal fold adduction	Interarytenoid Lateral cricoarytenoid
Vocal fold abduction	Posterior cricoarytenoid
Vocal fold tensing	Cricothyroid
Vocal fold relaxation	Thyroarytenoid

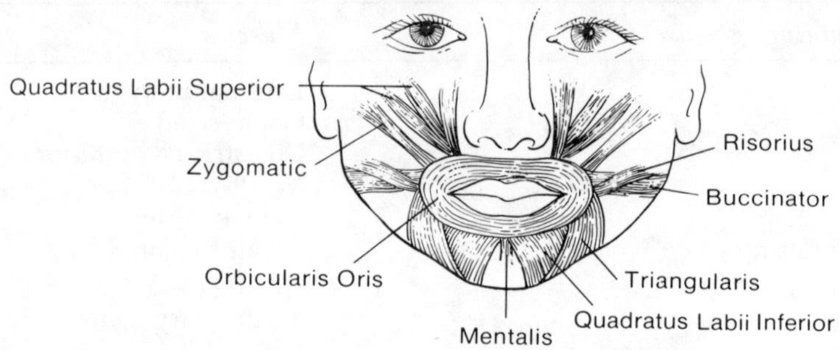

Fig. 1-10. Muscles responsible for labial gestures.

that the various portions of the tongue, although a single organ, can, within limits, move simultaneously in three directions and are therefore divided into the *tip, dorsum,* and *body* articulators, each of which can move forward, backward, and up or down in the oral-pharyngeal cavities.

Labial Gestures

Figure 1-10 shows a schematic drawing of the muscles that make up the bulk of the lips. The core of the upper and lower lips is a ring of muscular tissue. This muscle is called *orbicularis oris.* It has superior and inferior bellies that correspond to the upper and lower lips. When this muscle contracts, the lips close and protrude. The orbicularis oris is contracted when you pucker (round) your lips. You round the lips when you produce the back vowels [u] and [o]. The closing gesture is used to bring the lips together to produce bilabial and labiodental articulations as in production of [p] and [f].

A number of paired facial muscles attach to the lips. When these contract, they pull the lips in the direction of their fixed attachment to the facial skeleton. The two muscles labelled *risorius* and *buccinator* form part of the cheeks. They attach to Orbicularis Oris at the corner of the mouth. When they contract, they pull the corner of the mouth toward the side. This results in the lips being *spread.* In phonetic terms, this lip spreading gesture is the opposite of the rounding gesture produced by orbicularis oris. The lips are spread when producing vowels such as [i] and [I].

When the *quadratus labii superior* muscle contracts, it pulls upward, raising the upper lip. Similarly, the *quadratus labii inferior* muscle pulls down, lowering the lower lip. The opening gesture may be used to part the lips during production of sounds such as the vowel /a/.

The closing gesture produced by orbicularis oris may be aided by the *zygomatic* muscle, which approach the corner of the mouth from above. This muscle attaches to the lower lip and may pull it up against the upper lip.

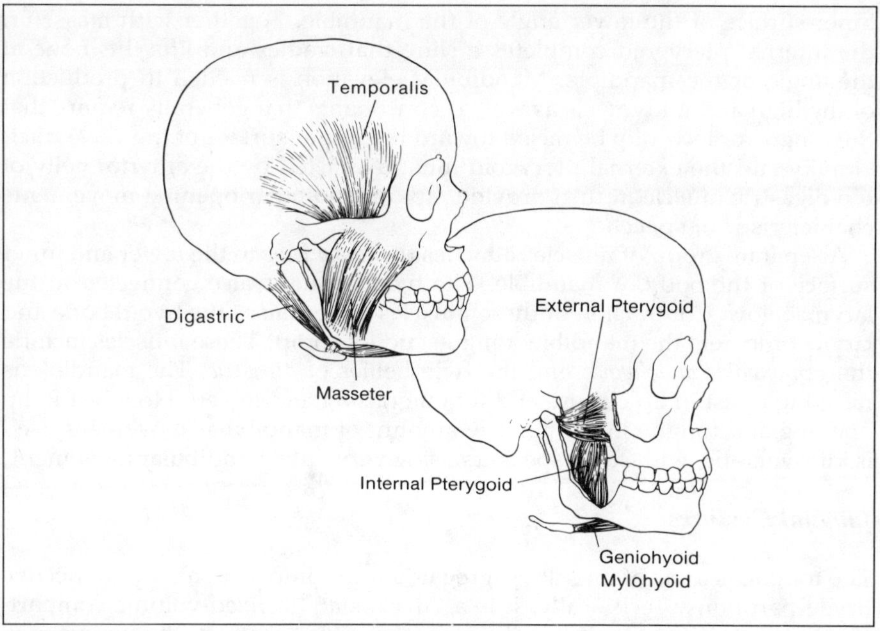

Fig. 1-11. Muscles responsible for mandibular gestures.

The muscle called *triangularis* attaches to the upper lip from below; it may also aid in the closing gesture by pulling the upper lip down against the lower lip. The muscle called *mentalis* pulls the skin covering the chin up to aid in raising the lower lip as well.

In summary, the speaker controls the muscle of the lips to produce two gestures: opening-closing and spreading-rounding. Lip opening ranges from fully open for the low vowels [æ] and [a] to fully closed for labial stops [p] and [b]. When the lips are fully rounded, the vocal tract is both longer and has a smaller labial opening. When the lips are fully spread, the vocal tract is shorter with a larger opening.

Mandibular Gestures

The lower lip and the tongue are attached to a large, horse-shoe shaped bone called the *mandible*. The mandible, the lower jaw, is pictured in Fig. 1-11. A series of muscles attach to the mandible from above and below. *Temporalis, masseter,* and the *internal pterygoid* are muscles whose contractions raise the mandible. Temporalis arises from the side of the skull to insert into the upper portion of the mandible. Masseter originates from the zygomatic arch (cheekbone) to insert into the lower angle of the mandible. The internal pterygoid runs from the base of the craniofacial skeleton to the inner surface of the lower angle of the mandible. Together with masseter, the internal pterygoid completes a sling that cradles and lifts this bone at the angle of the mandible. Mandibular elevation is needed in production of the high and midvowels as well as consonants that generally require that the tongue or lower lip be raised toward the upper surface of the vocal tract. Gravity and the external pterygoid muscle assisted by the anterior belly of the digastric muscle in turn provide rapid mandibular opening movements characteristic of speech.

A separate group of muscles attaches the *hyoid bone* to the lower and inner surface of the body of mandible. The hyoid bone is also connected to the larynx below. Contraction of these muscles either raises the hyoid bone and larynx or lowers the mandible, tongue and lower lip. These muscles include the *geniohyoid, mylohyoid,* and the twin bellies of *digastric.* The mandible is raised to assist in lip closure and tongue raising and lowered to assist in lip opening and tongue lowering. The amount of mandibular movement used is idiosyncratic, with some speakers using very little mandibular movement.

Lingual Gestures

The tongue is a sac of muscles segregated into compartments by connective tissue partitions. Technically, it is a "hydrostat," a fixed-volume compartment of watery tissues. When its internal muscles contract, the tongue may rise or fall, shorten or lengthen, or curl. The bulk of the tongue is made up of a group of four intrinsic (internal) muscles that create changes in the shape of the tongue. These changes of tongue shape alter the shape of the vocal tract and if tight enough create noise-producing constrictions in the vocal tract. These intrinsic muscles of the tongue are shown in Fig. 1-12.

The *superior longitudinal muscle* runs from the front to the back along the upper surface of the tongue. The *inferior longitudinal muscle* runs from front to back along the under surface of the tongue. Contraction of the superior longitudinal can cause the tongue tip to raise toward the alveolar ridge for production of alveolar sounds such as [t]. Further contraction of this muscle can curl the tongue tip up and back to produce a retroflex sound such as [r]. The inferior longitudinal can act to balance the force of the superior longitudinal in production of sounds such as [r] and [l]. It can also be used to rapidly pull the tongue tip down from alveolar constrictions.

The *transverse* muscle runs from the middle of the tongue toward the two sides—left and right. Contraction of this muscle narrows the tongue mass and protrudes the tongue tip. This narrowing gesture would aid in producing sounds such as [l] in which the tongue tip must be narrow for the passage of air around its sides.

The "vertical" muscle runs up and down in the central portion of the tongue. Contraction of this muscle causes the tongue to flatten and spread out toward the side. This gesture is useful in forming the tongue seals against the teeth that channel airflow down the center (not the sides) of the vocal tract for production of fricative sounds such as [s]. Contraction of the

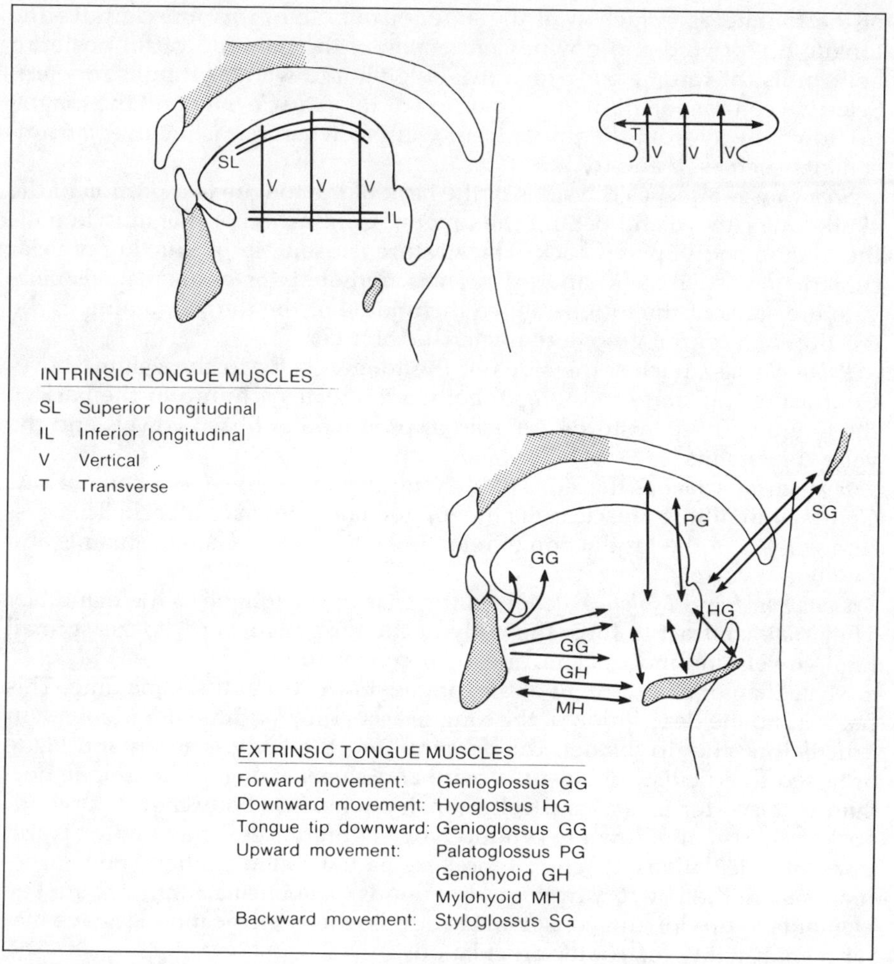

Fig. 1-12. Muscles responsible for lingual gestures.

middle-most fibers can create a groove in the upper surface of the tongue. This grooving action allows the establishment of a central pathway for airflows used in production of lingual fricatives [s] and [ʃ].

A group of extrinsic tongue muscles attach the tongue mass to the mandible and skull. These muscles move the tongue mass horizontally and vertically around the oral-pharyngeal cavities for the production of the vowels. They may also aid in the formation of differing tongue shapes associated with consonant production. They are also shown in Fig. 1-12.

Genioglossus attaches the front and center of the tongue mass to the inside of the mandible. Its fibers make up a large proportion of the central portion of the tongue. Contraction of the anterior bundle of this muscle pulls the tongue tip forward and down. Contraction of the more powerful posterior belly pulls the tongue body forward, bulging it upward as it pulls forward. Selective contraction of the front portion of this muscle may pull the tongue tip down, away from the upper front teeth as when releasing alveolar consonants such as /t/ and /d/.

Styloglossus attaches the sides of the back of the tongue to a portion of the skull that is above and behind the tongue. Contraction of this muscle pulls the tongue body up and back. This gesture is useful in production of velar constrictions such as [k] and [g]. Contraction of styloglossus may also elevate the sides of the tongue above the middle of the tongue, aiding in the creation of a central groove characteristic of /u/.

Palatoglossus attaches the sides of the tongue body to the velum above. Contraction can raise the tongue body and creates a hump in the back of the tongue. These gestures are used in production of back vowels and the velar consonants.

Hyoglossus attaches the sides of the tongue body to the hyoid bone below. Contraction of this muscle pulls the tongue body down and back. This gesture will aid in the production of releasing gesture for velar consonants and for all low vowels.

Geniohyoid and *Mylohyoid* connect the base of the tongue to the mandible. They may contract to force the body of the tongue upward, to assist in all high vowels and most palatal and velar consonants.

More than one movement of the tongue may occur at the same time. This has lead to the description of the tongue as a group of three interdependent articulators: the tip (blade), the dorsum, and the body. The tip and blade are used to articulate against the teeth and alveolar ridge. The tongue dorsum is raised for palatal and velar constrictions. The body moves forward, backward, up, and down to produce vowel differences. The tongue tip and dorsum articulations are crucial for consonantal sounds; tongue body articulations are the key to vowel-vocalic sounds. The intrinsic muscles are key elements in tip-dorsum-consonantal sounds; the extrinsic muscles have major responsibility for vocalic articulations.

Velar Gestures

The velum is a muscular extension of the hard palate. It functions as a valve between the oral and nasal cavities. As seen earlier in Fig. 1-6, the velum can either be raised or lowered. When it is raised, it contacts the pharyngeal wall, closing off the nasal cavities. When it is lowered, it allows air and sound to pass through into the nasal cavities.

Like the tongue, the velum is largely composed of muscle fibers, most of which connect to other structures. These are shown in Fig. 1-13. *Palatoglossus,* as we have already seen, connects the velum with sides of the tongue dorsum. You can see this muscle in a mirror. It forms the bulk of the structures called the *anterior faucial pillars,* which appear as drapelike structures

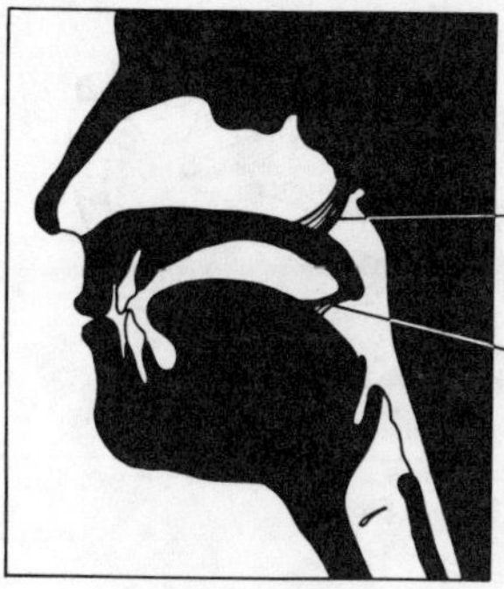

Fig. 1-13. Muscles responsible for velar gestures.

in the back of the oral cavity. This gesture is used in production of nasal consonants that must allow airflow and sound to move through the nasal cavities.

The *levator palatine* muscle connects the upper surface of the velum to portions of the skull above and behind the velum. When it contracts, it pulls the velum up. This gesture is necessary to trap air pressure in the oral and pharyngeal cavities for the obstruent consonants such as fricatives and stops, and to prevent leaking of acoustic vibration into the nose for vowel sounds.

Pharyngeal Gestures

The pharyngeal cavity is formed by a continuous wall of muscle that wraps around the funnel-shaped cavity. This wall is made up of three constrictor muscles: the *superior constrictor, middle constrictor,* and *inferior constrictor.* Each constrictor can narrow the width of the pharynx during contraction. This narrowing gesture assists the rising velum in sealing off the nasal from the oral cavity. Furthermore, the pharynx narrows for the voiceless sounds, making the air pressure above the folds higher to help stop the flow of air through the larynx. Muscles attached to the constrictor help to widen the pharynx, which aids in maintaining a flow of air through the larynx for voiced sounds.

Laryngeal Gestures

The *larynx* is a nest of cartilages sitting atop the trachea that forms the structural framework for the attachments of the vocal muscles and folds. The twin vocal folds consist of outer layers of ligament and membrane covering a body of muscle, the *thyroarytenoid.* The vocal folds can be stretched

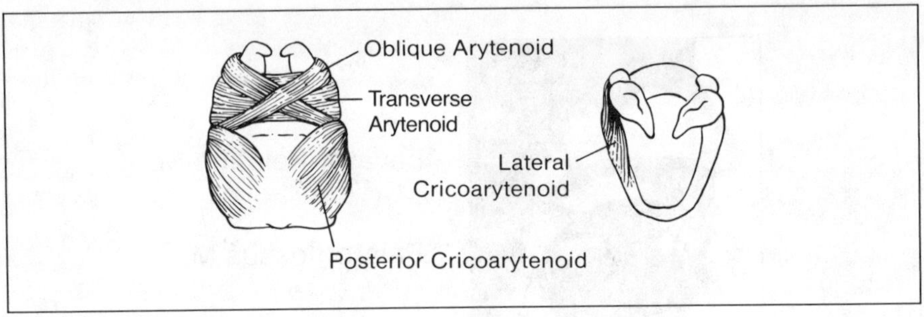

Fig. 1-14. Muscles responsible for laryngeal gestures.

(tensed), shortened (relaxed), moved apart (opened), and moved toward each other (closed) by contraction of muscles internal to the larynx. These are shown in Fig. 1-14.

The *posterior cricoarytenoid* muscle pulls the folds open, away from the midline. This gesture is useful in production of voiceless sounds, in which no laryngeal sound source is required.

The *lateral cricoarytenoid* and *interarytenoid* muscles push the folds together, a gesture used to create a periodic glottal wave for production of voiced sounds. The vocal folds are closed, and if a sufficient amount of air pressure from the lungs is forced against them, they will burst open and emit repetitive high-velocity air puffs. The elastic recoil of the folds and a drop in air pressure between the open folds as the air burst speeds through, together, pull the folds back together. As long as the muscles of the larynx steadily hold the folds together and air pressure is steadily applied, the vocal folds will repeatedly burst open and shut. The resulting stream of high-velocity air bursts crash into the much larger vocal tract air column, forcing it into sympathetic acoustic vibration.

The folds are stretched and tensed by action of the cricothyroid. The stretched folds are thinner and being more tense, the elastic recoil forces are higher; therefore, the lung pressure is pushing against a smaller mass per area under greater tension. This causes the vocal folds to open and close more rapidly, raising the fundamental frequency of vibration. The cricoarytenoid muscle shortens, thickens, and relaxes the folds, lowering the speed of their vibration. If both cricothyroid and thyroarytenoid contact, the resulting "isometric" increase of tension can also elevate fundamental frequency.

Table 1-4 lists the articulatory gestures discussed above and the muscles that aid in accomplishing each.

Each phonemic spatial (positional) goal for the vocal tract is achieved by a combination of articulatory gestures. For example, the vowel /i/ is described as a high front vowel. Attaining this articulatory configuration involves raising the tongue body, moving it forward, raising the mandible, raising the velum, opening the lips, spreading the lips, and so on. Spatial goals for the vocal tract are reached by selecting appropriate individual articulatory gestures and adjusting them to mesh with related gestures for preceding and following phonemes. For example, say the words *heat* and *hot*, and notice the amount of mandibular movement used in production of the /t/ sounds. You probably notice much more mandibular movement in producing *hot*. Both /t/ sounds use tongue tip to alveolar ridge contact as the primary target, which is achieved in both cases. In the word *heat*, the mandible has already been raised for the production of the high front vowel /i/. Thus, production of an alveolar constriction can be accomplished by a slight raising of the tongue tip. On the other hand, in the word *hot*, the mandible is lowered for the vowel /a/ and a larger tongue tip–raising gesture is needed. These two gestures—tongue tip raising and mandible raising—are coordinated differently in the two /t/s to achieve a fixed spatial goal—tip alveolar contact!

Folkins and Abbs (1975) produced evidence that if several articulatory organs can contribute to a single articulatory gesture, they *will*. For example, both mandible and lower lip contribute to lip opening and closing. During repeated productions of "ba ba ba" syllables, it has been observed that the "net" lip opening was nearly constant for each /a/ made. That is, the target "opening" was always achieved. However, the exact amount of lower-lip movement and mandible movement used by an individual speaker varied across successive productions. On one token the mandible was less open and the lower lip more active; on other tokens, vice versa. It is as if the brain were coordinating lip opening as follows:

Lip opening (c) = mandibular lowering (x) + lower-lip lowering (y)

Thus, c is a constant for a particular phoneme. It can be arrived at by addition of many possible combinations of x and y. On repeated productions, fluctuations in *mandibular lowering* were reciprocally offset by coordinated fluctuations of *lower-lip lowering* so that the sum total "lip-opening" gesture was very nearly constant.

Similar coordinations have been observed between the following pairs of articulators: lip-jaw, jaw-tongue, and lip-larynx. The brain swiftly, automatically coordinates two variable and cooperating articulators to achieve an invariant articulatory gesture. Speakers can use differing movement patterns and still achieve a *constant* articulatory target automatically.

Abbs, Gracco, and Cole (1984) also demonstrated a feed forward control system that compensates for motor errors in speech. These investigators had subjects repeat "ba ba ba" utterances. They then jerked the subject's jaw back without warning. The speakers rapidly and unconciously compensated by using a more vigorous lower-lip movement to achieve labial closure. Apparently, feedback from the temporomandibular joint receptors and

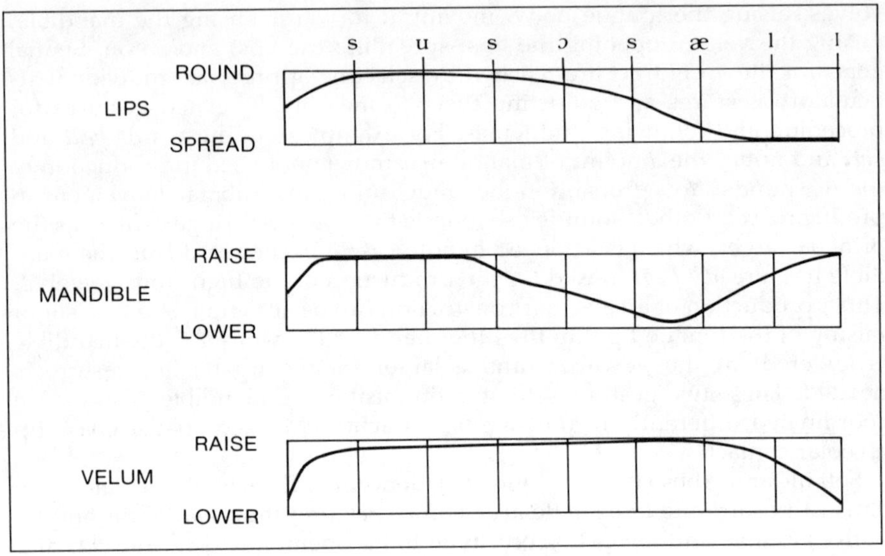

Fig. 1-15. Selected patterns of articulatory gestures during production of "Sue saw Sally."

muscles of the mandible rose to mid and upper brain, and within 30 milliseconds or so, an extralarge motor command was issued to the unrestrained lower lip to perform a compensatory movement. Information from one organ (mandible) was fed forward to another organ (lip). It might be thought that the 30 to 40 milliseconds it takes to send feedback to the central nervous system would be too slow to control sounds only 80 to 150 milliseconds in duration; however, speech sounds are 20 to 80 percent longer physiologically than they are acoustically. This is not unexpected since muscles must start contracting well before the resulting movements start and stop contracting slowly. Thus, phonemes are long enough at a muscle contraction level to make "online" feed-forward compensation for articulatory inaccuracies useful.

Figure 1-15 shows the movement patterns of some of the articulators during production of "Sue saw Sally." Each articulator moves smoothly from target position to target position, at a velocity determined by the target positions that must be approached. For example, the tongue tip must approach the alveolar ridge for each /s/. It provides a gesture for each /s/. On the other hand, the velum has a similar target position throughout this utterance and can remain raised. It essentially will be programmed to make one gesture.

The mandible aids in raising the tongue tip for /s/ and for raising and lowering the tongue body. Thus, it makes gestures for each of these purposes.

MUSCULAR ORGANIZATION

Each articulatory gesture can be achieved by contraction of a set of cooperating muscles. For example, both the internal pterygoid and masseter muscles can raise the jaw. The degree to which each contracts will determine the amount of force applied to the mandible. Individual speakers generally can use somewhat different combinations of muscle activity to achieve the same articulatory configuration goals.

Most articulatory gestures come as opposing pairs of gestures (e.g., lip rounding-lip spreading). The agonist-antagonist muscle sets involved are closely coordinated with one another. For example, when the muscles that round the lips are contracting, the muscles that spread the lips are relaxed. When this kind of "reciprocal inhibition" of muscle activity is not being properly coordinated, the movement can become stiff, slow, and jerky. As we will see, damage to the central nervous system can cause such speech errors.

Two general classes of movement patterns for speech articulation exist. "Ballistic" movement involves contraction of one set of muscles with little or no opposition from antagonist muscles. The resulting movement is rapid, ending only when the moving structure strikes another structure or can stretch or move on its joints no farther. In the word *hat*, the final *t* sound can be produced with a ballistic movement of the tongue tip in conjunction with movement of the mandible. Both move upward quickly until the tongue tip strikes and holds against the alveolar ridge.

"Controlled" movements involve a balanced contraction of agonist-antagonist muscle groups. For example, during the production of the [æ] in *hat*, the muscles of the tongue and jaw that raise and lower both structures co-contract, with the depressors contracting stronger to produce a smooth, accurate lowering of mandible and tongue rather than the simpler, more rapid, less accurate movement that agonistic contraction alone would produce.

Muscle contractions are controlled by the nervous system which can be divided into *peripheral* and *central* divisions. In this section we will examine the basic anatomy of the nervous system that is most directly related to control of the articulatory muscles. The later section describing a model of speech production will look at the types of control decisions that the nervous system is making during speech production.

Peripheral Nervous System

The peripheral nervous system consists of all of the components of the nervous system that are outside the cranium and spinal column. Twelve pairs of *cranial nerves* supply innervation to the head, neck, and thorax. Each of these peripheral nerves has its first nucleus in the mid- or hind-brain. The nerves then leave the brain, pass through the cranium, and branch out to the parts of the body they serve. Many cranial nerves have both sensory and motor fibers. Motor branches send commands to the individual muscles, directing how strongly the muscle fibers will contract. The degree of contraction in a muscle is controlled by motor nerve excitation rate. Each cranial nerve controls a group of muscles that are associated with movements of a group of articulators. Thus, the coordination of agonist and antagonist muscles for a particular articulatory gesture can be controlled by the action of a single cranial nerve or several nerves.

Afferent portions of a cranial nerve bring sensory information from the tissues and joints surrounding the muscles into the central nervous system. This "feedback" is used to control and integrate muscle commands. Information useful in controlling muscular contraction in speech includes tactile and proprioceptive feedback. Tactile information tells the brain which structures are contacting one another. For example, if you say the words *key* and *coo,* you will notice that the body of your tongue touches your teeth in a more forward position for *key* than *coo.* This sensation starts with the action of receptors embedded in the tongue that tell where pressure is applied to the surface of the tongue.

Proprioceptive feedback signals where an articulator is in space, even if it makes no contacts with other articulators. For example, if you say the words *fee* and *free,* you will probably find a difference in tongue-tip positions. Muscle spindle receptors relay information about muscle length to cortex and to the cerebellum of the hindbrain (unconscious level); receptors in joint capsules, tendons, ligaments, and cartilages relay information on joint angle and loading to the sensory cortex where we become conscious of position of body parts in space. In the remainder of this section we will present the *cranial* nerves, which are important to speech articulation. They are shown in Fig. 1-16.

The 12 cranial nerves are numbered by where the nerve fibers exit the central nervous system. Those nerves that exit at higher portions of the brain or brain stem are assigned lower numbers; those exiting from lower portions of the brain stem are given higher numbers.

The cranial nerve that directly serves speech production is the fifth, called the *trigeminal.* The trigeminal carries sensory information from the face, mouth, and lower jaw. It supplies motoric innervation for the muscles that raise and lower the mandible. It also supplies muscles that raise the soft palate.

The *facial* nerve, the seventh cranial nerve, receives sensory information about taste in the anterior two-thirds of the tongue and sensation from the pharynx. It is motoric for the muscles of the face, including those that control the lips.

The *glossopharyngeal* nerve, the ninth cranial nerve, supplies sensory information from taste in the posterior one-third of the tongue and sensation from the lining of the mouth. It supplies motor commands for one of the muscles of the pharynx.

The *vagus* nerve, the tenth cranial nerve, supplies sensory information

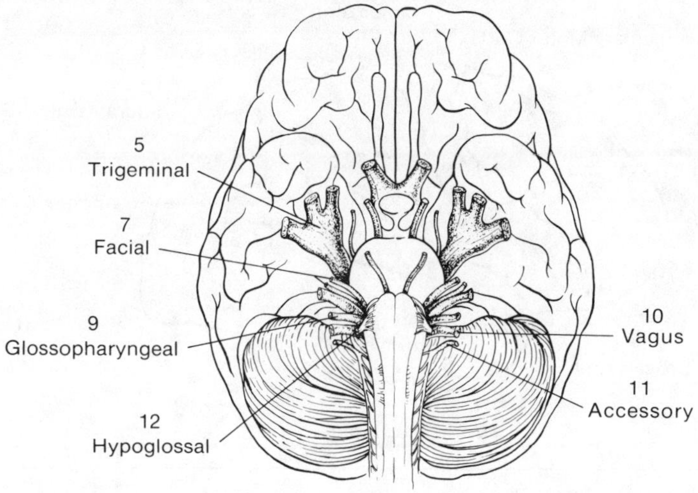

Fig. 1-16. Cranial nerves associated with speech production.

from the linings of the larynx and lungs. It supplies most of the motor control of the larynx.

The *accessory* nerve, the eleventh cranial nerve, is motoric in nature. It supplies commands to the soft palate. Muscles that both raise and lower the soft palate are controlled by this nerve.

The *hypoglossal,* the twelfth cranial nerve, largely controls movement of the tongue. It supplies motor commands for both the extrinsic and intrinsic muscles of the tongue.

CENTRAL NERVOUS SYSTEM

The neural structures that organize speech and language production and perception are known to be localized in the cortex of the left hemisphere of the brain for the great majority of humans. A diagram showing these areas is seen in Fig. 1-17. Neural areas serving speech production and perception are found along the length of the lateral fissure.

Auditory signals arrive at the primary auditory receptive area of the temporal lobe. This information is relayed to surrounding areas (planum temporale and angular supramarginal gyrus) that are collectively known as *Wernicke's area.* Damage to this area results in a severe disability for recognition of phonemes and jargonlike speech production. This area is crucial to phonemic perception and selection and ordering of words in production.

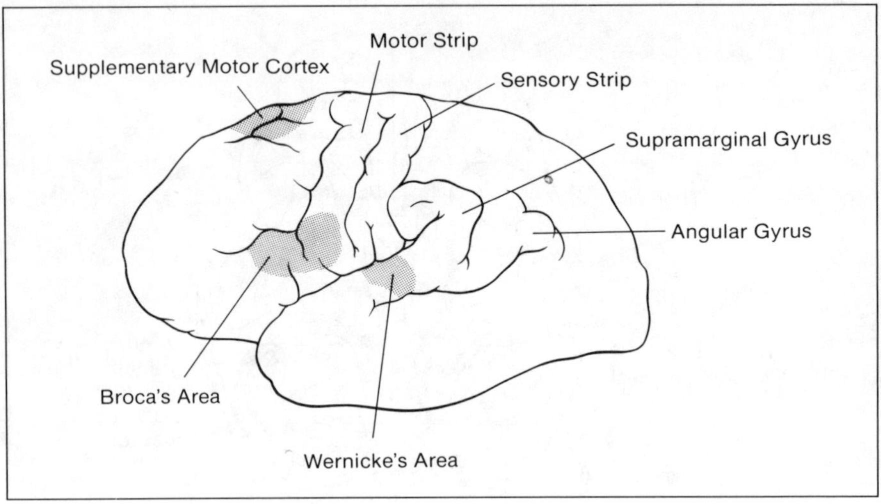

Fig. 1-17. Areas of cortex associated with speech production.

Wernicke's area is connected to *Broca's area* (BA) by a bundle of fibers known as the *arcuate fasciculus*. BA is an association area in front of the primary motor control region for speech production. Damage to BA produces effortful, telegraphic speech. Damage to the motor strip itself produces paralysis and weakness of articulatory muscles. A larger area of frontal cortex anterior and superior to Broca's area, the Supplementary motor association (SMA) region, is responsible for planning articulations in an utterance. Damage here causes phonemes and words to be misordered and fluency of speech to deteriorate.

Motor control is vested in the SMA area, Broca's area, and the motor cortex (Fig. 1-18). Fibers from the SMA area and BA project to the cerebellum and basal ganglia. The cerebellum and basal ganglia smooth the movements planned in BA and the SMA area. The smoothed movement patterns are sent back, via the thalamus, to the cortical planning areas, which modify the plan and forward it to the motor cortex. The motor cortex issues the motor commands to the peripheral nerve motor nuclei and to the cerebellum. The cerebellum then compares this plan to feedback from the joints and muscles so that real-time corrections can be issued to finetune the actual movement pattern.

The sensory information gathered during speech production is relayed to the cerebellum and to the neural centers of the forebrain such as the basal ganglia. Since the speech motor commands are also routed through these neural centers, it is clear that these centers are involved in adjusting the speech commands with regard to what has actually taken place in the vocal tract. For example, experiments have been conducted in which speakers were asked to say something like "ba ba ba." Closing the lips in this task is achieved by raising the jaw and contracting the muscles that close the lips. Without warning, a machine was used to stop the movement of the jaw. The speakers rapidly, and unconsciously, compensated for the decreased jaw movement by increasing their lip movement. To do this, the speaker must have been processing information about the positions of the mandible and lips. When the jaw failed to reach its anticipated target position, a compensatory lip movement was used.

The neural circuitry that so precisely and elegantly times the CV gestures of syllables has been called *coordinative structures* (Fowler, 1985) and *complex pattern generators* (CPG) (Grillner, 1982). A coordinative structure is a hierarchical network of neurons extending from association and motor cortex through basal ganglia and cerebellum. Grillner (1982) speculated that such a system of control can be erected by bringing individual, reflex-like neural control circuits for simple gestures such as lip opening, tongue raising, velar closing, and laryngeal closing under the control of higher "mediating" neuronal networks. Each of these coordinative structures guides the control of a coordinated set of movements called a *fixed action pattern*. As more gestures are added to a fixed action pattern, additional high levels of mediating neuronal networks are added until a very few high-level neurons can trigger a cascade of carefully cotimed movement.

In mechanical terms, the coordinative neural network takes a system with many degrees of freedom of movement and reduces the number of degrees of freedom of movement to a minimum. For example, given 7 articulators, each with movement possible in two directions, 14 degrees of freedom of movement are to be controlled. At least 14 control signals must be provided to make any sound, and the signals must be staggered in time and variable in strength to propel every organ properly. Each of these articulators is affected by contraction of a variety of opposing muscles. Thus, in order to control the 7 articulators, approximately 40 muscles must be co-controlled to make any sound.

It is well known that the simplest "coordinative neural networks" are those that co-time agonist/antagonist muscle groups that propel a single joint/limb in one direction (flexion) or the other (extension). This "coordination" is "hardwired", achieved by reflex arcs that are genetically determined. For example, in the knee jerk reflex the tap of a hammer extends the length of one muscle on the front of the leg. This extension triggers the action of another muscle on the back of the leg, which returns the originally stretched muscle to its resting length.

Higher-order reflex systems, the fixed action patterns, control many muscle pairs to enable crucial, more complex vegetative motor acts: lip closure, sucking, crying, and gagging. Coordinated cotiming of the many muscles involved in these actions had certain survival value for animals. For example, a failure to coordinate exhalation with laryngeal closing would lead to an inefficient cough reflex, which could be fatal.

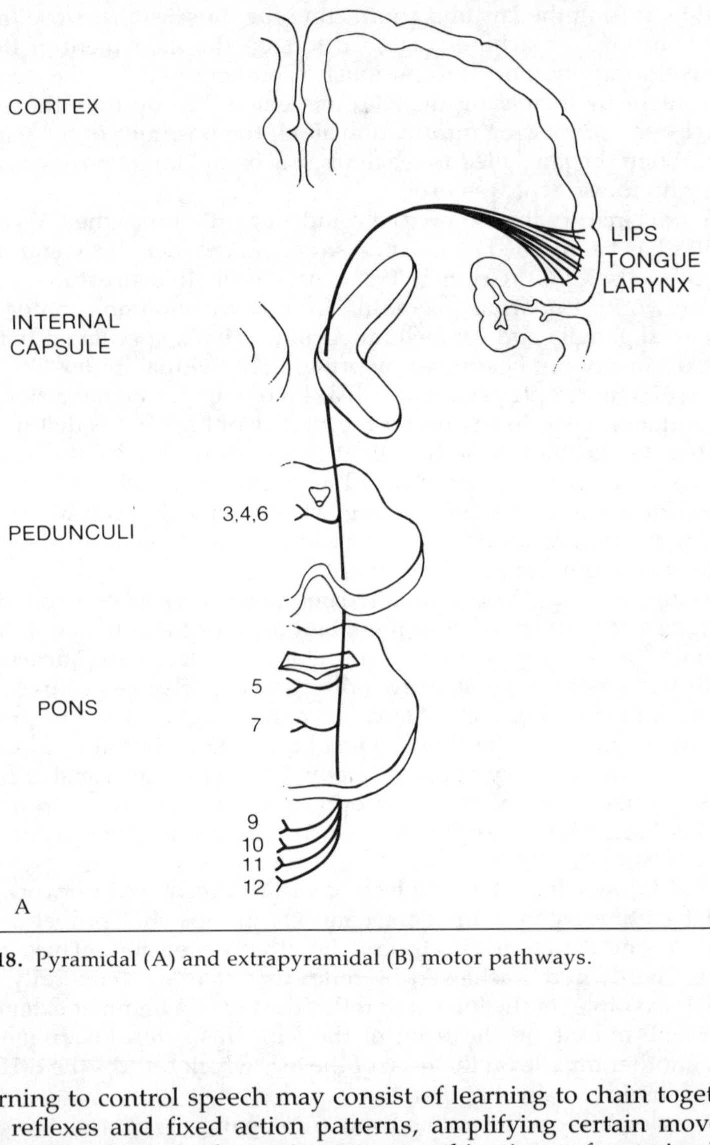

Fig. 1-18. Pyramidal (A) and extrapyramidal (B) motor pathways.

Learning to control speech may consist of learning to chain together differing reflexes and fixed action patterns, amplifying certain movements, suppressing others, and creating new combinations of entrained movements. As babies grow more and more skillful through practice and development, control of the coordinative networks is shifted higher and higher to fewer and fewer neural centers until the firing of just a few control neurons unleashes a cascade of commands, carefully cotimed and of proper amplitude to elicit control of segments and CV syllables.

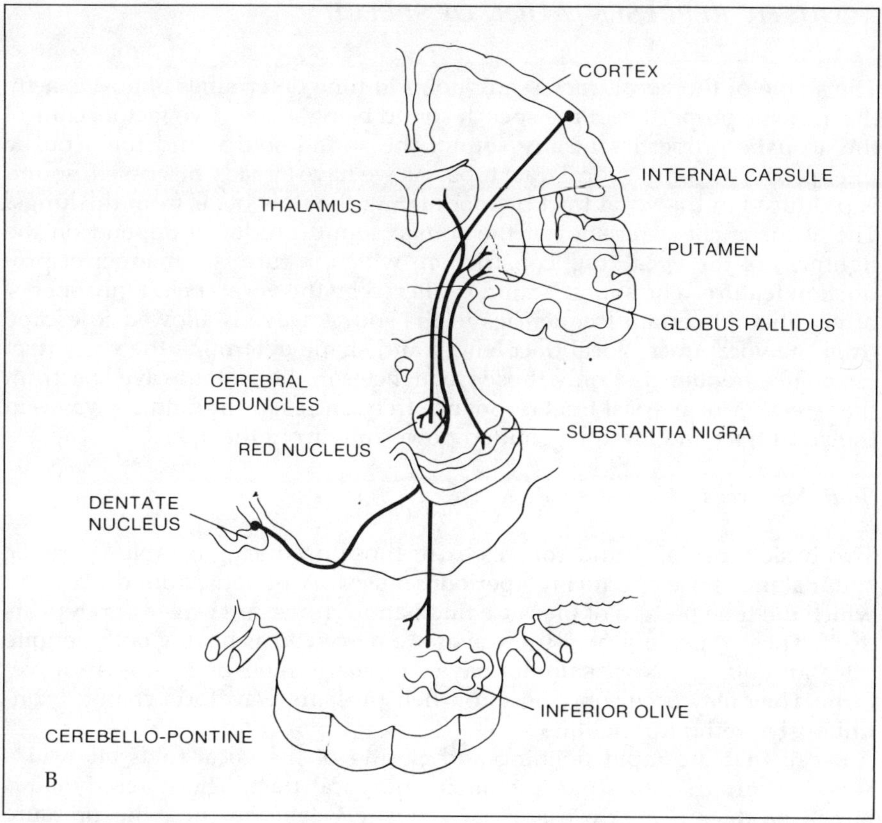

Fig. 1-18 (continued)

AUDITORY-PERCEPTUAL ASPECTS

Within this model of communicative ability, meaningful linguistic units, syllables, and phonemes consist of connections to perceptible features. Phonemes are developed by association of auditory, visual, and physiological features of speech sounds. In this section we will look at the acoustic characteristics of speech sounds. These characteristics must be organized by the language learner and attached to the higher levels of phonemes, syllables, and so on. In this section, we will first discuss how the vocal tract works during sound production. Next, we will discuss the basic acoustic characteristics of differing classes of speech sounds that will be detected and learned by the child. Finally, we present a model of speech perception within the overall model of verbal communication.

ACOUSTIC REPRESENTATION OF SPEECH

The shape of the vocal tract at any point in time determines almost exactly the acoustic properties of the speech sound being made. Two factors control the acoustic properties of any sound: the sound source and the acoustic filter properties of the vocal tract tube. As we have already discussed, sound is produced in the vocal tract by modulating the flow of air from the lungs. The acoustic characteristics of the source sound produced depend on the tightness of the vocal tract constriction, which in turn is a manner-of-production feature. The source sound is filtered by the vocal tract. Only energy of vibration at certain frequencies in the source wave is allowed to escape from the vocal tract. Vocal tract length and shape determine the vocal tract resonance frequencies; only those frequencies in the glottal wave spectrum that are at or near vocal tract resonance frequencies form standing waves in the vocal tract and are thus emitted powerfully from the lips.

Sound Sources

Two basic types of sound sources exist: those producing complex periodic sounds and those producing aperiodic noises. A periodic sound is one in which the time pattern of pressure fluctuations (pressure waveform) repeats itself. These repeating pressure waves are perceived as having both definite pitch and quality. Noises do not have a regularly repeating pressure waveform: They may occur only once, or their pressure waveform changes continuously, without repetition.

Recall that the rapid opening and closing of the vocal folds allowed a series of airbursts to strike the air in the vocal tract. These aerodynamic bursts produce a nearly triangular acoustic waveform (i.e., the pressure rises sharply to a peak and then falls sharply). Figure 1-19 shows the triangular pressure waveforms produced during vocal fold vibration at two fundamental frequencies: 100 Hz and 200 Hz. The triangular waveform for the 100 Hz fundamental frequency occurs in 0.01 second. The 200 Hz fundamental frequency involves a waveform that repeats itself twice as fast, each occurring in 0.005 seconds.

Each of these complex tones contains a lowest, or fundamental frequency, and higher frequencies that are integer multiples (harmonics) of that fundamental frequency. The amplitude of the higher harmonic frequencies smoothly decreases in power as frequency increases. The fundamental frequency is determined by the rate at which the vocal folds open and close. Figure 1-19 shows the power vs. frequency spectrum produced by vocal fold fundamental frequencies of 100 Hz and 200 Hz. A vocal fold vibration rate of 100 Hz is typical of an adult male speaker. Notice that energy is produced only at integer multiples of 100 Hz (i.e., 100, 200, 300 and so on). The amount of energy produced, shown by the height of the energy bars, is greatest at the fundamental frequency and gradually declines as frequency

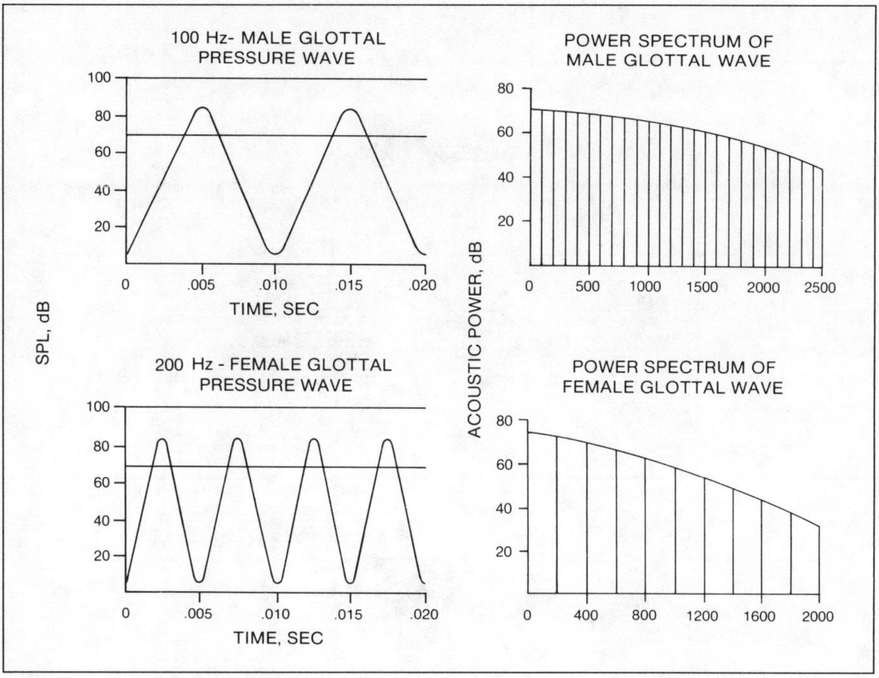

Fig. 1-19. Sound pressure waveforms and spectra produced by voicing at 100 Hz and 200 Hz fundamental frequencies.

increases. The 200 Hz rate of vibration is typical of adult female speakers, and the energy produced is more spread out than that of the 100 Hz pattern inasmuch as the integer multiples of 200 are 400, 600, 800, and so on.

In the following pages, spectrograms illustrate acoustic characteristics of speech sounds. In a spectrogram, time is the abscissa (from left to right) and frequency is the ordinate (from bottom to top). The intensity of sound energy at any time or frequency is shown by the darkness of the display. For example, Fig. 1-20 shows a spectrogram of a sentence, "We play ball on summer days," spoken by an adult male speaker. Each vertical stripe represents the energy produced when the vocal folds open and a burst of air from the glottis shocks the air in the vocal tract into vibration. The frequency at which the vocal folds are moving in this utterance is about 90 times per second, or 90 Hz. Thus, the triangular waveform produced contains energy at 90 Hz, 180 Hz, 270 Hz, and so forth. The darkness of these vertical lines decreases as one moves up in frequency, revealing that sound intensity is decreasing as frequency increases. This change in darkness is the spectrographic way of showing the decreasing amplitude bars in the spectra in Fig. 1-19.

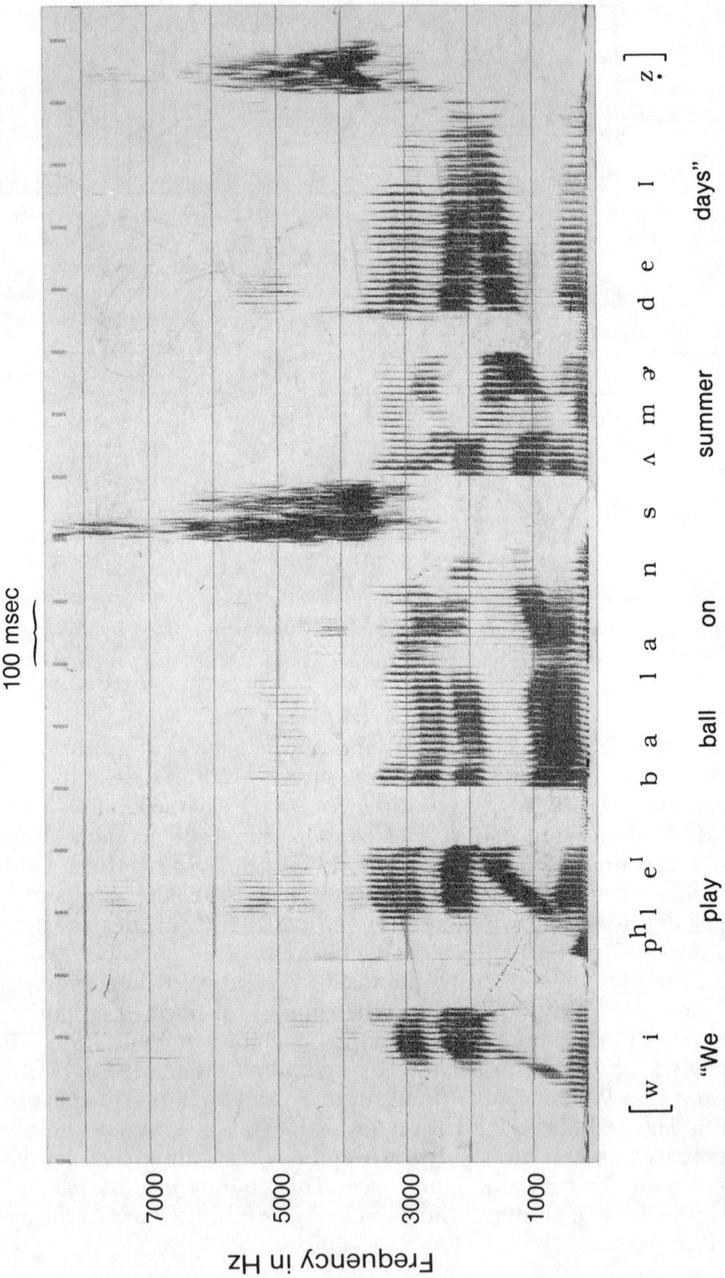

Fig. 1-20. Spectrogram of "We play ball on summer days."

Except for the /p/ and /s/ sounds, all of the sounds in this sentence are *sonorants,* sounds produced exclusively with a glottal vibration sound source. No other constriction above the larynx is tight enough to produce sound. In contrast, the /p/ sound involves a sound source at the lips, and the /s/ sound involves a sound source between the front of the tongue and the alveolar ridge. The sonorants include all vowels, the glides, the liquids, and the nasals.

In Fig. 1-20 the vertical "voicing" lines are absent only for the /p/ and /s/ sounds. The vocal folds were vibrating, opening, and shutting for all of the other sounds. The remaining differences in the spectrogram reflect changes in the vocal tract filter function attributable to articulator movements.

With a complete constriction of the vocal tract, air flows through the larynx into the tube behind the constriction, raising oral pressure until it is released. The sudden release of oral pressure shocks the air in the vocal tract beyond the constriction into vibration. The resulting sound is known as a *transient* because it is short-lived and is rich in higher frequencies of vibration. The transient starts out being relatively intense, but it dies out quickly. Transients are the popping sounds produced by air bursts . Stop consonants produce transient noises when the air pressure in the vocal tract is suddenly released. They contain a wide range of acoustic frequencies that are not harmonically integer related to one another. Thus, these sounds are perceived as noises rather than as having tonal qualities.

When a narrow constriction is made in the vocal tract, airflow pushed through it tumbles turbulently; the turbulent air "eddies" generate a "hissy" friction noise. Like the transient sounds, these turbulence noises exhibit a wide, often continuous range of noninteger-related harmonics that do not arouse a sensation of "tone." Such turbulence briefly follows the transient explosive release of voiceless stops as well as being the major component of fricative sounds.

Figure 1-21 shows a spectrogram of the word *east* produced by an adult male speaker. The first part of the spectrogram, from point A to point B, shows the vowel [i]. The sound source in this vowel production is the rapid opening and closing of the vocal folds in the larynx. Each time the vocal folds open, a puff of air strikes the air in the vocal tract and causes the air to vibrate. This vibration then dies out until a new opening of the vocal folds causes the air in the vocal tract to be excited again. Each new pulse of sound energy is seen on the spectrogram as a vertical line. These alternate with lighter areas that reflect the damping out of the vibration between glottal pulses. This repetitive shocking of the vocal tract air column creates the periodic sound characteristic of the vowel /i/.

The second portion of the spectrogram, between B and C, shows the turbulence noise produced for /s/. Hence, the regularly spaced vertical lines are absent, indicating no vocal fold vibration. Scanning the [s] segment from left to right, you can see that the exact frequency locations of the energy change from moment to moment. For example, look across the 3,000 Hz line and notice that sometimes energy is present and sometimes it is not.

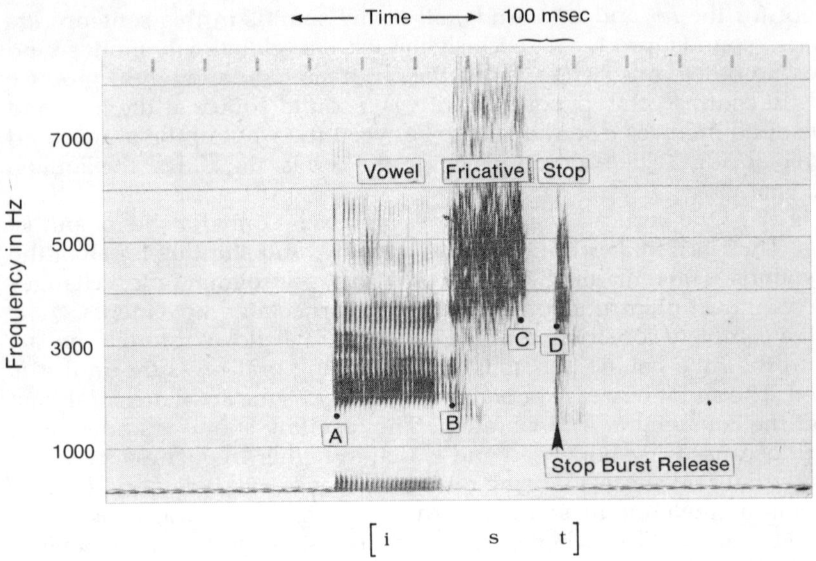

Fig. 1-21. Spectrogram of the word *east*.

This random fluctuation of energy from frequency to frequency is characteristic of turbulence noise sources.

The area from C to D is a period of silence resulting from the vocal tract closure and glottal opening for the voiceless /t/. At point D, the speaker's tongue tip was rapidly pulled away from the alveolar ridge, allowing pressurized oral air to burst through, creating a "transient" shock wave in the vocal tract beyond the alveolar ridge. This transient shock wave can be seen as a strong vertical line similar to the smaller shock lines produced by the glottal air bursts for vowel production.

Vocal Tract as an Acoustic Filter

The vocal tract contains a tube of air whose vibrations constitute the sounds of speech. The air bursts produced by laryngeal vibration shock this tube of air into "sympathetic vibration," the way a bell resonates after being struck by its clapper. With each burst of glottal energy, sound waves at many harmonic frequencies bounce back and forth along the length of the vocal tube at the speed of sound. When the waves reach the mouth opening, most of the energy reflects back into the tube toward the larynx, but some escapes to be heard as a speech sound. Figure 1-22 shows the pattern of acoustic

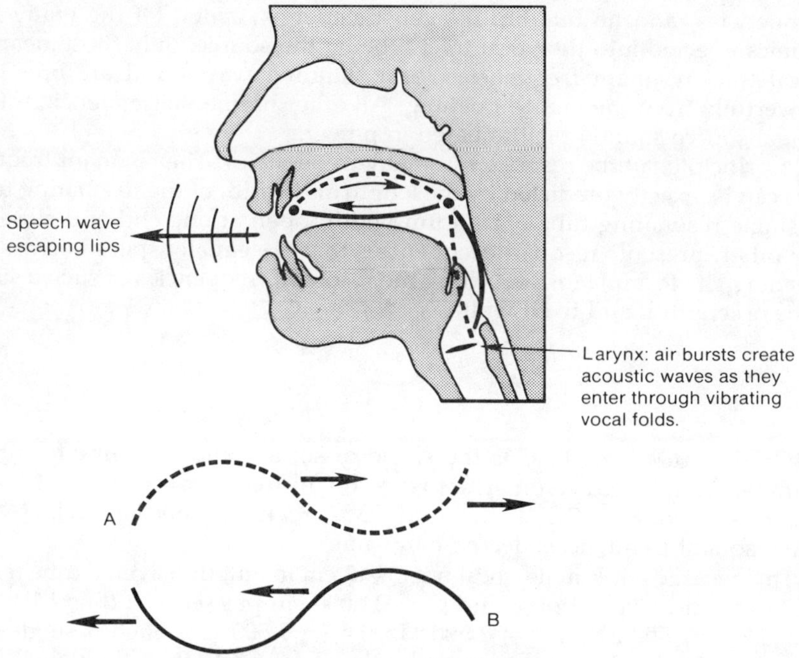

A. Speech acoustic wave propagating inward toward larynx from point of reflection at lip opening.

B. Speech acoustic wave propagating from larynx outward toward lip

Fig. 1-22. Acoustic waves reflecting between the larynx and lips during vowel production.

vibration of air in the vocal tract created by the impact of air bursts from the larynx.

Depending on the length and width of the tube, the "outgoing" and "reflected" acoustic vibrations create a pattern of "constructive interference" at the resonant frequencies of the vocal tract tube. At the resonant frequencies, the waves reflected from the lip arrive at the larynx in perfect synchrony with the onset of the next burst of air. The reflected energy and the energy being input from the larynx "add," causing a new, larger sound wave that travels to the lip, reflects, and again adds with a new, emerging energy pulse. The result is, at or near each tube resonant frequency, creation of strong vibrations, some of which escape the lips to reach the listener. If the tube length and width do not permit synchronous arrival of reflected and emerging sound waves, a standing wave is not created at those particular frequencies, and no buildup of acoustic energy occurs. Of the many harmonics injected into the vocal tract tube by the source, only those near the vocal tract resonant frequencies form standing waves and are broadcast powerfully from the mouth opening. All other harmonic frequencies of the glottal source sound are attenuated in power.

In principle, a tube resonates at many frequencies. The resonant frequencies can be exactly predicted by the length and width of the resonating tube. A single resonating tube of uniform width, open at one end and closed at the other, presents resonant frequencies that are equally spaced across frequency. The formula for predicting the resonant frequencies of such a single tube of length L and fixed width is

$$F = \frac{NC}{4L}$$

where *L* is tube length, C is the speed of sound, and *N* is an odd integer number, 1, 3, 5, and so on. The first resonant frequency would be F1 = C/4L; the second, F2 = 3C/4L; the third, F3 = 5C/4L. As tube length increases, the resonant frequencies decrease in value.

The average adult male vocal tract is 17 cm in length. Given a tube length of 17 cm and a speed of sound C = 34,000 cm per second, then F1 = 500 Hz, F2 = 1,500 Hz, F3 = 2,500 Hz, F4 = 3,500 Hz. Such a single-tube resonator is closely approximated by the vocal tract when the vowel /ɜ/ is articulated and the resonant frequencies of this vowel are close to those predicted above. Relatively long and short vocal tracts and their resonant frequencies are shown in the left side of Fig. 1-23. To the right of each tube is its resonance function. The peaks in each function represent the frequencies at which acoustic power in the glottal wave is emphasized and allowed to radiate from the lips. The low points in the functions represent frequencies that would be filtered out (rejected) of the glottal source and not radiated from the lips. Thus, a listener hearing the adult's vowel will hear energy at or near the frequencies 500 Hz, 1,500 Hz, and so forth. It is this pattern of energy across frequencies that will cue the listener as to the identity of the vowel intended by the speaker.

As vocal tract shape changes, the resonant frequencies also change. Figure 1-24 shows the simplified, effective tube shapes produced when the vocal tract is constricted to produce the vowels [i], [u], and [a]. When an [i] is produced the first resonant frequency is relatively low in frequency and the second resonant frequency is relatively high. A vocal tract constriction appropriate for [u] produces relatively low frequencies for both of the two lowest resonant frequencies. An [a] constriction produces resonant frequencies that are relatively close to one another, near 1,000 Hz. These patterns of resonant frequency locations serve as the strongest cues to the listener who is attempting to identify the vowels intended by the speaker.

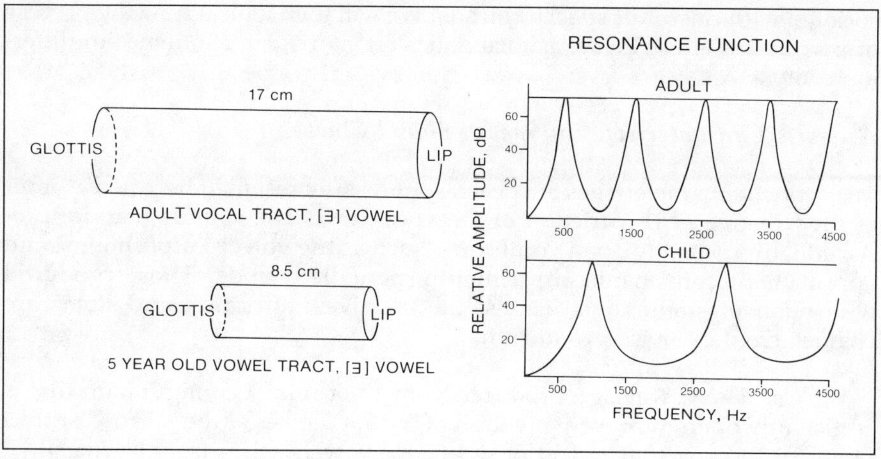

Fig. 1-23. Resonant frequencies of adult and child vocal tracts.

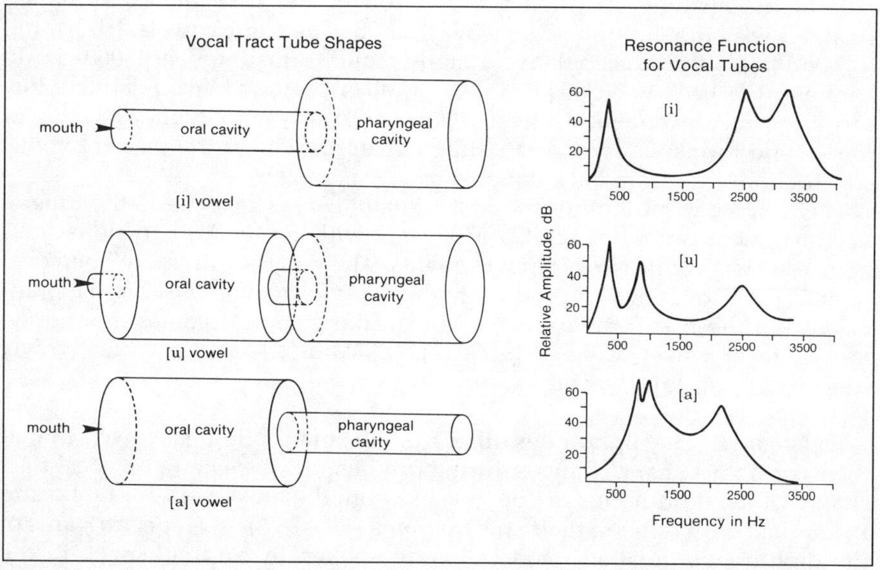

Fig. 1-24. Resonating tube models and spectra of the vowels [i], [u], and [a].

These sound source and filter characteristics of the vocal tract provide the basis for describing acoustic features associated with speech sound production. In the following discussion, we will describe the acoustic features associated with classes of speech sounds. We will then look at how the process of production alters these characteristics for particular phonemes in differing contexts.

Acoustic Characteristics of Speech Sound Classes

The acoustic characteristics of speech sounds are presented here in the order of their degree of constriction of the vocal tract. The sounds that are produced with relatively open vocal tracts such as the vowels, diphthongs, and approximant consonants are primarily periodic sounds. Those produced with relatively tight constrictions, the fricatives, affricates, and stops, are characterized by noise production.

Vowels. The vowels are produced with a vocal tract configuration that is sufficiently open to prevent creation of friction noises at the narrowest tract point for the vowel. The sound source for vowels arises from laryngeal vibration. This can be seen in the vertical striations of the spectrograms of the English vowels shown in Fig. 1-25.

Note the changes in frequency location of the two lowest formants* (marked with dots) in the vowels in Fig. 1-25. The front vowels, [i], [ɪ], [e], [ɛ], and [æ], all produce relatively high second formants, near 2,000 Hz. In contrast, the back vowels, [a], [ɔ], [ʊ], and [u], all produce relatively low second formant frequencies, near 1,000 Hz. Thus, the frequency location of the second formant serves as a strong perceptual cue to the place of vowel constriction, i.e., front/back dimension.

The frequency location of the first formant serves as a cue to the tongue height dimension. In general, the vowels with tighter constrictions (i.e., high vowels) produce lower first formants. The vowels with more open oval cavities (i.e., low vowels) produce higher first formants. Observe the gradual rise in the first formant as the vowel constriction becomes more open for the front vowel series—[i], [ɪ], [e], [ɛ], and [æ]—and the back vowel series—[u], [ʊ], [o], [ɔ], and [a].

Diphthongs. The diphthongs differ from the monopthongal vowels in that their vocal tract shape changes during production. The changing vocal tract shapes of the diphthongs can be inferred from the movements of F_1, F_2, and F_3 (marked with dots) in their spectrograms (Fig. 1-26). The spectrograms of the diphthongs [aɪ], [aʊ], and [ɔɪ] were spoken by an adult male in the words *buy, bow,* and *boy.*

---

*The resonant frequencies of vowel and consonantal vocal tract tubes are reflected by the regions of strong harmonics seen as dark "bars" or "formants" in the spectrograms shown herein. A formant is to its underlying tube resonant frequency as a spray of water is to the pin hole in a hose that releases it.

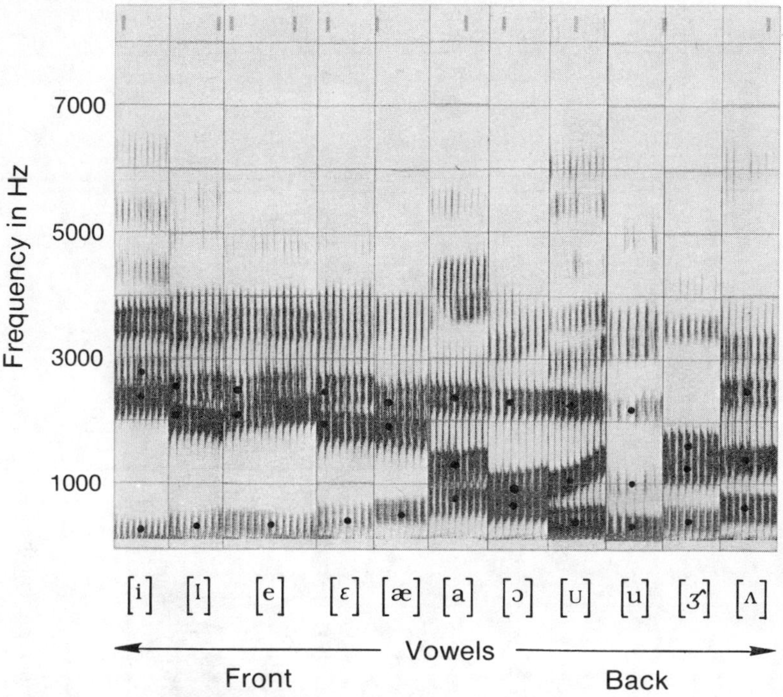

Fig. 1-25. Spectrograms showing formant frequencies of the vowels. (Dots represent the lowest three formant frequencies for each vowel.)

The diphthong [aɪ] starts with a low back constriction and ends with a high front constriction. Accordingly, F_2 rises as the constriction moves from back to front, and F_1 falls as the constriction moves from low to high. In /aʊ/, a low back constriction is moved to a high back constriction. As the tongue rises, F_1 falls. F_2 also falls because some movement of the tongue occurs farther back for /ʊ/ than /a/, but also because of lip rounding, which increases the length of the vocal tract, thus lowering all resonant frequencies. The diphthong /ɔi/ starts as a low back vowel and ends as a high front vowel. As the tongue moves from back to front, F_2 rises. As the tongue moves from low to high, F_1 falls.

Approximant Consonants. The approximant consonants include the glides, liquids, and nasals. Their acoustic properties are similar to the vowels. The glide consonants /j/ and /w/ are similar to diphthongs. They start with vocal tract configurations similar to the vowels /i/ and /u/ and then change shape to approximate the vowel that follows them in a word. Recall that /j/ and /w/ only occur at the beginning of stressed syllables. Figure 1-27

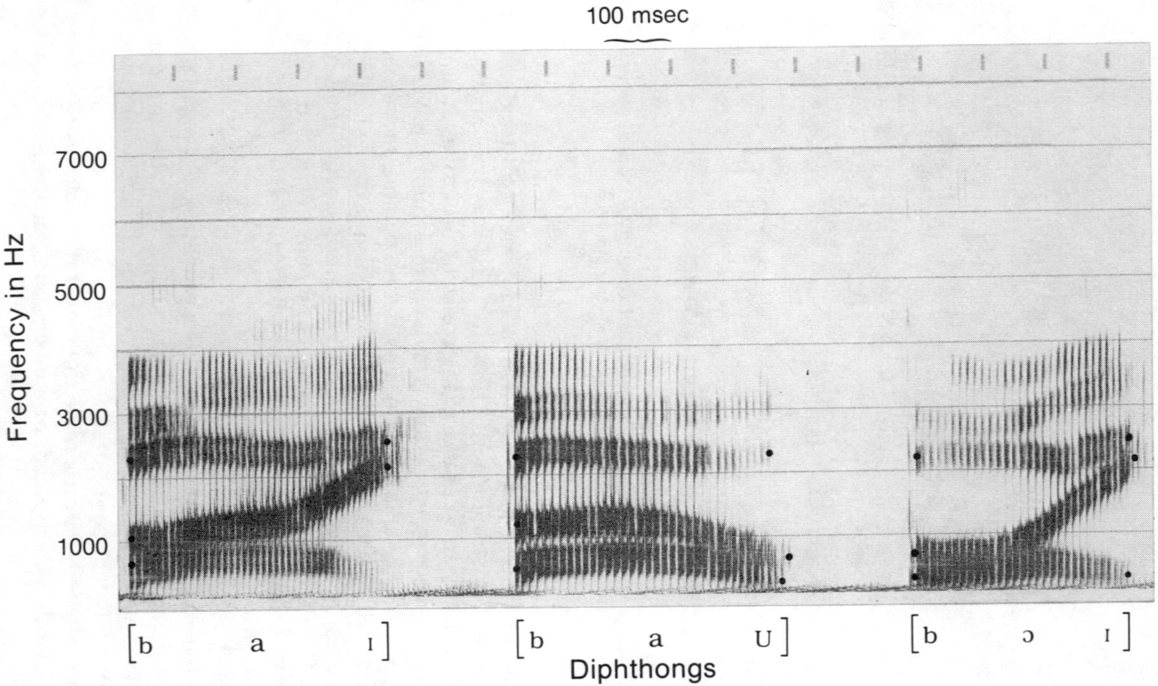

Fig. 1-26. Spectrograms of *buy* [baɪ], *bow* [baʊ], and *boy* [bɔɪ]. (Dots represent the starting and ending formant frequencies.)

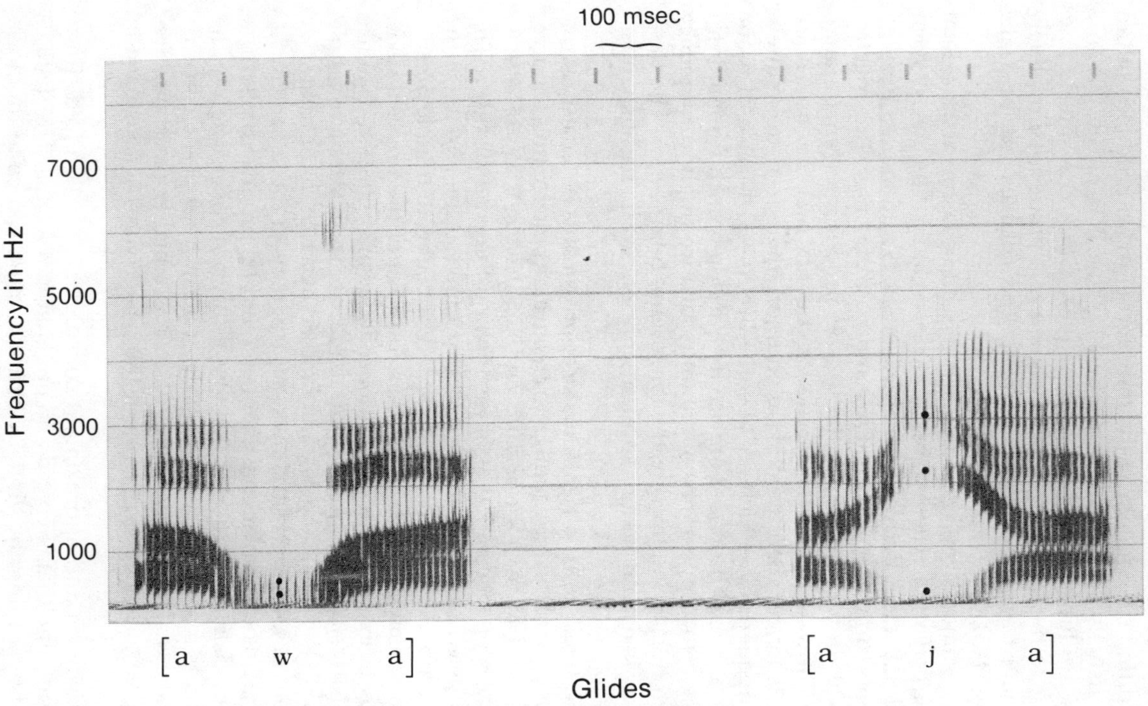

Fig. 1-27. Spectrograms of [awa] and [aja]. (Dots represent the lowest formant frequencies of the glide sounds.)

shows spectrograms of the syllables /awa/ and /aja/. Note that the relationship between the first two formant frequencies during [j] production is similar to that for /i/ (i.e., F_2 is high, indicating a front constriction; F_1 is low, indicating a tight constriction). The formant frequencies of /w/ are similar to those of /u/ (i.e., the first two formant frequencies are low).

The liquids /l/ and /r/ display acoustic representations that are similar to /w/ in that all produce relatively low first and second formant frequencies. However, they differ in frequency of the third formant: /w/ produces a third formant that is usually so decreased in intensity that it is not visible in a spectrogram; /r/ produces a third formant frequency that is relatively low, strong, and close to the second formant frequency; /l/ produces a relatively high third resonant frequency. Spectrograms of the syllables /ara/ and /ala/ are shown in Fig. 1-28.

The nasal approximants /m, n, ŋ/ are, like the stop consonants, made at three places of articulation. The oral cavity is closed at the lips /m/, alveolar ridge /n/, or soft palate /ŋ/. Both airflow and acoustic vibration pass through the open velar port into the nasopharynx and nasal cavities. The spectrograms in Fig. 1-29 show the nasals in the syllable productions [ama], [ana], and [aŋa]. Each shows a pattern of very low frequency first formants since the nasal cavity is longer than the oral. In addition, there is a strong attenuation of high frequencies, which are absorbed by the soft mucosal tissue lining the nasal cavities. The closed oral cavity is a side-branch resonator for the nasals, causing the appearance of an antiresonance (high in frequency for the short oral tube of /ŋ/; low, for the longer oral tube of /m/). The nasal antiresonance weakens and widens formants present in the nasal sounds.

Fricatives. Fricative sounds differ from the approximants because the constriction in the vocal tract is tight enough to create a turbulence noise source. The two varieties of fricatives are *sibilants* and *nonsibilants*. The sibilants /s, z, ʃ, ʒ/ show places of articulation at or just behind the alveolar ridge. The air stream is funneled smoothly in the groove formed in the surface of the tongue blade and tip. As the air picks up speed, it begins to tumble noisily. The tumbling, noisy air jet generally strikes the edge of the upper incisor, or edge of the lower lip, and creates additional "edge or spoiler" turbulence noise. These noises (sibilants) are long (up to 0.25 second), strong in amplitude (only a few dB less than vowels), and marked by a rich, high-frequency noise power spectrum. Figure 1-30 shows spectrograms of the syllables [sa], [ʃa], [za], and [ʒa]. The alveolar consonants [s] and [z] produce higher frequencies than the palatal [ʃ] and [ʒ]. The more forward constriction in the vocal tract produces a smaller vibrating body of air in front of the constriction for the alveolars. This smaller mass of air has a higher resonance frequency than the larger air mass in front of the palatal constrictions used in [ʃ] and [ʒ].

Although the vowels and approximant consonants are all voiced, fricatives come in pairs, one that is voiced and one that is voiceless. The distinction is produced by adding the glottal vibratory sound source to the noise

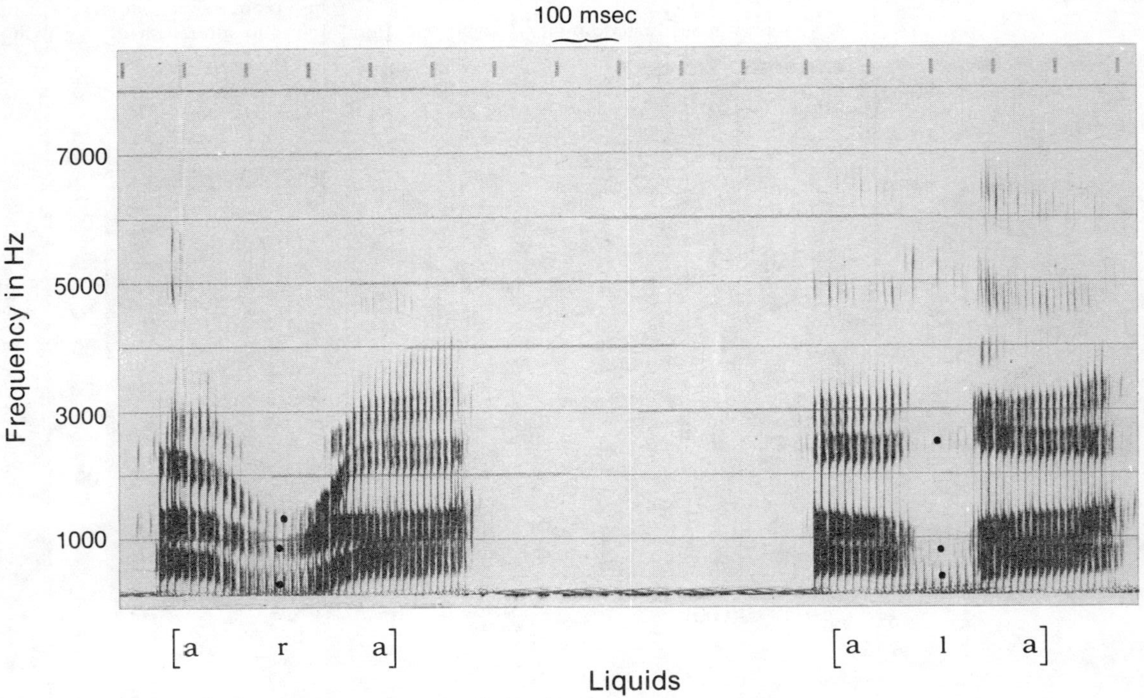

Fig. 1-28. Spectrograms of [ara] and [ala]. (Dots represent the lowest formant frequencies of the liquid sounds.)

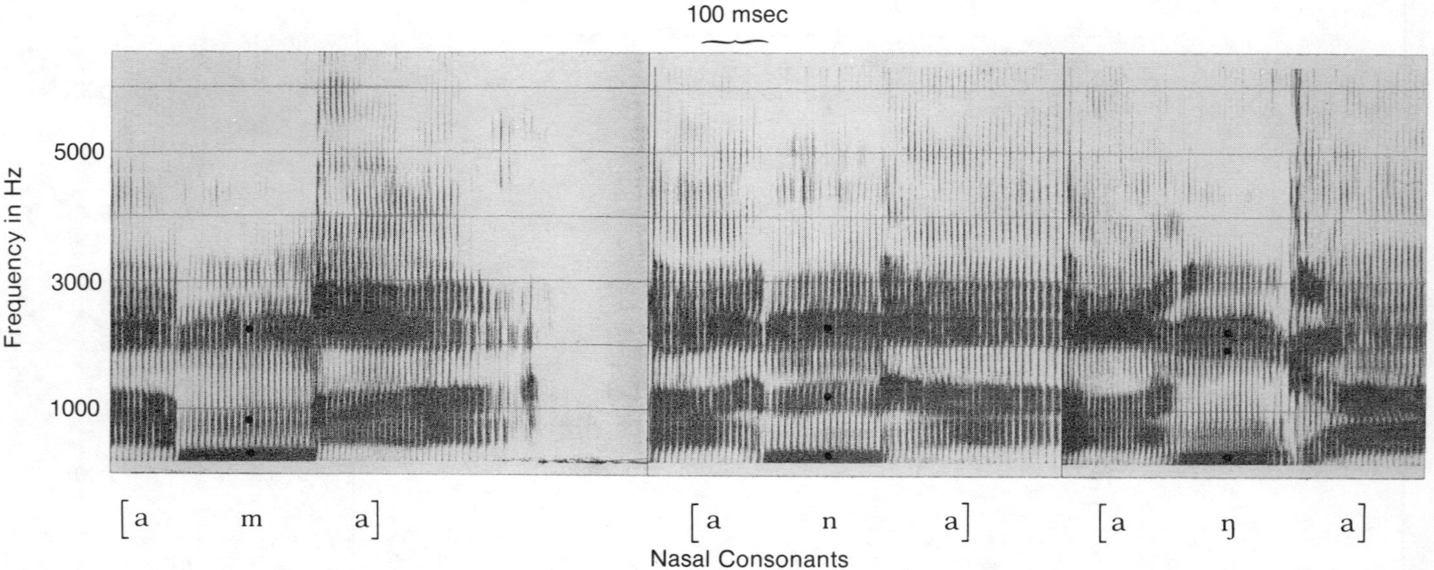

Fig. 1-29. Spectrograms of [ama], [ana], and [aŋa]. (Dots represent the lowest formant frequencies of the nasals.)

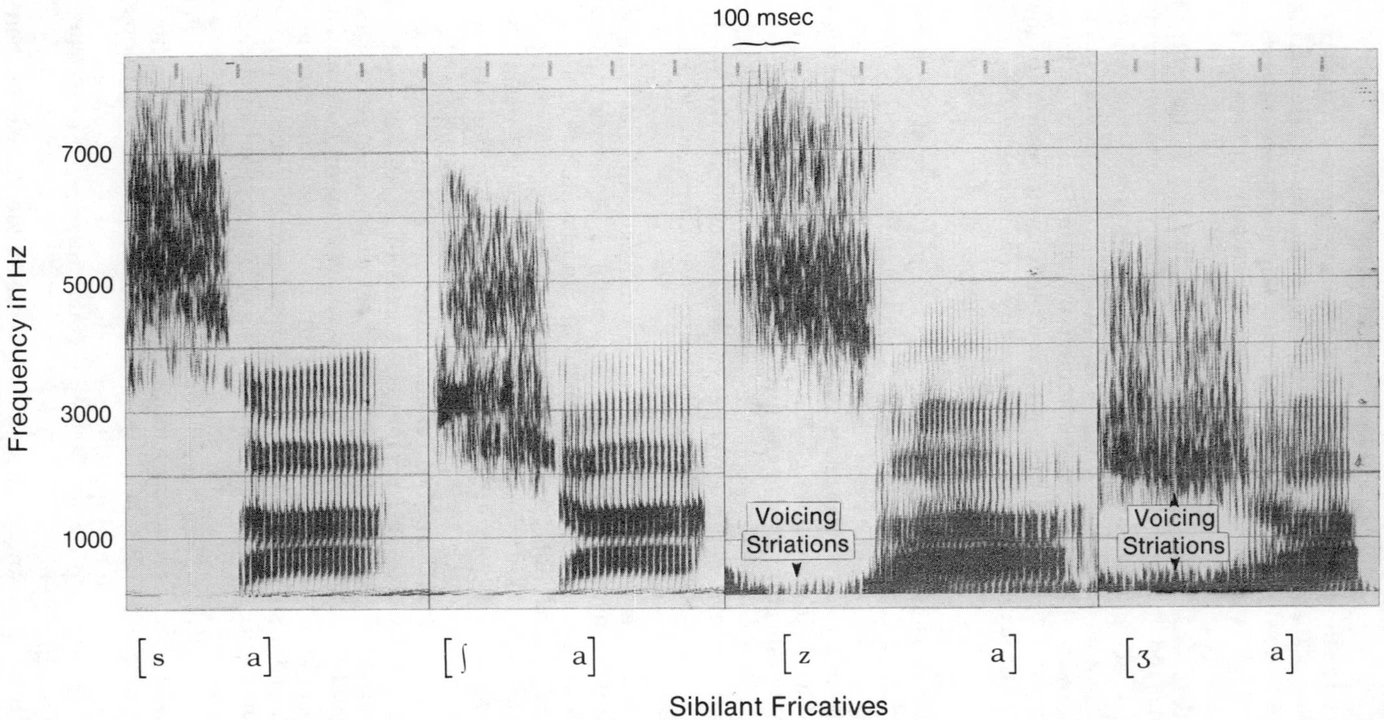

Fig. 1-30. Spectrograms of [sa], [ʃa], [za], and [ʒa], showing voicing striations for the voiced coguates.

source produced at the consonant constriction. Voicing appears in the spectrograms of Fig. 1-30 as vertical stripes mixed with the noise. The voicing stripes are especially strong at low frequencies, producing the characteristic "voicing bar" at the bottom of the spectrogram. Essentially, the voicing bar corresponds to the fundamental frequency of vocal fold vibration.

The nonsibilant dental fricatives /f,v/, /θ,ð/, shown in Fig. 1-31 are made with labiodental and linguadental constrictions. The soft lip or tongue tissue held against the teeth creates an abrupt, narrow constriction that generates a weak turbulence noise whose energy is spread to very high frequencies. The noise is so weak that listeners often derive the acoustic clues for identification not from the noise but from the prominent CV transitions of the labial fricatives. The presence of voicing is readily seen in the spectrograms of [v] and [ð].

Stops. Stop consonants must include a complete closure of the vocal tract. During this time period, air pressure rises inside the oral cavity until the stop is released. Pressure rises rapidly and high because of airflow through the opened folds for voiceless stops; it rises less rapidly and high because of reduced air flow through the vibrating folds for voiced stops. Figure 1-32 shows spectrograms of the utterances "a cab," "a cap," and "a gab." Note that in each the vowel [ə] is followed by a period of silence. A similar silent period follows the vowel [æ] in each spectrogram, again indicating the vocal tract closure period for production of the word-final consonants.

Each of these silent periods is followed by a transient noise associated with release of the consonant constriction. The point of release for the first stops in the words *cap* and *gap* are marked in the figure with an *R*.

Voicing of the syllable-initial stop consonants is cued by *voice onset time* and aspiration. Voice onset time refers to the length of time between the release of the vocal tract closure and the onset of voicing for the following vowel. This time is quite short for the /g/ in *gap* (about 20 msec) and longer for the /k/ in *cap* (about 70 msec). In general, voice onset times of less than 30 msec represent voiced stop consonants whereas those greater than 30 msec cue voicelessness. Upon release of the constriction, a surge of high pressure airflow for voiceless stops produces a burst-explosion noise and a following turbulence noise; the lower air pressure for voiced stops does not support such a noisy surge of airflow upon release of the closure. The explosion and turbulence (aspiration) noise are important supplemental cues for voicelessness.

At the ends of syllables, stop consonants need not be released nor followed by a vowel. Thus, a voice onset time cue for final-consonant voicing will not be available. The difference between voiced and voiceless final stops is cued by vowel duration and transition speeds. Voiced stop consonants, such as the [b] in *cab,* are preceded by longer vowels than are the voiceless stops, such as the [p] in *cap.*

Stops differ from nasal and glide sounds in terms of the velocity of their

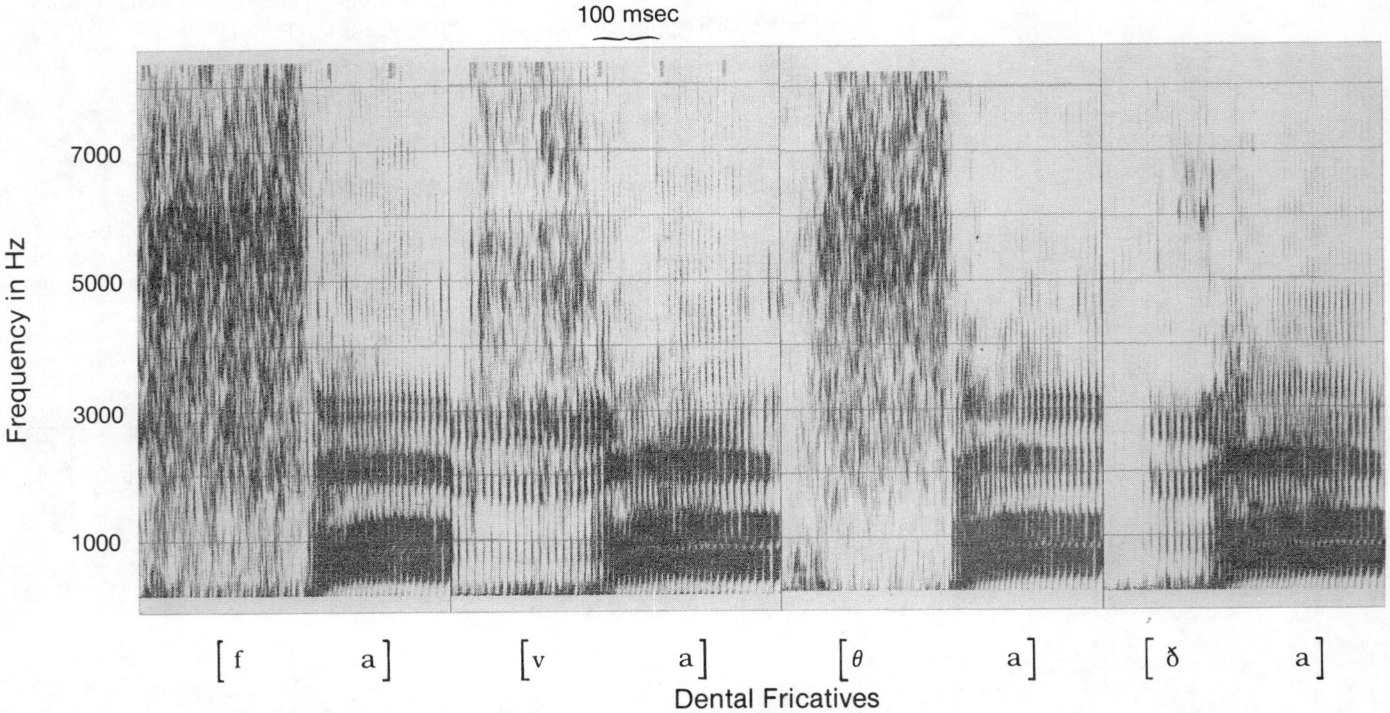

Fig. 1-31. Spectrograms of the dental fricatives [fa], [va], [θa], and [ða].

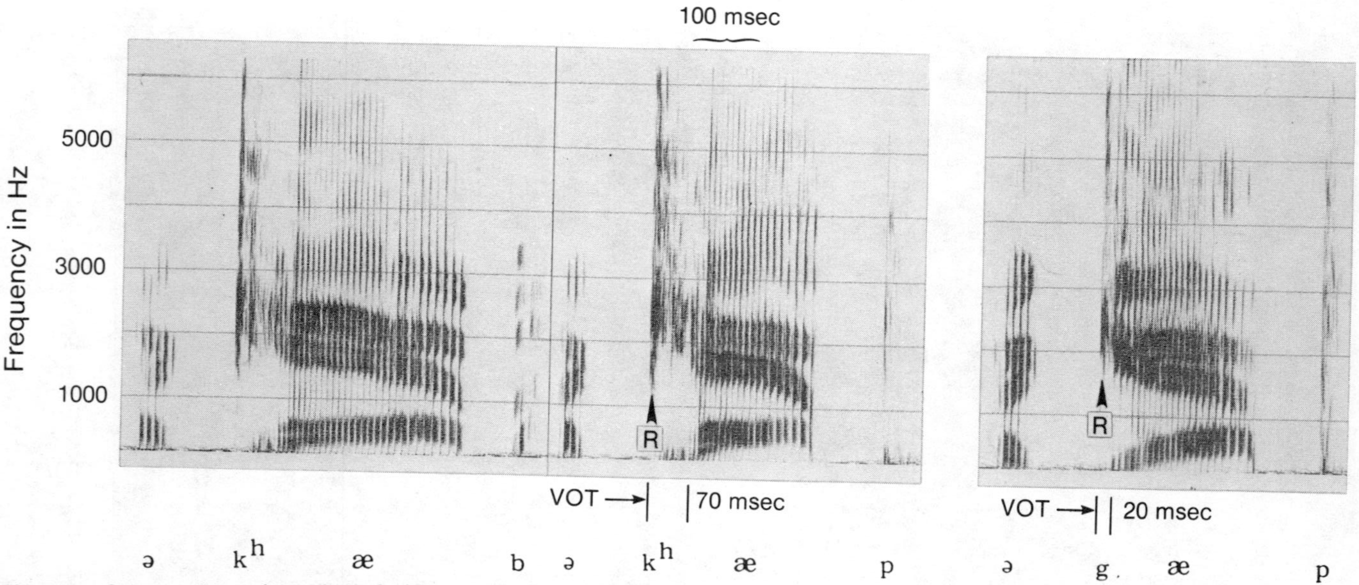

Fig. 1-32. Spectrograms of "a cab" [ə kæb], "a cap" [əkæp], and "a gap" [əgæp], showing consonant release (R) and voice onset time (VOT).

transitions. Stop consonants are produced with very rapid transitions, nasals with slightly slower CV transitions and glides [w,j] with even slower transitions.

Place of articulation of stops is cued by the initial formant frequencies and their transitions to the following vowel. The transition contains information about both the consonant and the vowel. For example, Fig. 1-33 shows spectrograms of the syllables /aba/, /ada/, and /aga/. The basic difference between these stops is seen in the positions of the second and third formant frequencies, marked with dots at the point of consonant constriction release (the time point marked with a *B*). In /aba/ the second and third formant frequencies remain relatively constant because the tongue position for /a/ can be maintained throughout the labial closure. In /ada/ the second formant rises from the first /a/ and then falls back toward the second /a/, while the first formant moves in an opposite direction, falling from the first /a/ and rising to the second /a/. The /aga/ transitions differ in that the third formant approaches the second for the /g/ and then diverges from the second formant for /a/.

Affricates. Like the stops consonants, affricates /tʃ/ and /ʤ/ require a stop-like closure period followed by rapid release into a friction noise. Figure 1-34 shows spectrograms for the syllables [atʃa] and [aʤa]. Note the silent period produced by the consonant closures and the noise produced after release of the consonant closure.

Acoustic Effects of Coproduction

As speech production processing progresses, articulatory gestures smoothly move from one target position to another. The phonemic targets are adjusted in time and space by coproduction processes. Thus, phoneme targets shift as their neighboring phonemes (targets) are changed. These differing vocal tract targets cause variations in the acoustic patterns for the phoneme as well. Coproduction spreads the acoustic cues for a particular sound over several neighboring sounds within the utterance. The following are examples of the acoustic effects of coproduction.

Figure 1-35 shows spectrograms of the utterances [gi, gu, ga]. As we have discussed, the place of articulation of the consonant /g/ is cued by the relative positions of the first three formant frequencies of the vocal tract. Notice the changes in the starting frequency of the second formant as [g] is coproduced with these differing vowels: It is near 2,000 Hz preceding [i], around 1,300 Hz preceding [u], and near 1,800 Hz preceding [a]. These changes reflect the movement of the constriction for [g] from palatal (preceding [i]) to velar (preceding [a] and [u]). The extra lowering of the formant frequencies preceding [u] are in part caused by lip rounding.

The velum tends to be moved relatively slowly so that vowels that follow and precede nasal consonants are produced with opened velums. Figure 1-36 shows spectrograms of the names *Dan* and *Nan*. Compare the two vowel

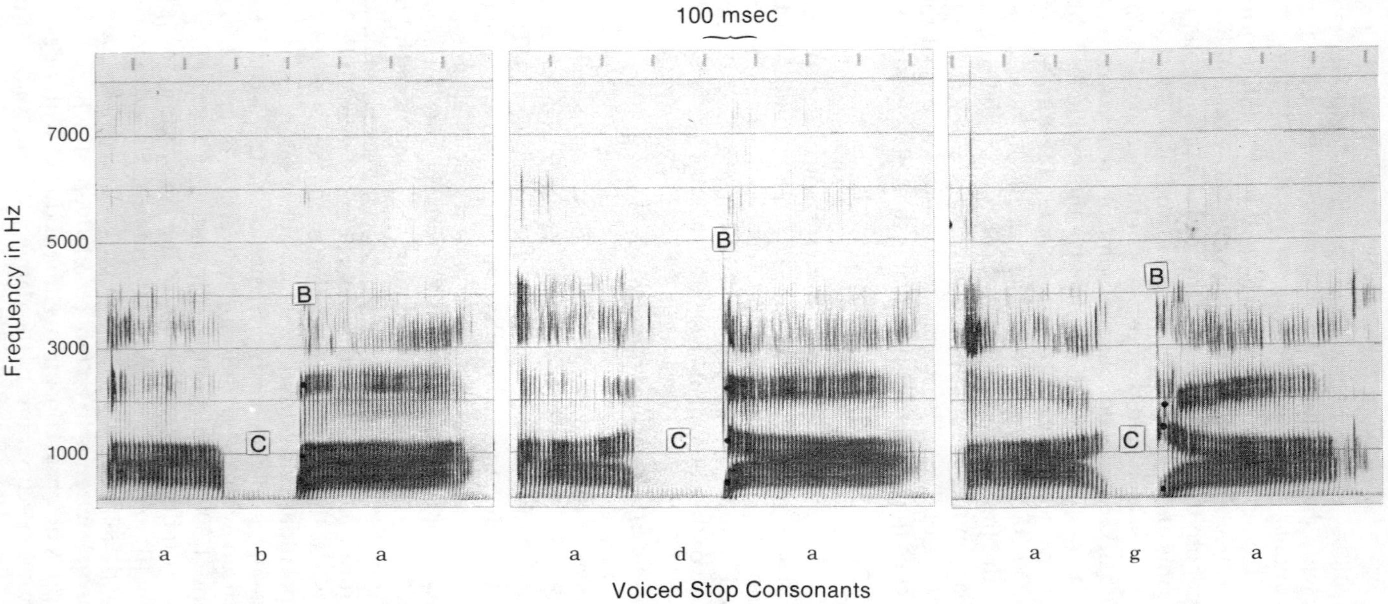

Fig. 1-33. Spectrograms of [aba], [ada], and [aga], showing the consonant burst (B) and consonant closures (C).

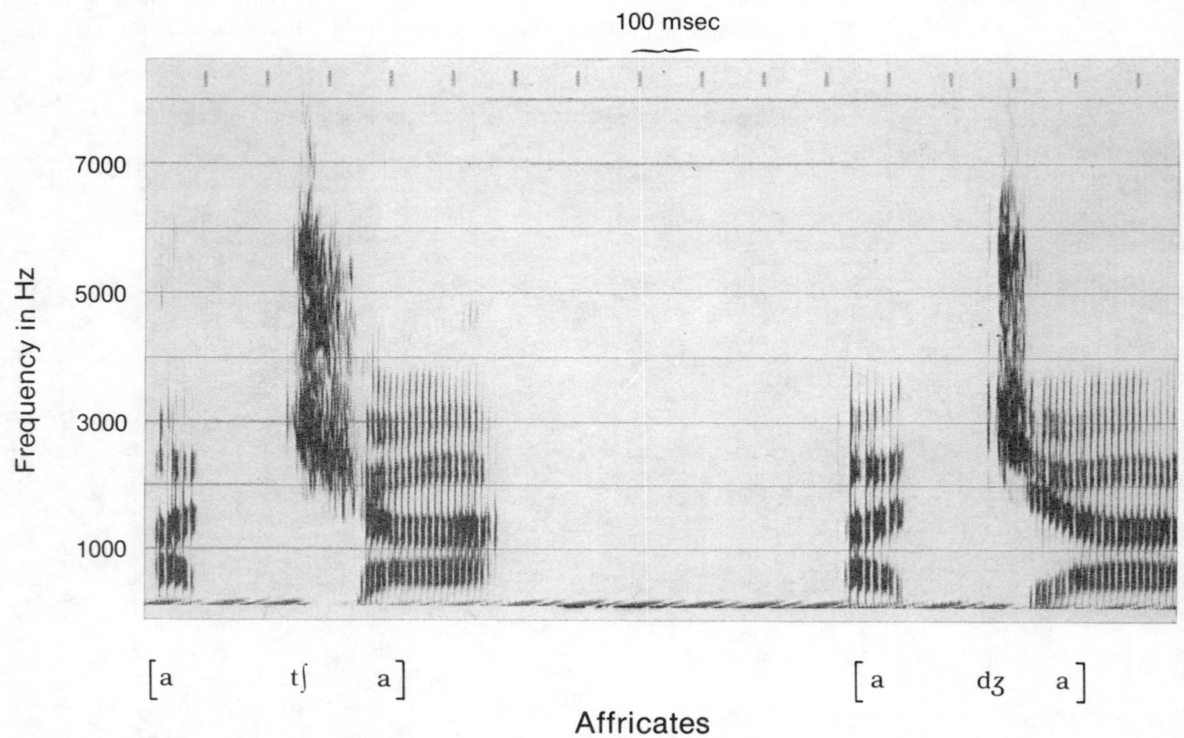

Fig. 1-34. Spectrograms of [atʃa] and [adʒa].

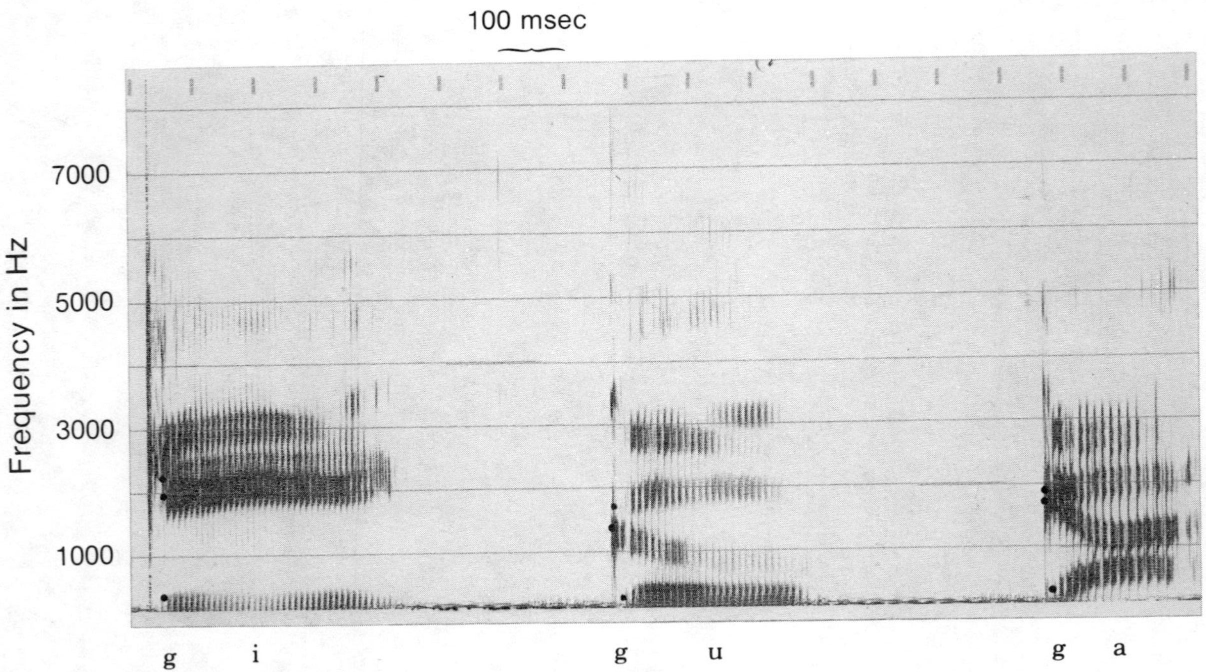

Fig. 1-35. Spectrograms of [gi], [gu], and [ga]. (Dots represent the formant frequencies at consonant release.)

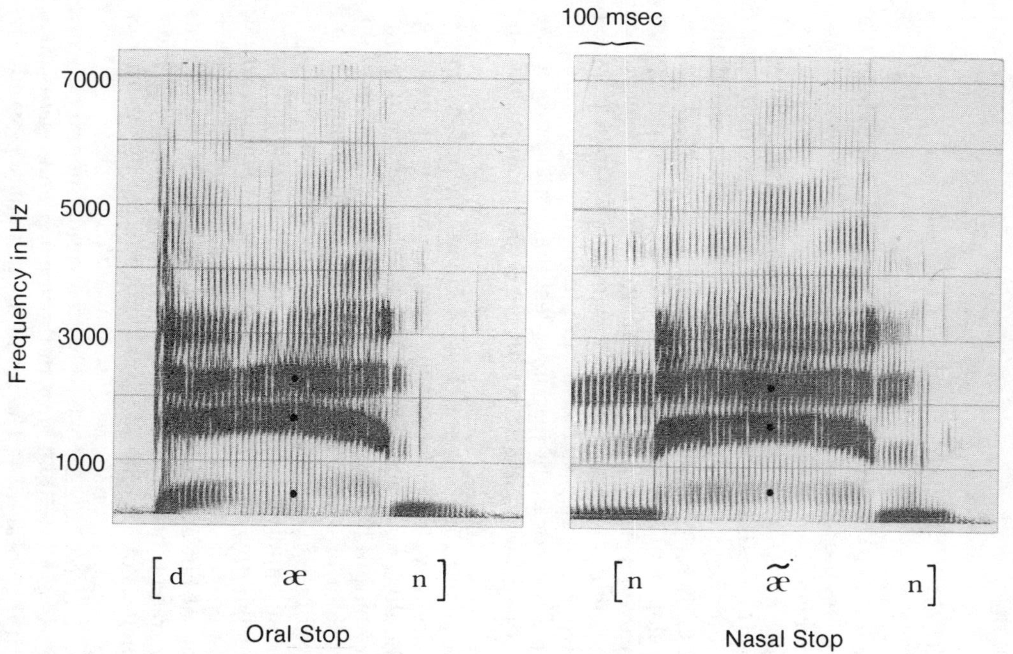

Fig. 1-36. Spectrograms of the vowel æ in the words *daen* and *nan* showing differences in vowel nasalization.

spectra and you will see in *Nan* that the vowel is relatively weak in intensity throughout, indicating full coproduction of nasalization throughout [næn]. For /dæn/, coproduction is more limited, with nasalization occurring well into the vowel.

Figure 1-37 shows the effect of lip rounding on /s/ production. Observe that the energy concentration (shown by arrows at the lowest frequencies of energy present) in the /s/ of /usu/ is much lower in frequency than in the utterance /isi/. This is due to the lengthening of the vocal tract when the lips are rounded throughout the /s/ production. The perceptual system must factor out this difference in deciding that the utterance contains an /s/ and not an /ʃ/, which would also have lower-frequency energy.

MODEL OF SPEECH PERCEPTION

In this section, we will describe a model of speech perception in which the perceiver ultimately infers the articulatory gestures used by the speaker and does so in a swift, sophisticated, automatic manner.

Consider the evolutionary forces that shaped human hearing abilities. In the animal world, hearing is used to find prey, avoid predators, and attract mates. In accomplishing these tasks, the function of hearing is to recruit the motor systems of the body for pursuit, flight, and social behaviors. This was accomplished by development of strong neural linkages between perception of particular auditory events and actions of the motor systems. Detection of high-frequency sounds might indicate a smaller animal that is to be pursued as food. Hearing lower-frequency sounds might indicate a larger animal, which should invoke a fight or flight response, lest the hearer become the food. In either case, the hearer must detect, localize, and evaluate the auditory event rapidly.

Fodor (1986) has claimed that when a class of environmental signals is vital to survival, nature may "modularize" the neural analysis of these signals. The module should be fast acting and error-free and produce immediately useful sensory output. Consider the food-locating mechanism of the barn owl. A flash of light or a small noise leads to a rapid pounce on an unlucky field mouse. Investigators have found that the owl's nervous system integrates visual and auditory stimuli into a three-dimensional map of space with particular neurons responding to either type of stimuli arising from a given point in space. The spatial representation is amodal: It is neither auditory nor visual but a form of "something in that location." This analysis is relatively free of interference from cognitive processing. It must provide a truthful analysis of the stimuli that are not affected by whether or not the owl is hungry, excited, or sleepy at the moment.

The speech perception mechanism may rely on a similar neural network that combines auditory and visual features of the speaker and relates them to motoric features of the vocal tract. The result of such analysis would de-

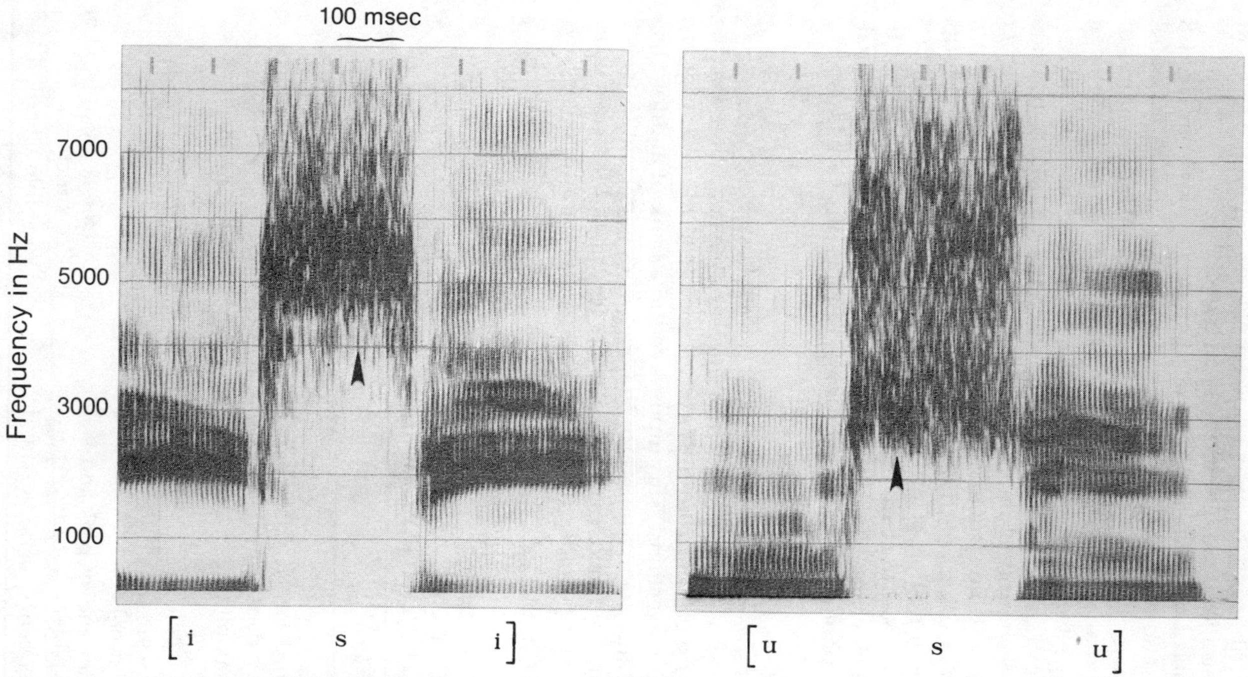

Fig. 1-37. Spectrograms of [isi] and [usu]. The arrows show the lowest frequencies present in the [s] noises.

termine where in vocal tract space a speech sound was produced. In the case of speech, this means inferring the vocal tract gestures that produced the vocal configuration responsible for the speech sound. In the pages that follow, we will describe how this may be accomplished within the levels of the verbal communication model we have been exploring.

The lower portion of the verbal communication model shown in Fig. 1-8 connects the basic auditory and visual input features to the tactile-kinesthetic features of basic articulatory gestures. Auditory and visual features of the speech input are analyzed simultaneously and unconsciously matched to the articulatory gestures most likely to have produced them. These features are analyzed by reference to the same, gestural, stored, phoneme units that are used in speech production. Simultaneously, in parallel, the listener seeks to derive the syllable structure, meaningful linguistic unit structure, and underlying propositions of the speaker. Essentially, the feature inputs serve as cues to the intention of the speaker at all of the levels simultaneously, including the vocal tract shapes intended to represent phonemes. In the following sections we will look at some of the characteristics of this analysis at the feature, phoneme, and higher levels of perceptual analysis.

Feature Level

The basic auditory processing provided by the ear delivers a time-varying spectral analysis of the input sound that is analogous to the spectrograms presented in previous sections. This input is fed to a bank of auditory feature detectors that analyze the sound for characteristics important to speech perception. For example there may be detectors for each of the cues listed in Table 1-5. Each cue provides information about the vocal tract gestures that produced the sound.

Table 1-5. AUDITORY CUES AND ASSOCIATED ARTICULATORY GESTURES

Cue	*Articulatory gesture*
Intensity rises F_1 frequency location rises Vocal fold frequency rises	Vocal tract opening
Decrease in sound amplitude F_1 frequency falls Vocal fold frequency falls Presence of frication noise Presence of transient noise	Vocal tract closing
F_2 falls as constriction moves back and cavity in front is larger	Size of cavity in front of constriction
Presence of low-frequency, periodic sound	Vocal fold vibration

Because the features of particular phonemes are coproduced and spread over time, it is necessary for feature processing to occur over a stretch of speech—perhaps as long as a second. To accomplish this, McClelland and Elman (1986) suggested that repeated sets of feature detectors exist. The sound is input to the first set and then progressively passed on to the later sets. This allows the higher-level processing units to gather information on the speech signal over a certain time by accessing the feature patterns in adjoining sets of feature detectors. This is analogous to the screen of an oscilloscope, which shows a stretch of time by repeating the movements of a beam of electrons across the face of the scope.

We suspect that an auditory feature analysis is one of the first stages of speech perception because studies have shown that when listeners make errors in the perception of speech, the errors are usually only one feature away from the intended sound (Miller & Nicely, 1955). Miller and Nicely had listeners identify words with increasing background noise. When the noise forced the listeners into error, the errors involved sounds that were close to one another in feature composition. For example, [s] would be heard as /z/ but would probably not be heard as /m/ or some other sound that was many features different from /s/.

One of the major principles of speech perception is that each speech sound is cued by many features. In a pioneering study Slis and Cohen (1969) demonstrated that more than 12 acoustic cues were important to the perception of stop consonants. This richness of auditory cues helps the listener, who can miss one or a few cues due to background noise or inattention and still have enough cues to identify the phoneme.

A second aspect of speech perception is that the auditory cues for identification of a particular phoneme may be traded for one another. For example, the stop consonant /p/ may be cued by a silent period, followed by a burst transient, followed by an aspiration noise. If the aspiration noise is shortened, the sound is perceived as /b/. However, experimenters have weakened some of these cues and found that by strengthening others they can maintain a perception of /p/. For example, the burst noise can be eliminated if the silent period is made longer, and the listener will still perceive that /p/ has been produced. This ability to trade cues is one mechanism for coping with poorly articulated speech produced in noise. It does not appear that the listener is trying to match a perfect set of auditory cues to the incoming speech to find the phonemes signalled within. Rather, the listener uses the cues available to try to predict the phonemes that were intended by the speaker.

Another aspect of speech perception that suggests that the listener used auditory cues for predictions is the normalization that must be accomplished across speakers. Vocal tracts differ in size and shape from speaker to speaker, resulting in different vocal tract formant frequencies. Therefore, the absolute acoustic cues produced by one speaker are different from those produced by other speakers. Furthermore, different speakers employ different habitual strategies for speech production, which result in differing cue sets being associated with phonemes. Listeners are able to swiftly accommodate the changes in absolute values of the cues produced by different speakers.

The listener is confronted with both visible and auditory features of the speaker's utterance. We hypothesize that these cues are interpreted with reference to the vocal tract gestures that produced the speech sounds. This is a rather strong claim and suggests that speech perception is basically different from auditory perception of nonspeech events such as music. This type of theory of speech perception has been called a "motor theory" because it involves using motoric features in the perception of speech (Liberman & Mattingly, 1985). The following are some reasons why we suspect that such a mechanism exists.

Combining Auditory and Visual Features. One form of evidence that listeners use gestural features in the interpretation of speech signals comes from studies in which visual information changes a person's perception of auditory events. McGurk and McDonald (1976) had adult listeners identify the speech sounds they heard as they watched a videotape of a person saying the syllable /ba/. The visual cues associated with this syllable include an obvious lip-closing gesture. When the sound track associated with this video image was also a /ba/ syllable, the listeners unerringly called it /ba/. However, when the audio was changed to /da/, the listeners did not generally report hearing /da/. Rather, the listeners heard the speaker say /va/! The listeners altered their perception of the auditory /d/ and visual /b/ to yield /v/, whose place of articulation (dental) is intermediate between labial /b/ and alveolar /d/. They apparently melded the acoustic and visual place features together into a combined audio-video perception of /v/, a sound neither heard /d/ or seen /b/. This appears to be a process similar to the barn owl's melding of sight and sound to produce a perception of place in space. In the speech perception case, the listener melds sight and sound to produce a perception of place in the vocal tract.

The conjunction of auditory, visual, and gestural features appears to be something that is innate to the human brain. Kuhl and Meltzoff (1982) simultaneously presented two video recordings of a woman saying the vowels /i/ and /u/ to 3-month-old children. That is, one video display would show lip spreading, /i/, while the other showed lip rounding, /u/. When the audio track carried a /u/, the children looked at the rounded lips more often and vice versa! If both visual displays were incorrect (i.e., the woman had spread lips and the auditory image was a /u/) the children did not look at the video displays nearly as often. Furthermore, when visual and auditory events were presented appropriately matched, the children babbled more often! These data point to a strong, innate linkage between the visual and auditory systems in relation to the speech gestural system.

Making Reference To Gestures. Evolution has provided a progressive elaboration of the human nervous system from lower forms of animals. Some

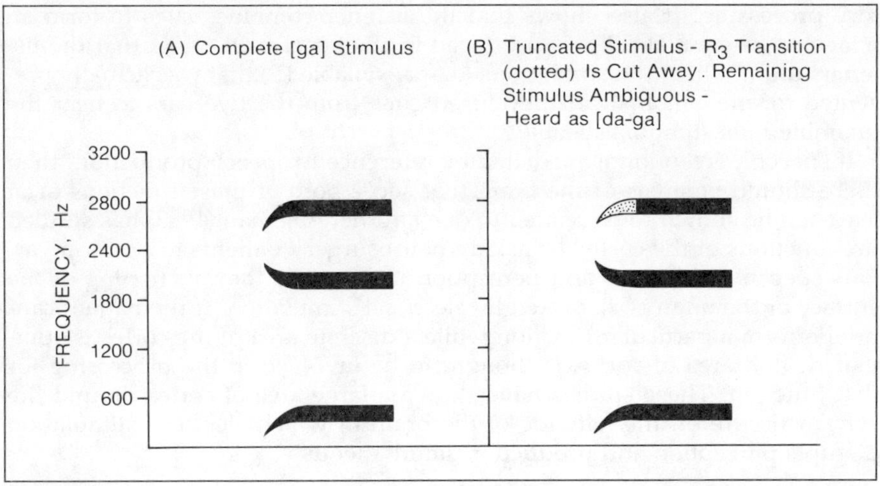

Fig. 1-38. Schematic spectrograms of two syllables heard as [ga] (stimulus A) and as an ambiguous [da] or [ga] (stimulus B).

of these animals show auditory-gestural linkages in their sound-producing and-perceiving systems. Williams and Nottebohm (1986) studied the song production and perception of finches. These investigators found that the songs of this bird were composed of small mini-themes of notes. Longer songs were made up of combinations of these mini-themes, and each mini-theme was controlled by a particular region of the motor nervous system. They found that when the finch hears one of these mini-themes, the motor region associated with its production was active! Thus, the finch appeared to be using the motor nervous system to interpret melody!

The *motor theory of speech perception* suggests that humans use two modes of auditory perception: one for speech and one for other sounds. Best, Hoffman, and Robson (1981) have demonstrated these two types of auditory processing by cleverly manipulating speech stimuli. Figure 1-38A shows a schematic spectrogram of a computer-generated syllable that is consistently heard as [ga]. Figure 1-38B shows the same syllable with the transition of the third resonant frequency eliminated. When the second syllable (B) is presented without the third resonant frequency transition, it is heard half of the time as /da/ and half of the time as /ga/. When just the third resonant frequency transition is presented, it is heard as a "chirp."

To show the two types of perception, Best and colleagues played the altered syllable (B) to one ear and put the F2 transition into the other ear. The listeners simultaneously heard the chirp and the integrated syllable, which was identified as [ga] (syllable A). This phenomenon has been called *duplex perception*. It shows that the listener uses both speech and nonspeech auditory processing. It also shows that the listener combines cues to form an image of where a syllable is produced in the vocal tract. Note that the listeners did not hear the ambiguous /da-ga/ syllable (B) that was actually presented to one ear. Instead they fused cues from the two ears to hear the unambiguous stimulus syllable.

If speech perception is mediated by reference to speech production, then there should be areas of the brain that serve both of these functions or at least can be shown to be related to one another. Ojeman (1983) has studied the functions of the cortex by asking neurosurgery patients to perform various speech production and perception tasks while the functioning of the surface of the brain is disrupted by electrical stimulation. If the patient cannot perform a particular function while a discrete area of the cortex is stimulated, that area of cortex is thought to be involved in the processing for that function. These studies have shown a large area of cortex around the sylvian fissure on the left side of the brain in which electrical stimulation disrupts perception and production simultaneously.

Phonemic Level

At the next higher level, the listener determines the phonemes represented by the changing feature complexes over a stretch of speech. In order to do this, the listener must undo the alterations in acoustic features of a phoneme that were caused by the speaker's coproduction of phonemic targets. Each phoneme can appear in thousands of different phonetic environments, each of which causes differing feature sets to appear. At this level, the various forms of a phoneme must be categorized as belonging to a particular phoneme. This process has been called *categorical perception*.

Categorical perception is the opposite of continuous perception. When auditory stimuli are continuously perceived, each change in an acoustic pattern is detected as a stimulus of differing quality. For example, listeners are able to tell that two pure tones that differ in frequency by as little as 1 Hz are different sounds. They are able to discriminate pure tones in this fashion across a wide area of the frequency domain. If we perceived speech sounds continuously, we would be able to discriminate all of the thousands of allophones of a particular phoneme.

In fact, listeners do tend to hear vowel sounds continuously. Figure 1-39 shows schematic spectrograms of synthesized vowels whose formant frequencies differ in steady increments, changing from /i/ to /æ/. When asked to tell if pairs of these stimuli differ, listeners succeed more if the stimuli are farther apart in resonance frequencies. That is, they would be more likely to succeed in saying that stimulus 1 is different from stimulus 3 than they would in saying that stimulus 1 is different from stimulus 2. The more different the sounds are acoustically, the more likely one can tell they are different.

However, for many speech sounds, listeners do not improve their ability to discriminate stimuli solely by how far apart their acoustic cues are.

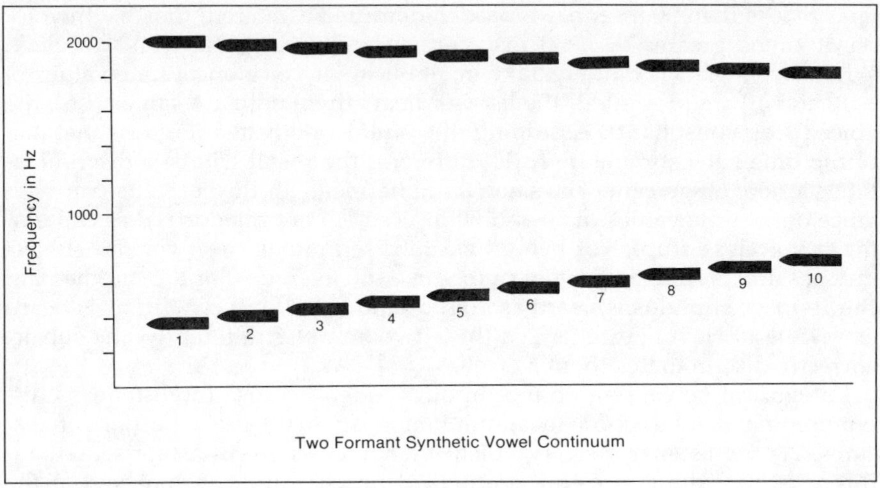

Fig. 1-39. Schematic two formant spectrograms of continuously discriminated vowels from [i] to [æ].

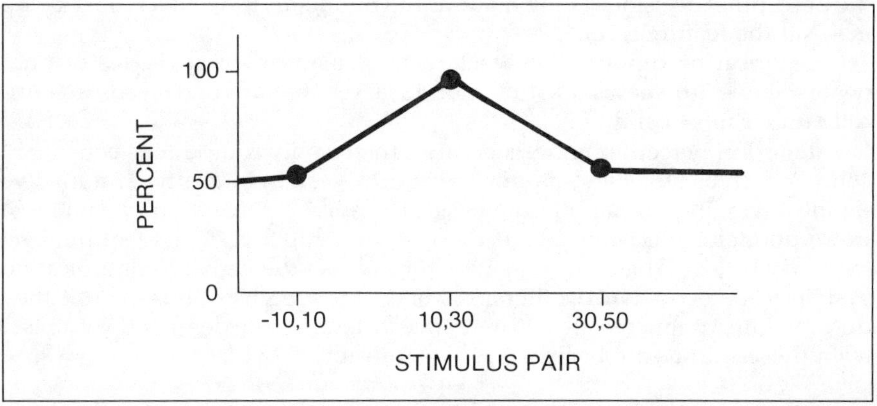

Fig. 1-40. Percentage of correct discrimination of syllables that differ in voice onset time showing categorical perception.

Rather, two speech sounds are heard as different only if the listener can categorize them into different phoneme classes. This limitation of discrimination ability by categorization ability is categorical perception.

Figure 1-40 shows a typical result from an experiment showing categorical perception. The ordinate shows the percentage of times that a subject correctly says that two stimuli presented in succession are "different." The x axis in this figure shows the voice onset time values of stop consonants paired together for judgment. Stop consonants whose voice onset time values are less than 30 msec are typically identified as voiced; those with voice onset times greater than 30 msec are typically categorized as voiceless. When two syllables that are alike in all but their voice onset time values of −10 and 10 are presented, the listener hears them both as "same" (i.e., the voiced stop consonant). Assuming the adult is motivated to guess that half of the time such stimuli are really different, the result will be a discrimination score of 50 percent. The same thing happens for the stimulus pair with voice onset time values of 30 and 50 msec. Both are categorized as containing a voiceless stop. Not being able to discriminate the two, the subject guesses and is right 50 percent of the time, on average. For the middle pair, the 10-msec stimulus is heard as voiced, and the 30-msec stimulus is heard as voiceless. Having categorized these two syllables differently, the subject correctly discriminates them as well.

Categorical perception occurs, in our model, because the listener is discriminating among phonemes simultaneously with the detection of features. As the listener decides which phoneme is present, nonessential auditory feature differences are ignored. As each feature is analyzed at the lower levels, the possible phonemes are positively stimulated, and the others are inhibited. The positively stimulated phoneme units inhibit the nonrelated features as well. This is a clear case of top-down processing in which the perceptual decisions being made at the phonemic level affect those being made at the feature level.

Categorical perception is characteristic of many natural classes of phonemes. Table 1-6 shows a list of sound classes that are perceived categorically under most conditions.

Categorical perception occurs because the heavily coproduced consonant sounds such as stops and liquids are short, weak in intensity, and involve rapidly changing resonant frequencies. The speech perception system must make phonemic decisions about these sounds rapidly, or the feature level cues may be lost. This longer analysis time allows the verbal communication system to detect detailed differences between speech sounds even if they do not differ phonemically. When speech is rapid or degraded by noise, even these sounds are heard more categorically.

Table 1-6. PHONEMIC SOUND CLASSES THAT ARE PERCEIVED CATEGORICALLY

Sound classes	*Auditory cue*
Consonant place of articulation	Frequencies of formants F_1, F_2, F_3 onset and transitions
Stop consonant voicing	Voice onset time
Fricative versus affricate manner	Amplitude rise time
Stop versus glide manner	Transition rate

The tendency to hear speech sounds categorically is apparently not a totally learned phenomenon dependent on the acquisition of a set of language dependent phonemes. Rather, children as young as 2 to 3 months and mammals such as monkeys and chinchillas have been shown to discriminate some speech sounds categorically.

Higher Levels

The human listener is not just "pulling together" features to identify a string of phonemes. As often stated in this chapter, processing at the higher levels of syllabic organization, meaningful units, and propositions is occurring simultaneously with the lower levels of feature and phoneme processing.

One set of experiments showing the effects of higher-level processing involves the phenomenon of phonemic restoration. Warren (1970) deleted parts of the speech signal and inserted plausible environmental noises such as coughs and hisses. Listeners readily recognized the missing phonemes as part of words, phrases, and sentences. Often, the listener was actually unaware that part of the speech signal was missing.

Within our model, phonemic restoration takes place because the processing at the meaningful unit level is also activating the appropriate units at the phonemic level. For example, as a listener decodes the phrase "A man was happy" before actually hearing the /n/ sound, he or she has partially activated all of the words known that contain the beginning sounds /m/ + /æ/ (e.g., *map, man, manage*). If the /n/ were eliminated, the listener would already have a smaller set of words to consider. As the listener moves on in the utterance, knowledge of sentences and phrases can be used to predict that the missing sound was part of a noun, and it should be a word that expresses a concept that can be associated at a propositional level with happiness.

As you might suspect, phonemic restoration occurs most often when more information is available to the listener. It is more likely to occur at the end of an utterance rather than the beginning and in longer utterances rather than shorter utterances.

Miller (1951) has shown that speech perception in noise is better as the utterance contains more information that can be used to make predictions about the speaker's intended message. Listeners made fewer perceptual errors when a smaller list of words was being recognized. For example, if you were listening for two words, *captain* and *say*, some fairly minimal cues would suffice to allow you to tell which word was spoken. Listeners made fewer errors when asked to identify meaningful words rather than meaningless words. This effect is accounted for by processing of meaningful linguistic units, which can feed information about the shapes of known words down to the phonemic level.

In summary, perception of a speaker's verbal messages is an active process involving a number of levels of activity. The lowest level involves innately interrelated feature complexes. Higher-level decisions about phonemes, syllable structures, and meaningful units are all made with reference to higher and lower levels of processing information.

SUGGESTED CLASS ACTIVITIES

The following activities are suggested for class discussion. Each is intended to help the student actively organize the concepts presented so that they will become a useful part of the student's knowledge system.

1. Look at the first drawing in Appendix A. Write 10 *descriptive* sentences, 10 *inferential* sentences, and 10 *interpretive* sentences that relate a story about this picture.
2. Each class member should pick a consonant phoneme. Generate minimal pairs demonstrating that this phoneme contrasts with the other phonemes in word-initial and word-final positions.
3. Describe the typical vocal tract shape for your phoneme. Describe how the individual gestures used to reach that target shape change as you produce it in the following phonetic contexts: iCi, aCa, uCu, and aeCae.
4. Class members taking courses in a foreign language should make a list of the speech sounds used in that language that are not used in English, or sounds used in English that do not occur in the foreign language. Instruct the other members of the class in the characteristics of the non-English sounds in minimal pairs of words.

CHAPTER 2

Acquisition of Phonetic Ability

Topics in this chapter include

- Cognitive-Linguistic Development
  - Prelexical Stage
  - Conceptual Stage
  - Semantic Stage
- Auditory-Perceptual Development
  - Prelexical Stage
  - Conceptual Stage
  - Semantic Stage
- Sensory-Motoric Development
  - Prelexical Development
  - Conceptual Stage
  - Semantic Stage

The preceding chapter presented a model of the cognitive knowledge and physiological mechanisms involved in production and perception of speech sounds. In that model, visual, auditory, and tactile-kinesthetic sensations related to speech sound production were assumed to be basic features. These basic features are organized through experience into language-related cognitive categories of phonemes, syllable structures, meaningful linguistic units, concepts, and propositions. The present chapter describes how this organization is accomplished during children's normal language development. The structure of this chapter is similar to that of the last. Cognitive-linguistic development is presented in overview to set the background for discussion of the development of speech sound production and speech sound perception.

Children progressively approximate adult speech and language performance by developing cognitive categories similar to those of the adults with whom they interact. Within social interactions a child is exposed to models of the phonemes, syllable structures, and linguistic meaning units that must be organized. Children are constantly given opportunities to express their desires using this language code. In an effort to enhance communication with adults, children organize cognitive categories to match those of adults. This organization occurs as the child interprets and produces speech acts. These actions of speech perception and production increase the strengths of the connections among those units of the different levels of the communication system that occur in the speech acts heard and produced by the child. For example, features of speech sounds that occur together in segments heard by the child are bound together in the child's cognition to form phoneme classes. Words that occur together in phrases and sentences used to express propositions are similarly associated with one another and the expressed conceptual relationships to form the child's syntactic and semantic knowledge of the parent language.

The child's anatomical and neurological systems are not blank slates at the beginning of this learning process. Rather, at birth, the child possesses certain visual and auditory perceptual capabilities that allow formation of cognitive categories regarding speech sounds and linguistic units. Within our model of communication, these capabilities exist as neurological connections among tactile-kinesthetic, auditory, and visual systems that are basic to all normal newborns. In the second section of this chapter, development of speech sound perception particular to the parent language is presented.

Although able to detect and coordinate many of the auditory and visual features of speech sounds at birth, the newborn's vocal tract structures are ill-equipped to produce speech sounds. Development of speech production must interact with physiological maturation of the vocal tract during the first year of life. Later development of speech sound production is directed by cognitive categories that are developed through the child's social interactions. The third section of this chapter discusses development of the ability to produce speech sounds.

COGNITIVE-LINGUISTIC DEVELOPMENT

Language development is driven by the child's need to communicate with others in the social environment. Development of language occurs as the child adds information about the outside world to a conceptual knowledge base and continually reorganizes information already available. Conceptual development includes development of linguistic meaning units that efficiently code the child's experiences and actions. At later stages of development, the linguistic code may be manipulated mentally so that the child can create relationships that may or may not exist in experience.

The child's progressive reorganization of knowledge occurs as a result of social interaction. The child interprets the environment, including language forms used by others, acts on the basis of these interpretations, and is reacted to by others. Reactions of the persons around the child show which of the child's behaviors are communicative and provide models for learning socially accepted symbols of the parent language. Children refine their communication systems by associating basic meaningful linguistic units such as words and their hierarchical arrangements into phrases and sentences with appropriate concepts and propositions. A basic feature of the young human is to be a social creature, one who needs to communicate with others.

Development of phonemic and syllabic categories occurs within the overall development of language use and structure. The following discussion uses Nelson's (1985) stages of language development: *prelexical, conceptual,* and *semantic.* The *prelexical stage* starts with the infant's reflexive facial expressions, bodily movements, and sound productions. This stage ends with acquisition, at about 18 months, of the first 20 to 50 words. These words are used within particular action routines and cannot be separated from the action itself. The *conceptual stage* begins when the child starts to use words to label concepts referring to classes of objects or actions. This conceptualization allows production of novel combinations of word symbols expressing a variety of relationships among concepts within the context of language use. In the *semantic stage,* beginning around age 6 or 7 years, the child develops increasingly more abstract concepts based on other concepts, rather than on real objects or events. This development allows the child to view language much the way a linguist does, as arbitrary symbols that can be analyzed for characteristics such as number of syllables or speech sounds, rather than strictly for use in social settings.

PRELEXICAL STAGE

In the *prelexical stage,* the child learns to express intentionality using verbal symbols and develops nonverbal concepts that continually become refined with respect to those of the adult community. With reference to the model presented in Chap. 1, the child is developing *concept* categories based on interactions with objects and persons. At the end of this period, the child will start to develop use of words to refer to these concepts. The following sections describe development of the use of language symbols to express intentions and the process of altering concept categories to more closely approximate those of the adult community.

Developing Expression of Intentionality

In Chap. 1, a speech act was defined as the expression of a proposition for some purpose. That is, speech acts contain an intended effect on a listener. One of the first cognitive aspects of speech acts developed is *intentionality*. The use of speech to affect a listener develops from reflexive to intentional and from nonverbal to verbal. This development is guided by adults with whom the child interacts in social interchanges.

The infant's first actions are reflexive in nature and are related to internal and external stimuli. For example, the discomfort of a wet diaper may be reflexively reacted to with a fixed action pattern that results in leg kicking. However, the caretaker will not react to these actions as though they were simply reflexive. Rather, the adult will impose meaning on these reflexive activities and react to them as though they were intentional. Having heard the child cry and seen the leg movements, the parent will likely change the child's diaper. While changing the diaper, the adult will comment on the child's actions and internal feelings (e.g., "Oh, you're kicking because you're wet. You must be uncomfortable"). From such episodes the child learns that kicking and crying may serve as indices of wetness, which cause an attentive adult to come and relieve the wetness. The child learns to use these indices in the future to affect adults in the environment. The adult has also supplied examples of utterances that may accompany this event so that the child is exposed to language symbols that may be used to replace more primitive reflexive indices. The child may learn to apply the word *wet* to this event with the same intent as the earlier kicking responses. The linguistic symbols used become associated with the whole event of being wet, kicking and crying, and having the diaper changed. The child's earliest cognitive system consists of connections among such commonly occurring perceptions within particular events.

As the child develops, use of nonverbal indices will become intentional and more refined. Rather than crying in an uncontrolled manner, the child may learn that one sharp cry is sufficient to rouse an adult to check for a wet diaper. The child will also develop use of gestures, such as pointing, to obtain objects from adults or to have adults perform some action. Later expression of needs will incorporate use of words that have been associated with particular events. These verbal symbols tag the developing concepts. At this early stage, the child's concepts are quite different from those of the adult and are primarily organized by immediate perception. Indeed, infants may not know that an object exists once it is no longer seen and heard. Such sensory inputs are organized into concepts by developing connection strengths. For example, visual characteristics of the family dog become associated with the dog's bark, smell, feel, actions the dog produces, and actions the child can use with the dog. The child's concept of *dog* is based on these characteristics. The child's concept obviously contrasts with the adult notion of *dog* as a class of animals that shares certain physical features and is different in certain features from other animals such as *cows* and *cats*.

Typically, the child's first words are closely related to objects and actions that are close at hand. It makes sense that children would first talk about those things whose perception and manipulation have repeatedly formed connections within the child's system. Because they are communicating about things and actions present in the environment, the child's communicative intention is supported by the adult's perception of not only the child's vocalizations and gestures but of other aspects of the situation. Adults continue to act as facilitators of language growth by fulfilling the child's requests and modeling language forms (e.g., "You want me to bring you the doll? Here's the doll").

At about 8 months, children start using speechlike vocalizations to affect behavior of others. Examples of this type of utterance use can be seen in early spoken forms produced by Halliday's (1975) son Nigel. These early word forms were apparently not based on the child's attempt to produce adult words but were phonetically novel forms produced as part of particular events. These utterances were bound to particular events in which they occurred and appeared to serve a number of purposes. Halliday categorized utterances produced during the first 18 months according to purposes they served and found an approximate order of appearance for these during that period. Table 2-1 lists these language functions.

The first function exhibited was called *Interactional*. The intent of these is to establish and maintain social interaction with an individual. Examples include greetings, responses to greetings, and use of a person's name to establish contact. Halliday described an interesting version of establishing contact in which Nigel would sometimes name and point to an object, with the apparent intention of focusing an adult's attention. This "Let's play with the ball" kind of utterance was apparently used to establish personal contact with the listener through joint focus of attention. An example of an utter-

Table 2-1. LANGUAGE FUNCTIONS REPORTED BY HALLIDAY (1975) DURING THE AGE RANGE FROM 8 TO 18 MONTHS

Function	*Purpose*
Interactional	Establishing social contact
Regulatory	Directing action of a particular person
Instrumental	Request for action not directed to a particular person
Personal	Expressing opinion

ance that was consistently used to attract the attention of an adult was production of the syllable [en]. This shared focus of attention had previously been attained without vocalization, through pointing alone. Now, this "old" function was expressed in a "new" verbal form as associations were built between intentions and verbal forms.

The second use of sound production developed by Halliday's son was called *regulatory*. Halliday referred to this as the "Do as I tell you" function. The child's purpose here is to direct the actions of a specific person. For example, he used the utterance [e], accompanied by a gesture, to direct a person to repeat a particular action. The gesture would typically be made toward the object involved in the action.

The third function, appearing at about age 10.5 months, was called *Instrumental*. Halliday called this the "I want" function of language. In short, the child produces sound in order to be supplied with goods or services by some listener. Included in this category would be various cries and verbalizations that are used to attract the attention of a listener to change a diaper or bring a bottle. Use of sound production in this manner has an obvious, immediate, reinforcing payoff for the child. An example from Nigel Halliday's repertoire is the utterance [bo], meaning "Give me my toy bird."

The fourth purpose, called *Personal,* was involved in expressing the child's personal feelings about things and activities. Verbalizations were apparently expressing the child's opinion, usually interest or disinterest in an activity or object. For example, the child may have been expressing ideas of not wanting to start some activity or wanting to quit a current activity. Nigel used the utterance [do] to say something such as "Look, it's moving" to express interest in a particular thing.

Developing Concepts

The infant builds nonverbal concepts of objects in the environment through active manipulation. Until about 3 months, objects are purely sensory events that are known by the child only while they are being observed or manipulated. The infant will form relationships among objects by associating the objects with actions such as stacking and piling. Relationships between objects and the child are formed through actions such as combing or drinking using appropriate objects such as combs and cups.

Later, the child will combine a variety of relationships among objects and actions to recreate complex activities such as feeding a doll, an action routine involving setting the doll up, getting the food, getting utensils, and so forth. At about 12 months a variety of objects can be used in a particular role. For example, one doll can be used to feed another rather than the child taking the feeding role.

The adult aids in this process of development by modeling the exchangeability of roles in nonverbal games. Adults engage in many repeatable activities with their infants. Bruner (1983) has analyzed the gamelike events that parents structure for their infants. For example, in the game of peek-a-boo, the adult and child take turns hiding eyes and being surprised by the others' unveiling of eyes. These nonverbal interactions form the training ground for later communication development. In particular, such games teach the child that standard action slots within event routines can be filled by either the child or the adult. Thus, the child is starting to learn that events can be analyzed into components. A game of rolling a ball back and forth includes an "actor" (the person who rolls a ball), an "object" (any ball), and a "recipient of action" (the person who catches the ball).

Nelson (1985) described the conceptual development occurring from the first words to about 18 months of age as *prelexical* because the words produced appear to be part of the child's actions rather than referring to cognitive categories of particular actions or objects. In other words, the first words spoken by a child are part of an overall activity without being used to refer to parts of that activity. Nelson proposed that the words refer only to *event representations.* An event representation initially contains unanalyzed perceptions of a sequence of actions or changes in state. For example, the child may originally have unanalyzed event representations for eating lunch, playing pattycake, or ball rolling. In the ball-rolling activity, the child may utter "ba," but this utterance does not refer to the adult object concept of "ball" but rather to the whole activity itself. The word appears to be activated by its connection strengths with the whole activity. The words are functional (i.e., used intentionally) but do not have meaning in the sense of adult reference to concepts that can be independently brought together into relationships with one another.

Adults continue to model referencing nonverbally and verbally for their children during this stage. Bruner (1983) described a series of stages through which adult and child learn to refer to particular objects first nonverbally then verbally. At the end of the child's second month, adult and child will achieve sustained eye contact with one another. Next, the parent can draw attention to some object by bringing it between adult and child during eye contact. This will typically be accompanied by some utterance such as "Look at the block!" Another means of focusing a child's attention is to pick up some object to which the child is already attending and highlight it through some utterance. In a later stage, the parent will get the nonattending child to look at an object that is introduced with an utterance such as "Zack" (spoken with a rising intonation) or "Look what I have." Between approximately 8 and 12 months, the child will be able to follow the parent's line of sight to some distant object. At first this will be accompanied by alerting utterances such as "Oh, look." The child will then check the adult's gaze to see where she is looking and then will follow that gaze. Having adopted a shared focus on some object or action, the child can express his or her desires with regard to the object using gesture or vocalization. By checking one another's visual focus, parent and child are agreeing on the topic that will be commented on by the actions and vocalizations that follow. In this way, the adult helps the child to parse experience into component concepts that can be associated with appropriate verbal symbols (words).

CONCEPTUAL STAGE

In the prelexical stage, word productions were part of events or referred to whole events. Nelson (1985) proposed that the next stage, the *conceptual stage,* occurs as the child learns to parse event representations into discrete conceptual parts. This process of conceptualization is aided by the caretaker's speech during events that highlight the words used to refer to objects, actions, and changes of state within the event representation. For example, an "eating lunch" event representation would contain a number of caretaker utterances highlighting individual concepts.

"*Put* the *cereal on* the *spoon.*"
"*Drink* the *milk in* the *cup.*"
"Oh, *you spilled* the *milk.*"
"*Baby*'s *getting full.*"

From such utterances the child is exposed to labels for objects such as spoons, cups, cereal, and milk. Reference is made to the child. The actions of drinking and eating are referred to. And a change in state (i.e., "getting full") is labelled. The adult also models some basic relationships between concepts, including spatial relationships (e.g., "in" and "on") and indications of past and present time (e.g., "spilled" and "getting").

At the beginning of the conceptual stage, children learn that words can be used to denote individual elements of an event representation (i.e., the actors, actions, and objects). Nelson (1985) proposed that this development occurs at about 18 months when children typically show an explosion in their rate of vocabulary development. At this time, the child recognizes that a particular concept (e.g., "ball") can occur in a number of event representations. This allows the child to form a concept of a ball that crosses a variety of event contexts, freeing it from any particular context. For example, a child may initially use the word *cookie* in a lunch event. Then, *cookie* may be used in a shopping event in which a box of cookies is requested from the shelf. In this way, the concept and label for *cookie* can be liberated from their original event-related context.

The child's earliest action words are likely to refer to actions that can be asserted on a variety of objects. For example, giving and taking, mouthing objects, throwing, banging, and so forth. These may be used in a variety of contexts for a variety of objects and thus are more likely to be used prior to other words.

As the child's vocabulary expands, words are added, and the meanings of old and new words are constantly adjusted to approximate those of the community. Words that refer to actions and objects are used by adults to refer to concepts based on features of the referents. In large part, these perceptual features are actively used by the observer to organize perception of the world. Children's early words often involve "overextended" meanings because they apply the best available label for a novel object or action. For example, children often start using a word such as *doggie* to refer to the family pet. Later, the child may overextend the use of this label for other animals (e.g., a cow). The overextension occurs because the child has yet to learn a label that distinguishes between these animals. A similar overextension occurs when the child refers to all adult males as "daddy," an available word label that will later be replaced by "man" or "adult" or some other term.

Children's earliest verbalizations are single-word utterances that are apparently attempts to express semantic relationships for some purpose. For example, the word *shirt* might be expressed to get an adult to bring a shirt, or take a shirt off. These single-word productions do not contain enough information to completely express these relationships, but parents interpret them as though the relationship were specified and supply expansions of their interpretation (e.g., "Oh, you want to put on the shirt"). Early produced propositions express basic relationships between concepts such as actor-action-recipient of action. Analysis of children's single-word utterances has shown that actor-action-object relationships are presented in linear strings of children's single-word utterances. For example, Scollon (1979) found the following single-word sequences in the speech of a 19-month-old child: "finger ... touch," and "cook ... say." These single word utterances combined to express actor-action relationships.

Next, children produce two-word utterances that more completely specify the intended conceptual relationships. Brown (1973) described the earliest two-word utterances as expressing a limited set of meanings. Some of these are listed in Table 2-2.

As the children's language development continues throughout the preschool years, they will learn to linguistically encode their perceptions of relationships between objects and actions. Blank, Rose, and Berlin (1978) described this as a process in which children's language becomes further and further separated from the child's immediate perception of the world. They described four levels of development in the separation of language from perception. These levels are shown in Table 2-3.

Table 2-2. SEMANTIC RELATIONSHIPS EXPRESSED IN TWO-WORD UTTERANCES (BROWN, 1973)

Semantic relationship	*Example*
Agent-action	mommy push
Action-object	hit ball
Agent-object	boy ball
Action-location	jump bed
Possessor-object	baby bottle
Entity-attribute	car red

Table 2-3. LEVELS OF LANGUAGE ABSTRACTION (BLANK, ROSE & BERLIN, 1978)

Level	*Example*
I. Immediate perception	Labels an object or action that is present
II. Selective analysis of perception	Describes particular aspects of present object or action
III. Reorganizing perception	Labels an object described by perceptual characteristics it does not possess
IV. Reasoning	Makes predictions of future events from present experience

In level I, the child expresses something that is directly observable in the situation. For example, children are often asked to label an object or action, which requires that the child perceive what the adult is referring to and supply an appropriate label. As we have discussed, joint visual focus should have developed early. The ability to produce the label will depend on the child's vocabulary development (i.e., what words the child has been exposed to and the conceptual categories associated with the word). The child may also be required to label objects for which only partial information is available from perception (e.g., labeling an object that is only felt, or only heard moving). This ability can be tested in a way that is removed from immediate perception by asking the child to recall objects that were seen a short time back. In this first level children are showing the ability to attach word labels to appropriate sets of perceptual features.

Level II demands require selective analysis of perception. The child is required to attend to particular perceptual aspects of the situation. Language demands in this category include looking for an object that is described by its characteristics ("Which one is hot?"), recalling information from a previous statement ("What happened when Goldilocks tasted the father bear's porridge?", asked after the adult has told this part of the story), naming characteristics of objects ("Tell what you do with a ball"), identifying differences ("What's different about these two things?"), and citing an example in a category ("Name some animals"). To answer these questions, the child must align his or her definitions of the vocabulary involved using the perceptual characteristics that are important to the adult. They also require that the child be able to use language to express relationships among objects and actions distanced in time and space.

Although level I demands may often be responded to with labels of objects, level II demands more often require a descriptive level of utterance. The child must be able to relate the object labels to actions and descriptors. Thus, the development of surface linguistic characteristics such as the development from single-word utterances to two-word utterances is related to cognitive development and the increasing demands placed on the child's utterances by the social environment.

Level III demands include those that require the child to reorganize his or her perception of the situation. For example, a child may be asked to name something that does *not* have some characteristic ("Which one is not sharp?"). This task requires that the child look for something that contrasts with the most salient aspects of the utterance. Or a child may be asked to describe all of the things that are *different* about two objects. Again, the child must reorganize a tendency to look for similarities between two objects that may be quite similar (e.g., two small toys that are both the same shape but are of different color). An even higher-level task in this group includes demands to define words. Now the child is asked to rely almost completely on memory and organization of information about the thing that has been labeled.

Level IV demands that the child reason using language. This category includes making predictions ("What will happen to the milk if I punch a hole in the glass?"), identifying causes ("What might make milk leak out of a carton?"), and justifying a response ("Why do you think that this happens?"). Constructing utterances to answer these questions requires that the child be able to extrapolate beyond the information given in the question in putting together a response.

Being able to address the relatively complex relationships between perception and language cited above requires that the child develop the use of linguistic markers that express changes in the time and place of event occurrence. Brown (1973) also described the development of syntactic devices that modulate basic meanings expressed by agent-action-object expressions. These devices are called *grammatical morphemes.* The children studied by Brown showed a relatively stable developmental order for the following: simple spatial prepositions, ("in" and "on"), present progressive verb marking ongoing action ("walking"), plural morpheme ("cats"), Irregular past tense ("ran"), possessive morpheme ("dad's car"), copula ("he is here"), articles ("the boy is here"), regular past tense ("he walked home"), third-person present verb ("the boy walks"), and auxiliary verbs ("he has walked"). Development of these usually starts when the child reaches the two-word stage and continues through age 3 or 4 years. An approximate ordering of the acquisition of these linguistic units is shown in Table 2-4.

The child will also learn to linguistically express time, space, and causality relationships between more than one proposition. For example, the utterance "We will go for a walk after you have finished your dinner" expresses a relationship between otherwise unrelated experiences of walking and eating dinner. These are brought together in a time relationship by the speaker inasmuch as the first activity will occur after the second is completed. This is expressed in a fairly complex way linguistically. The first activity stated is put in the future tense relative to the second activity, which is put in the past tense. However, at the time of the utterance, the second activity is

Table 2-4. APPROXIMATE ORDER OF ACQUISITION OF ENGLISH MORPHEMES EXPRESSING TIME AND SPATIAL RELATIONSHIPS (BROWN, 1973)

Simple spatial markers	"in," "on"
Ongoing action	—ing
Irregular past	"ran"
Possession	—'s
Regular past	—ed
Present action	—s

ongoing. To understand this time relationship, the child must distance him- or herself from the immediate perception. This utterance may also be expressing a causal relationship (e.g., going for a walk may be a reward given by the parents for completion of an activity by the child who does not want to finish eating).

Linguistic devices used to express complex relationships are typically function words that have meaning only in the context of other words. Examples include the following:

I like him *because* he does nice things for me.
I do nice things for you *so that* you will like me.
After you do nice things for me, I will like you.

These linguistic markers can only be learned through the child's social interactions with others who mark these time, space, and consequence sequences with appropriate words.

SEMANTIC STAGE

In the preceding stage, the preschool-age child has developed the ability to label concepts and to compare concepts using principles of alikeness, difference, inclusion, and other logical relationships. These abilities are seen within contexts of language in use, that is, as the child is actually using terms such as *before, after,* and *because* for some purpose. In such usage, the child's understanding of these terms and the conceptual relationships they express is supported by the context of their use. The child does not necessarily understand the full meaning of these terms in the adult sense. During the *semantic phase* children learn about language as an abstract system. They start to use language to learn about things they have not experienced.

Children at the conceptual stage do not completely separate their words and concepts. Prior to 5 years of age, words are inseparable from their referent concept (Papandropoulow & Sinclair, 1974). To children in the conceptual phase, a word is not an arbitrary sound pattern that is used to label a concept: The word is a part of the concept. The word exists as connection strengths with perceptual features and the language structures and situations in which it has been used before. For example, when asked to name a long word, such children respond with words that are not long with respect to their syllabic structure or number of phonemes but rather with referents that are long (e.g., a train).

Further development occurs as the child learns to use language as a tool for thinking. This occurs as the child creates new concepts by relationships among old concepts. For example, the concept of "planning a day" involves temporally ordering a number of otherwise unrelated complex events: getting up, school, play time, dinner, bedtime. Each of these events has a number of subcomponents (e.g., school involves classroom activities, lunch time, recess, library time, gym time, and so forth). These higher concepts are not related to specific actions, times, or persons: They are related to one another by a hierarchical categorization created by the child's mental activity.

Further development in word meaning will occur as the child arranges hierarchies of meaning for classes of words based on comparisons of similarities and differences. For example, the hierarchical term *mammal* is a class of animals that is never directly experienced by the child. Rather, individual cases are experienced and classed together according to certain features that are common across various animals in this group. Much of this type of language use is the object of classroom activities in formal education settings.

The following sections of this chapter discuss the development of speech sound perception and production against the backdrop of language development. Most of the development of speech perception and production occurs during the first two stages of development: prelexical and cognitive.

AUDITORY-PERCEPTUAL DEVELOPMENT

Learning of linguistic meaningful units and structure of propositions in adult speech requires that children be able to decode and organize auditory and visual features of adult speech productions. The child's categorization of these features is continually refined to approximate those of the adult language users. As indicated in Chap. 1, infants' nervous systems appear to be structured to detect and interrelate auditory and visual aspects of speech production. This section discusses development of this basic ability and looks at some of the research that has described how children learn to perceive speech signals. In particular, we are interested in development of the ability to identify phonemes and words in the speech of adults. Research into these developments is discussed within Nelson's (1985) developmental stages.

PRELEXICAL STAGE

The *prelexical stage* extends from birth through approximately 18 months when children are producing more than 50 words and are combining words to express a variety of meaning relationships. Studies of children's speech perception abilities in this time period suggest that children are born with remarkable abilities to discriminate auditory and visual features associated with speech sound production.

At about 12 months, children's discrimination ability appears to be tuned toward the phonemes of the parents' language. Speech sound discriminations that used to be made by the infant are no longer made if sounds do not contrast phonemically. This suggests that by this age the child's interaction with environmental stimuli has formed perceptual categories approximating those of adult phonemic targets.

Near the end of this period, ability to discriminate phonemes appears to be related to word knowledge. Children are able to discriminate among phonemes better in words they know compared to novel words. Thus, the child is apparently developing phonemic categories in unison with development of meaningful linguistic units. As suggested in the verbal communication model, these different conceptual levels are developed in parallel. In the sections that follow, development of these perceptual abilities is discussed in two sections: "Acoustic Cue Discrimination" and "Developing Phonemic Categories."

Acoustic Cue Discrimination

During the first week of life, infants have been shown to prefer to listen to speech as opposed to nonspeech sounds. This implies that the child's nervous system is prewired to distinguish those aspects of sound that are characteristic of speech. In our model, this prewiring occurs as associations among auditory, visual, and sensory-motor features important to speech sound production and perception. Not only do children choose to listen to speech sounds, they tend to vocalize more while they listen, suggesting an innate auditory-motor linkage in the nervous system.

In experimental settings, DeCasper and Fifer (1980) have shown that newborns prefer to listen to their own mother's speech rather than that of other women. This is an important characteristic given the strong interdependence of social and language development. The child is born ready to attend to human speech, especially that of the mother.

The core of the verbal communication model presented in Chap. 1 is a network of connections among auditory, visual, and tactile-kinesthetic features of speech sounds. A number of experimental observations have led us to suppose that this network is available for use at birth. First, such discriminations have been demonstrated among lower animals, and second, very young infants show such discriminations.

Animals Discriminate Speech Sounds. Human behaviors, including speech production and perception, have been influenced by evolutionary forces. Behaviors and abilities that are useful for survival are selected and passed on to future generations. In the animal world, rapid perception of changes in background sounds was crucial to survival. A snapping twig or a rustling bush were indications of approaching danger or potential food. The animals who produced more rapid and appropriate motor responses of flight or fight were those who survived.

Ability to detect and rapidly analyze such transient sounds by animals may allow them to hear differences in rapidly changing characteristics of speech sounds. A number of studies of animal perception have shown just such abilities in other mammals. Kuhl (1981) showed that chinchillas discriminate *voice onset time* differences much like a human speaker of English. Obviously, it is not possible to ask a chinchilla to say whether two syllables are "same" or "different." Rather, the animals were trained to move from one side of a cage to another when they detected a difference in speech sounds. The animals were deprived of water so that they would normally stay on the side of a cage that had a water supply. A background syllable would be repeated (e.g., "ba ba ba"). At a predetermined time the syllable would be changed (e.g., "pa pa pa"). When the syllable changed, the chinchilla was given a short time to move to the opposite side of the cage before being subjected to an electrical shock and a loud buzzer. The animals learned to cross the cage whenever they detected a change in speech sounds. Using this procedure, it was found that the animals could hear a difference in voice onset time if the two syllables were from opposite sides of a 30 msec boundary. That is, a change from 10 to 40 msec would be detected because the two are on opposite sides of the boundary. However, a difference from −10 to 20 or from 40 to 60 msec would not be detected. This corresponds to the voice onset time boundary for English voiced and voiceless consonants!

Obviously, the chinchilla has not formed language-specific phonemic categories that are responsible for this behavior. Instead, some aspect of the hearing mechanism of this mammal detects such sound changes. Inasmuch as the human ear behaves in many respects like the ears of lower-order mammals, it is expected that the newborn child will have similar capabilities.

Newborns Discriminate Speech Sounds. The process associated with articulation development that appears to develop first is a portion of the auditory perceptual system having to do with discrimination of acoustic cues used to distinguish speech sounds. As discussed in the preceding chapter, adult listeners appear to discriminate these acoustic cues in a categorical fashion. That is, adults tend to hear acoustic cue changes that alter the phonemes they are listening to, while ignoring acoustic cue changes that do not signal a phonemic difference. But children are not born with a knowledge of phonemic classes. If they were, they would be predetermined to speak a particular language. Rather, infants appear to be endowed with an ability to discriminate many, if not all, of the acoustic cues to phonemic identity.

Studies of infant speech discrimination abilities have typically used some known reflexive behavior as a measure of the child's perception. One such reflexive response is called the *orienting response.* When young children detect a difference in sounds in the environment, they tend to stop present activities and attend to the new stimulus. This kind of behavior can be seen in animals who will stop eating and look up if background sounds change around them. A subtle, but readily measurable, aspect of this orienting response is a deceleration or slowing of heart rate.

Idealized results of an experiment using this response to test speech sound discrimination ability are shown in Fig. 2-1. The first stage would entail measuring the child's heart rate with no auditory stimulation. The measured heart rate, about 130 beats per minute, would form a baseline from which deviations would be measured.

In the second stage, a repeating speech signal would be played in the background. For example, a string of syllables such as "ba ba ba" would be introduced. This change in auditory background should cause the orienting response to occur, and the child's heart rate will slow down relative to the baseline, dropping by 15 to 20 percent. After some time, the repeating [ba] syllable will no longer be new to the background: It will become old. The child will no longer orient to the sound, and the heart rate will return toward baseline.

Fig. 2-1. Infant heart rate changes during an experiment in which syllable [pa] was discriminated from syllable [ba].

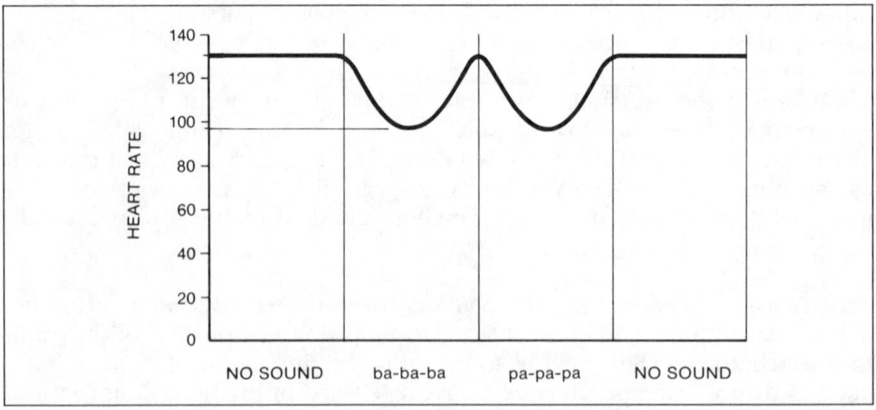

Once the child's heart rate has returned to normal, the third, and crucial, part of the experiment is started. At this point, the experimenter will do one of two things: change the repeating speech sound (e.g., to [pa]) or continue the first stimulus. When the experimenter changes the speech signal to [pa], a change will have occurred in the child's background. If the child hears this new stimulus as different from the old background, the orienting response should reoccur, and the heart rate will decelerate. If the child does not discriminate between the old [ba] stimulus and the new [pa] stimulus, the orienting response will not occur, and the heart rate will stay at the base rate. During this third segment, the experimenter makes a statistical judgment of a child's ability to discriminate two stimuli by comparing the percentage of times the orienting response occurred when the stimuli shifted from [ba] to [pa] with the number of times it occurred when the stimuli stayed the same (i.e., [ba] continued throughout the period of time in which heart rate was measured).

Another experimental procedure, or paradigm, that is useful in gathering infant perceptual data involves measurement of the child's sucking behavior. A special nipple that is electronically wired to count the number of sucks is inserted into the infant's mouth. The child will naturally suck the nipple. In the first phase of the paradigm, the experimenter will measure the child's baseline rate of sucking. Next the child is reinforced for sucking by playing a tape recording of a syllable each time the child sucks on the nipple. This auditory stimulation will typically cause the child to increase the rate of sucking, presumably to control onset of these interesting sounds. After some time, the child is apparently less interested in this repeating syllable, so the sucking rate reverts back toward the baseline. In the third phase of the experiment, a new syllable is substituted for the first. If the child detects a difference between the first syllable and the second, he or she should be motivated to suck more often to hear this novel sound. And so the sucking rate should increase for a while after introduction of the new syllable. If the child does not detect the difference between the first syllable and the second, the rate of sucking should remain low. Again, the experimenter will make a statistical decision regarding how often the child responded to the new stimulus and how often he or she did not.

Using these techniques, experimenters have shown that children below the age of 6 months, some as young as 1 month, can discriminate a variety of acoustic cues to phonemic identity. These include voice onset time and *formant frequency* cues to place of articulation of stop consonants, liquids, and vowels. Other cues, such as the frequency locations of fricative noises, indicative of fricative place of articulation, do not appear to be discriminated as well. Thus, the newborn infant has the ability to detect certain acoustic cues while not detecting other acoustic cues to speech sound identity.

Children not only hear these acoustic differences, they have some understanding of the relationship between vocal tract shape and sound produced. Kuhl and Meltzoff (1982) demonstrated that 18- to 20-week-old children would look for a longer period of time at a face that fit the sound they heard being produced. When these children were exposed to audio recordings of the vowel [u], they looked more often at a video recording of an adult with rounded lips than one with spread lips. They looked to the video of an adult with spread lips more often when they were exposed to audio recordings of the vowel [i].

Findings such as these suggest that children are born with nervous systems that are already connected in patterns that detect auditory characteristics of speech sounds and associate these to visual characteristics of speech sounds. These innate connections form the basis for learning the phonemes, syllables, and higher-level concepts of the verbal communication system.

Developing Phonemic Categories

Infants do not discriminate among all points along each of these acoustic dimensions. Instead, they show peaks of discrimination ability, such as those seen in adult speech discrimination and illustrated in Fig. 1-40. That is, particular regions of a continuum in which they cannot discriminate stimuli and particular regions across which they can discriminate stimuli exist. The best example of this occurs with voice onset time. A variety of studies, conducted in more than one language environment, have shown that infants can discriminate syllables with voice onset times of less than 20 msec from voice onset times of more than 20 msec. They were not able to detect differences that did not cross this boundary.

One explanation for this apparent ability to discriminate stimuli in one portion of an acoustic cue dimension and not in others suggests that these differences are due to the makeup of the auditory system. Aslin and Pisoni (1980) suggested that ability to discriminate voice onset time around a 20-msec boundary is dictated by a particular response characteristic of the auditory system. In particular, people respond to auditory events that occur more rapidly than 50 per second as though they formed a tone. That is, the person hears a periodic sound that has tonal quality. Below this rate, persons tend to hear individual pops, clicks, or bursts of noise. This cutoff rate of 50 events per second coincides with the 20-msec boundary (1 second/50 events = 20 msec/event).

Aslin and Pisoni (1980) reviewed studies of infants' discrimination abilities for a variety of acoustic cues. They proposed a logical model of how phonemic perception develops. Part of this model is shown in Fig. 2-2.

At birth, the child is endowed with certain abilities to discriminate acoustic parameters important to speech perception. Some cues will be discriminated well at birth (e.g., voice onset time), and others will not be discriminated well (e.g., fricative noise frequencies). The newborn's perceptual endowment at birth is independent of the language environment into which the child is born.

After birth, two forces act to shape the child's later perceptual development. The first of these is a continuing maturation of the nervous system serving speech perception. The second is the influence of the child's lan-

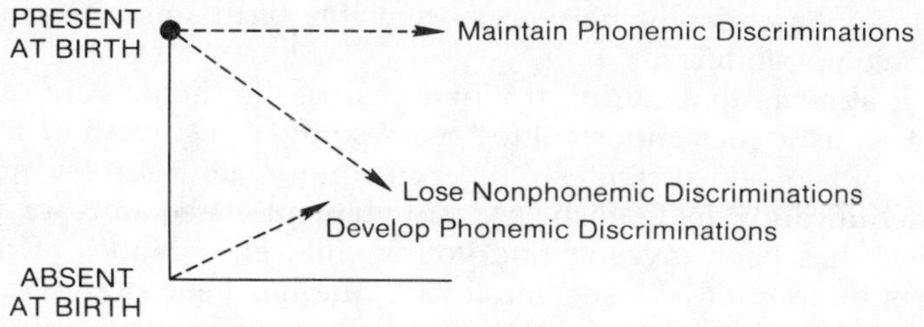

Fig. 2-2. Model of development of speech sound discrimination.

guage environment. If a particular discrimination ability coincides with the language stimulation the child receives, the child will maintain that ability, or improve on that ability as part of development. Within our model, these feature differences will be connected to differing phonemes, which enhance differences at the feature level. For example, the ability to discriminate voice onset time at a 20-msec boundary is useful in English because this boundary distinguishes voiced stops from voiceless stops. The young infant learning English apparently comes into this world well prepared to perceive this English contrast. Through maturation and practice in perception and production of phonemes differing in this feature contrast, this discrimination will be enhanced.

Discrimination abilities present at birth that do not quite coincide with the parent language will require adjustment. Aslin and Pisoni called this process *atunement.* The young infant born into a Spanish-speaking community needs to make adjustments in the endowed voice onset time boundary because the difference between voiced and voiceless stop consonants in Spanish is cued by a difference around 0 msec voice onset time. In this case, the child entered the learning situation with a system that is sensitive to an appropriate acoustic cue (voice onset time), but the discrimination point needs to be altered.

Some discrimination abilities are not needed in particular languages. For example, infants have been shown to discriminate [r] and [l] in syllables (Eimas, 1975). American adults show similar discriminations, but Japanese adults do not. (Miyawaka, Strange, Verbrugge, Liberman, Jenkins, & Fujimura, 1975). Apparently, the speaker of English maintains this distinction through production and perception of the phonemic contrast. The speaker of Japanese no longer discriminates the formant frequency differences of these sounds because his or her phonemic level does not contrast these sounds. The process that accomplishes this may be called *loss.*

Discrimination abilities not present at birth must be acquired. For example, infants do not appear to be able to discriminate among places of articulation of fricative consonants (Eilers, Wilson & Moore, 1977). Either this ability must be learned through language input stimulation or it requires further development of the nervous system after birth, or some combination of these two possibilities.

Thus, it appears that during the first year of life, infants are capable of detecting acoustic cues important to speech sound categorization. However, a number of acoustic attributes of speech sounds are not relevant to phonemic identification in English (e.g., fundamental frequency of voicing). Kuhl (1980) has been investigating young children's abilities to recognize phonemes in spite of acoustic variability. She has been doing this with a visually reinforced head turn paradigm. In this experimental situation, an infant is held in his or her mother's arms while facing one experimenter. This experimenter engages the child's attention with some toys. A background syllable is played repeatedly (e.g., "ba ba ba"). This background syllable is changed to a contrasting syllable (e.g., "pa pa pa"). The child is trained to look at the loudspeaker when the change occurs by activation of an interesting mechanical toy reinforcement. An example of this visual reinforcement is a toy monkey that plays cymbals. After the child has learned to look to the loudspeaker when the syllable is changed, the experimental trials are started. As in the heart rate paradigm, two types of trials exist, trials in which the repeating sound or syllable changes, and trials in which the sound remains constant. Ability to discriminate a sound contrast is seen when the child turns toward the reinforcer more often when the syllable is changed.

Using this paradigm, Kuhl taught 5- to 6-month-old children to look at the visual reinforcer when they heard a vowel change from [o] to [a]. The two vowels were spoken by the same speaker with the same fundamental frequency contour. After the infant correctly distinguished these two vowels, the experimenter systematically introduced acoustic variability. In the second phase of the experiment, the two vowels were produced with different fundamental frequency contours. The children were able to quickly learn to respond to the vowel difference rather than the difference between rising and falling fundamental frequencies. In later stages of the experiment, the children continued to distinguish the vowels in spite of changes in speaker sex and fundamental frequency contour. Thus, infants appear to be able to learn to attend to the important spectral acoustic dimensions representing phonemic categories while ignoring speaker-related variables.

Hillenbrand (1983) used a similar paradigm to demonstrate that 5- to 6-month-old children can be taught to categorize phonemes according to dimensions such as place, manner, and voicing. They taught children to make the head turn when one natural class of sounds was heard (nasals) as opposed to others (stops). Thus a particular child would learn to turn his head for reinforcement when a sequence of stops such as "ba da ga" was changed to a sequence of nasals such as "na ma na."

An important degree of phonemic categorization appears to develop in normal children by about 12 months. Recall that at this age, children are using verbal symbols for a variety of intentions and are also learning their first words based on adult words. Werker and Tees (1984) found that at age 12 months, children no longer discriminated nonnative phonemic contrasts that they were capable of discriminating earlier. They demonstrated this by asking children from three different language environments to discriminate phonemic contrasts from their own language and from the other two languages. All of the children were able to discriminate the contrasts from all of the languages at age 6 months. However, at 12 months they apparently lost the ability to discriminate outside of their own language's phonemic categories. Apparently, ability to discriminate speech sounds is in the process of becoming categorical in the sense that it is dictated by the strength of the connections of features to the phoneme level.

Waterson (1971) has developed a theory of speech development during this period that is based on increasing perceptual skill. She emphasized the differences in adult words *attempted* by individual children during this time period. Her data indicated that different children attend to different adult word forms. She theorized that adult words that children try to produce contain some feature that is perceptually salient to that child. For example, one of her subjects paid particular attention to adult words that contained nasals. When this child attempted to produce such words, they were produced with a NVNV pattern (nasal + vowel + nasal + vowel). Waterson theorized that the child had formed a perceptual representation of words with this NVNV format. The child was more likely to pay attention to and to attempt to produce words that were similar to this perceptual representation. Within our model, such perceptual representations would exist as connection strengths from a CVCV syllable structure to nasal consonant units at the feature level. Connections that happened to be formed early would be more likely to be attempted in production.

CONCEPTUAL STAGE

During Nelson's (1985) conceptual stage, children learn to elaborate their conceptual knowledge and attach appropriate language forms to these concepts. This development occurs within the framework of language use. That is, children can be shown to understand and produce language forms in situations in which children are experienced but not in novel situations. Experiments testing children's speech perception abilities have showed similar biases. The child in this stage is becoming more attuned to the phonemic structure of the language but is doing so within words that are commonly occurring in the environment.

Barton (1980) has studied young children's ability to recognize words. When the words being recognized are minimal pairs, that is, they differ by only one speech sound, this ability can be termed *phonemic perception*. The typical experimental paradigm used to assess phonemic perception is a word identification task. The child is presented with a pair of pictures or objects. The labels of these objects differ within one phoneme (e.g., *pea* and *bee*). The experimenter asks the child to do something with one of the objects (e.g., point to, pick up). If the child responds to the correct object, the phonemes presented have apparently been discriminated.

Barton (1980) investigated phonemic perception abilities of children in the age range of 1.8 to 2.0 years. He chose as stimuli, minimal pair contrasts that had been shown in earlier studies to be later acquired by normally developing children. These involved voicing contrasts between [b]-[p] and [k]-[g]. On the first day of the experiment each child was given objects representing these phonemic contrasts and then asked to perform actions with them. The items were a bear, a pear, a goat, and a coat. The child's understanding of these words was tested in nonminimal pair contrasts (e.g., the bear and the coat). If the child did not perform correctly with response to requests to manipulate a particular item (e.g., "Put the coat on the bear"), the name of the item was taught until the child responded reliably. On the second day of the experiment, all four objects were presented, and the children were requested to remove them from a bag or put them into a bag one at a time. Of the 10 children studied, 8 were able to reliably perform the task with one of the contrasts. Many of the children experienced some difficulty with the task. However, most appeared to be able to perform these tasks. A large proportion of errors made by these children involved words that they did not understand prior to the start of the experiment (i.e., the words that the experimenter had to teach the child).

Thus, the ability of 2-year-old children to discriminate consonant speech sounds of English appears to be fairly well developed. However, this ability interacts with the child's knowledge of the word units. This interaction between phonemic perception and word knowledge points to an important characteristic of phonologic development, namely that phonemes are not acquired separate from words. The child's phonemic knowledge may be derived from a need to phonetically distinguish important linguistic meaning units that are representative of important conceptual differences.

The 2-year-old child has considerable ability to distinguish the acoustic phonetic cues that are used to express phonemic differences. This does not mean that the 2-year old is perceptually analyzing phonemic strings in an adult manner. A large number of acoustic features cue any particular phonemic contrast. For example, the primary acoustic cue used by adults to discriminate [r] and [w] is the frequency location of the third formant. The third formant is lower in [r] than [w]. These sounds also differ in the overall amplitude of higher-frequency energy because of the lip rounding of [w]. A child may succeed in a phonemic discrimination task contrasting these two by responding to the loudness level rather than the frequency location. To become a more efficient perceiver and to become fully adultlike in perceptual ability, the child may have to focus on those perceptual cues that are most salient to a phonemic contrast.

To test such differences, experimenters have been examining children's responses to synthetic speech stimuli in which these acoustic cues can be controlled. Strange and Broen (1980) asked 3-year-old children to identify 10 synthetic stimuli that altered the frequency location of the third formant. This acoustic change results in adults hearing a shift from /r/ to /l/ as the third formant comes closer to the second formant in frequency. Both the adults and the children showed a change in identification of the phoneme at about the same stimulus in the sequence. That is, adults and children had developed the same phonemic boundary for this contrast. However, the children did not identify stimuli as consistently as the adults did. This implies that the children have not reached an adultlike categorization of these auditory features into phonemic classes. Rather, the children appear to be approaching adultlike performance in a progressive manner.

Further evidence regarding children's perceptual adaptation toward acoustic feature values employed in the parent language can be seen in children's responses to phonemic contrasts not employed in their language. Oller and Eilers (1983) asked English-speaking 2-year-olds and Spanish-speaking 2-year-old to identify a phonemic contrast from their own language and a contrast from the other language. The English-speaking children identified the native contrast /w/ versus /r/ in the *rabbit* and a nonsense word *wabbit*. They were also asked to identify the Spanish contrast between the tap [ɾ] in *ladder* and the trilled /r̃/ in [læɾ̃əɾ̃]. The Spanish-speaking children were asked to identify the English /w/ versus /r/ contrast in the word *huevo* and the nonsense word [reβo]. They also identified the Spanish contrast between trill /r̃/ and the tap /ɾ/ in the word *carro* and the nonsense word [kaɾo]. Both groups of children identified their native phonemic contrast at much better levels (around 85% correct) than the nonnative contrast (around 55%).

In summary, the prelexical infant is endowed with abilities to perceive acoustic phonetic cues to phonemic differences and to categorize speech sounds into perceptual sets. The infant's task is to learn which perceptual sets are used to express meaningful differences in word production. This process is in progress by at least age 12 months and no doubt sooner.

SEMANTIC STAGE

Development of speech sound perception and organizational abilities becomes entwined with academic learning in the semantic phase. Spelling, writing, and reading are often taught as skilled behaviors to be attained in discrete steps. Since English spelling developed to capture the sound structure of words using letters that are approximately related to individual sounds, spelling lessons often involve analysis of words for number of sounds, syllables, and so forth. For example, in one reading program, the child is taught to contrast vowel sounds [æ] and [I] by marking spellings for pictured nouns such as "bib bad," "him ham", "six sat," and so forth. In another lesson, the child is asked to supply missing consonants given a picture and a partial spelling of a word (e.g., shown a picture of a pig and given the partial spelling "pi_"). Children are also taught to tap out the number of syllables in words and to make up rhyming words. All of these behaviors are based on the child's learning of the sound structure of English in the previous phase. Their intent is to teach the child to look at language forms abstractly, consciously, rather than using language symbols as they have in the past.

The influence of the child's knowledge of the sound structure of English in learning spelling was demonstrated by Read (1971). He analyzed the spelling ability of preschool children who had received no formal training by asking them to spell words using lettered toy blocks. Most of the spelling errors produced were predictable from common speech production patterns such as the *deletion of final consonants* or *consonant cluster reduction.* Learning to read may well just be a continuation of the developmental process that directs development of speech perception and production from the conceptual phase. The child has already proved adept at connecting the visual aspects of speakers with their auditory impressions of speech. In learning to read, the child connects visual aspects of letter symbols with already established sound and word categories. This academic learning starts early for the child who is often exposed to books while sitting in the lap of a parent.

SENSORY-MOTORIC DEVELOPMENT

The newborn infant has certain oral structures and fixed action patterns that are designed to keep the child alive but that also hinder speech production. During the preverbal period, much of speech sound development apears to be related to the child's changing physiology. During the cognitive phase, the child shows development of conceptual categories of syllabic shapes and phonemes that are changed toward the adult usage as the child develops. During the semantic stage, a child's motor coordination continues to improve until puberty, at which time adultlike motor control for speech production appears to be achieved.

PRELEXICAL DEVELOPMENT

During the first half of the prelexical stage, speech sound production is largely dictated by the changing physiology of the infant. The anatomical restructuring that occurs during the first 6 months makes production of a wide variety of speech sounds possible. It is these sounds that are used in the child's first meaningful utterances as described by Halliday (1975).

Anatomical and Physiological Restructuring

Although the newborn appears to have considerable abilities to detect speech sound differences, the same cannot be said of the ability to produce speech sounds used in adult languages. In fact, the vocal tract of the newborn presents a number of anatomical obstacles to production of many speech sounds. The vocal tract of the newborn does not have the same shape as that of an adult, dictating that the vocal tract of the infant will not have the same properties of resonance as the adult. More problematic is that the newborn's oral cavity is separated from the larynx in a resting state and thus cannot be acoustically stimulated via phonation. Differences in vocal tract anatomy at birth make it impossible for the newborn to produce many of the sounds used in adult speech. Figure 2-3 shows schematic drawings of an adult vocal tract, that of an ape, and that of a newborn.

As seen in the last chapter, the adult vocal tract has three major divisions: nasal cavities, an oral cavity, and a pharynx. The oral cavity and the pharynx are joined by a right-angle bend in the vocal tract. This vocal tract shape allows a variety of tongue movements to produce speech sounds. Notably, the tongue can be moved forward and up to produce the vowel [i] and a variety of consonant sounds. The distinctive acoustic quality of the vowel [i] is due to the geometry of the vocal tract: in particular, a large cavity behind the constriction and a small cavity in front of the constriction. The tongue can be moved posteriorly to produce the vowel [u], whose distinctive acoustic pattern is due to cavities in front of the constriction and behind the constriction, which are approximately equal in size. By lowering the tongue constriction, the vowel [a] is produced. All of these sounds depend on a fairly large pharyngeal cavity. The adult vocal tract geometry that allows these differences is quite different from the infant's vocal tract shape. The newborn, like the ape, has one relatively straight cavity leading from the mouth to the esophagus. There is little or no bend, and thus, no pharyngeal cavity. Not being endowed with a two-tube vocal system, the infant is not capable of producing a full range of vowel sounds.

An even more critical difference in the newborn's anatomy is the contact of the epiglottal cartilage of the larynx with the velum when the child is at rest. This contact forms a seal between the oral and nasal cavities. Thus, the oral cavity leads directly and securely to the esophagus while the nasal cavity leads directly to the trachea alone. This anatomic situation produces functional consequences. The infant cannot inhale liquids or food into the trachea and lungs, and the newborn must breathe air through the nose because no direct connection between the oral cavity and the trachea exists. Also, important in terms of speech sound production, the infant is limited to production of nasal speech sounds because the air from the lungs can only escape through the nasal cavity. This functional linkage can apparently be broken during the child's effortful utterances such as yelling and crying.

The newborn's oral cavity is also relatively flat compared to the adult's, giving the tongue little room to maneuver for sound production purposes.

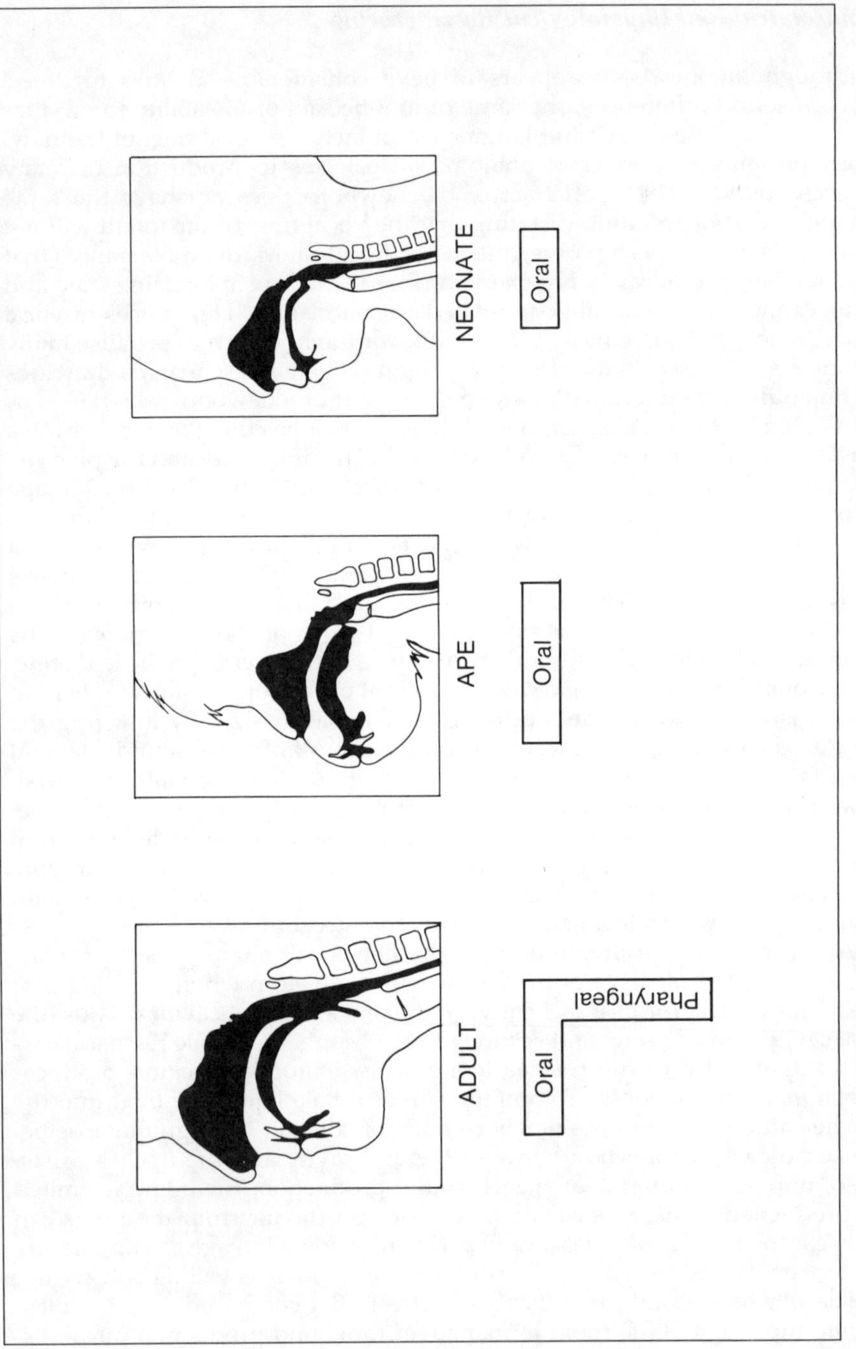

Fig. 2-3. Vocal tract shapes of an adult, ape, and neonate.

Much of the movement of the infant's tongue is in an anterior-posterior dimension. These characteristics limit the child's ability to produce the tongue height dimension, which is important to adult production of vowels. Without this ability, the child could not produce vowels that differ in the way that [i] differs from [æ], and [u] differs from [a].

Oller (1980) has described a series of stages in the speech sound production capabilities of the prelexical infant, which are shown in Table 2-5. The first stage is called the *phonation stage*. This stage occurs from birth through the first month. During this time, speechlike sounds are judged to be produced only rarely. Those that are produced are called *quasi-resonant nuclei* (QRNs). The QRN is produced with laryngeal phonation. Because of the joining of the newborn's larynx and velum, this phonation is forced to resonate through the nasal cavities. These sounds are described perceptually as being either syllabic nasals or high, mid-nasalized vowels. The infant appears to phonate with the mouth closed or nearly closed.

This is followed, between the ages of 2 to 3 months, by the *goo state*. During this time, the QRN is still the most often occurring speechlike sound. However, consonantlike sounds produced with constrictions in the back of the vocal tract are added to these nuclei. The timing of these consonantlike gestures has been shown to be slower than consonants produced in adult speech.

The third stage, starting at about 4 months, is called the *expansion state*. This is often described by adults as a period of vocal play. The infant develops a large repertoire of sound productions during this time. Kent (1982) has related this stage of development to the changes in vocal tract anatomy discussed above.

Table 2-5. OLLER'S (1980) STAGES OF PREVERBAL SPEECH SOUND DEVELOPMENT

Stage	*Approximate age*	*Types of utterances*
Phonation	Birth–1 mo	Quasi-resonant nuclei
Goo	2–3 mo	Quasi resonant nuclei Back constrictions
Expansion	4–6 mo	Fully resonant nuclei Raspberry Yells Squeals and growls Marginal babbling
Canonical babbling	7–10 mo	CVCV with mature timing
Variegated babbling	10–12 mo	Wider variety of consonants and vowels Gibberish

One change involves the production of *fully resonant nuclei.* These are oral vowellike sounds, typically quite open (e.g., [a] -like). In order to produce this type of sound as opposed to the earlier occurring QRN, the child must be able to separate the oral and nasal cavities and allow the sound produced during phonation to radiate through the oral cavity rather than the nasal cavities. Both of these characteristics of true vowels become possible at about 4 months when the larynx lowers in the neck. Again, this lowering of the larynx allows for the separation of the larynx and velum. In turn, this allows for air from the lungs to travel through the oral cavity, rather than through the nasal cavities. The lowering of the larynx also increases the size of the pharynx, allowing the production of vowels whose quality will be more adultlike than sounds produced with a single-tube vocal tract.

Since air from the lungs can flow into the oral cavity, and the oral cavity can be sealed off from the nasal cavities, it becomes possible to impound air pressure in the oral cavity. This ability to create positive air pressure in the oral cavity underlies the child's production of a class of sounds called *raspberries.* The raspberry is a labial trill produced by forcing the lips to open and close rapidly by blowing air through them. The process is similar to the mechanism by which the vocal folds are forced to open and close during phonation. The sound produced is quite similar to a "Bronx cheer."

Another sound class that requires a good seal between the oral and nasal cavities is *yells.* Yells also require good coordination between the respiratory system, which is supplying the air pressure, and the larynx, which supplies the sound source. Two other sound classes, *squeals* and *growls,* also attest to the infants development of laryngeal phonation. Squeals involve rapid upward shifts in fundamental frequency, as high as 1,000 Hz in some cases! Growls are produced by lowering fundamental frequency. Kent (1982) suggested that both of these are made possible by the lowering of the larynx in the neck. From this new anatomical position, the strap muscles of the larynx are able to raise and lower the larynx, causing it to tilt, and alter the tension on the vocal folds.

Near the end of the expansion stage, around 6 months, the child starts to produce *marginal babbling.* Marginal babbling consists of consonant closures alternating with fully resonant nuclei. Again, these productions are noticeably slower than the consonant vowel transitions involved in adult speech.

The next major stage is called *canonical babbling.* Children usually enter this stage between 7 and 10 months of age. The hallmark of this time period is that the transitions from consonant to vowel productions start to occur with adultlike-timing characteristics. The child now produces more rapid openings of the vocal tract into vowel sounds. Since these syllable productions are more noticeably speechlike, it is common for parents to report that during this time period, their children first talked. Another characteristic of canonical babbling is that it involves a lot of *reduplication,* or repetition, of the same syllable. Typical utterances include series of syllables such as "bababababa."

The final preverbal stage is called *variegated babbling.* This stage expands on the canonical babbling stage by including a wider variety of consonant and vowel sounds. Children aged 10 to 12 months are often heard to produce long strings of syllables that include a variety of stress and intonation patterns. These utterances are called *gibberish*. Gibberish appears to sound like sentence productions that have no identifiable words.

Throughout this developmental sequence, the predominant syllabic shape is CV or CVCV. During the first year children tend to produce syllables that move from a constricted vocal tract to an open vocal tract. By the end of the first year, the child will also be producing VC and CVC syllables.

Another general tendency in preverbal phonetic development has to do with the place of articulation of consonants that are produced. Irwin (1947a) transcribed the consonant productions of children from 1 to 30 months. At 1 month, the highest proportion of consonants (nearly 90%) are glottals. These were heard as fricative [h] or stop [ʔ] productions. At the end of the first year, the proportion of glottal productions had fallen precipitously to about 35 percent. The next highest proportion of productions at 1 month was due to velar productions. This is consistent with the earlier description of the goo stage. Velar productions remain relatively constant at around 10 percent throughout the first year. As the glottals decrease in proportion during the first year, the percentage of alveolar consonants increases dramatically. At the end of the first year, the child is producing as many alveolars as glottals. Labial consonants also increase throughout the first year. Thus, a dramatic shift occurs in preverbal place of articulation from the earliest speech sound productions to those used when the child starts to attempt adult word forms.

Irwin (1947b) also found a systematic shift in the manner of production of consonant sounds during the first year. The earliest consonant productions at 1 month, [h] and [ʔ], cause the fricative and stop categories to be dominant at the beginning. These both decline somewhat as the child introduces other consonants starting at 6 months, in particular nasals and glides.

Locke (1983) compiled data from a large number of studies of variegated babbling to see if a common core of speech sounds existed that children babble regardless of language environment. The studies he cited cover a variety of languages as well as studies of the babbling of deaf children, who presumably are not influenced by the language spoken around them. Locke found that 90 percent of the speech sounds produced by children between the ages of 11 and 12 months can be accounted for by a limited set of speech sounds that he called the "core" sounds. This core includes glides [h], [w], and [j]; the stops [p], [b], [t], [d], [k], and [g]; the nasals [m] and [n]; and a fricative [s].

Phonetic Characteristics of the First Meaningful Utterances

An early theory of the passage from preverbal sound production to production of the first words was formulated by the linguist Roman Jakobson in the 1940s and printed in English in 1968. Jakobson theorized that children's babbling included all of the speech sounds used in any natural language. He also suggested that no continuity existed between this preverbal sound production and true or meaningful speech. In fact, he cited a silent period between babbling and production of the first words as evidence of a reorganization or shifting to a linguistic mode of operation.

One of the first major studies that disproved Jakobson's discontinuity hypothesis was conducted by Oller, Weiman, Doyle, and Ross (1975). These researchers argued that if discontinuity existed between the babbling of infants and their first words, then babbling should not contain the same patterns of production seen in children's later productions of adult words. In essence, these investigators transcribed the sounds babbled by two groups of children, one between the ages of 6 and 8 months and one between 11 and 12 months. They predicted that the syllable structures and speech sounds found in babbling would contain (1) fewer syllable-final consonants than syllable-initial consonants, (2) fewer consonant clusters than singleton consonants, (3) fewer voiceless initial-stop consonants than voiced initial-stop consonants, and (4) fewer initial fricatives than stops and other expected patterns. They found that their predictions were true, showing that babbling shared a number of characteristics with children's later word productions.

As discussed in the preceding section, the 1-year-old child is likely to be producing consonants from among a core consonant set. Children use these in their first words. This use reflects a tendency to use connection patterns that are strongest at any particular time.

Between the production of the first words at about 12 months and the production of the fiftieth word at about 18 months, children appear to be learning to produce whole words rather than attempting to divide words into phoneme units. Ferguson and Farwell (1975) made this discovery when they attempted to determine the phonemic contrasts used by children in their early words. They repeatedly sampled the children's speech over a period of months. At each sample, they plotted the consonant sounds that occurred in word-initial position. They found that defining children's phonemic contrasts was difficult because the children often produced the same word with different initial consonants. For example, an individual child used both word-initial [p] and [b], which may indicate that these two sounds contrast phonemically. But the word *papa* was produced as both [papa] and [baba], indicating that these two sounds do not contrast phonemically.

Ferguson and Farwell (1975) also found examples of "progressive idioms," which had first been reported by Moskowitz (1971). In a progressive idiom, a particular word is produced with phonetic accuracy that is unlike the other words produced by the child. The classic example of this type of organization is the production of the word *pretty* by Hildegard Leopold, whose father transcribed her early utterances in a diary study (Leopold, 1947). Moskowitz (1971) showed how this word was produced well at age 10 months, [prItI], at a time when Hildegard did not produce other clusters or other two-syllable words that began with different consonants. Thus, at 10 months this production appears to be "progressive." Apparently *pretty* has been learned as a phonetic whole.

During the conceptual stage, at age 21 months, Hildegard's production of *pretty* regressed to [bɪdɪ], matching the syllabic structures and features of the rest of her vocabulary. In particular, other consonant clusters were not produced, and syllable-initial stop consonants were voiced instead of voiceless. Within our model, the earlier, advanced form of the word occurred because the word at the meaningful linguistic level was connected to a sequence of features in a syllabic shape that happened to be an accurate production. As the child strengthened other connections, such as CV rather than CCV syllables, and voiced instead of voiceless initial consonants, production of this word changed. At a later time, she reorganized the structure of the word again to be adultlike when other words containing these syllabic shapes and phonemes also appeared.

Like Waterson (1971), Ferguson and Farwell (1975) found that children in this age group appeared to be selective in the word forms they attempted. For example, one of their children appeared to favor adult words beginning with initial fricatives. These words would be attempted whereas others were not. Such tendencies appear to be quite individualistic as seen in Leonard, Newhoff, and Mesalam's (1980) study of 10 infants in this age range. Even a pair of twins were found to use somewhat different sets of sounds and to chose somewhat different structures to produce.

To systematically study children's perceptions of word forms, Schwartz and Leonard (1982) presented novel object and action words to children who were just beginning to produce their first words. The words presented were chosen as being either "in the child's phonology" or "out of the child's phonology." A word was considered out of phonology if it contained consonants or syllable shapes that the child had not been observed to produce. Each object or action and its label were presented an equal number of times in play sessions. The investigators counted the number of times each word was attempted by the children. It was found that the children learned object labels before action labels. They also learned more of the in-phonology words than the out-of-phonology words. Schwartz and Leonard (1982) theorized that the child constructs a set of perceptual representations called *schemas*. These schemas are similar to perceptual filters, which allow certain syllable forms and phonemes to be processed while others are not. At this age, the schemas are quite large, perhaps word size or longer.

A similar investigation by Camarata and Schwartz (1985) found that children's early object labels were better articulated than their action words. That is, the adult consonants contained in a word are more likely to be maintained during this early lexical acquisition period if the word is an object label than if it refers to an action.

Rather than viewing such findings as evidence of passive filters, we choose to look at this finding as evidence of the organization of the conceptual system at syllable, phonemic, and feature levels at a particular time. A child more rapidly learns to perceive new words that can share connection strengths at the syllabic and feature levels with words that have already been learned. In other words, *conceptual connections that have already been established operate more readily than those that have not.* This includes connections between features and phonemes, phonemes and words, and words and concepts, making certain types of words more likely to be produced.

CONCEPTUAL STAGE

In the *conceptual stage,* from 18 months to about 4 or 5 years, the child's vocabulary increases rapidly, and linguistic patterns expressing complex propositions are developed. The child's repertoire of speech sounds also increases as the child develops syllabic shapes and phonemic categories that fall in line with those of the parent language.

In the preceding stage, children attempted to produce words whose adult forms were similar to patterns existing in the child's system. Obviously, the child cannot continue this pattern without severely restricting potential word forms. Leonard, Schwartz, Folger, and Wilcox (1978) found that such restrictions do not appear to be operating in the conceptual child. They found that children past the 50-word stage attempted to produce as many in-phonology words as out-of-phonology words. As children attempt new, more complex word shapes, they produce error approximations. The errors produced by children in this stage are quite similar across children, suggesting that all children develop similar organizations.

Common Error Patterns

Ingram (1976) has described speech sound development during this age as the successive suppression of innate phonological processes. The phonological processes act to neutralize certain syllabic or phonemic distinctions in the adult phonology. Table 2-6 shows some of the phonological processes discussed by Ingram. These are divided into the three major classes: *syllable structure processes, assimilation processes,* and *substitution processes.* Each type is presented below with a discussion of how they are described within the verbal communication model.

Syllable Structure Processes. Children progress from an organization at the syllabic level that represents words primarily as single CV syllables or reduplicated CVCV syllables as produced in babbling to more complex syllable structures with final consonants (e.g., CVC), consonant clusters (e.g., CCV), and multisyllabic words. The more basic CV syllable may be an innate sensory-motor pattern that develops out of the child's reflexive sucking and swallowing. In order to suck, the child makes a lip closure around a nipple and presses the nipple up against the alveolar ridge with the tongue.

Table 2-6. PHONOLOGICAL PROCESS RULES USED BY INGRAM (1976) TO DESCRIBE NORMAL PHONOLOGICAL DEVELOPMENT

SYLLABLE STRUCTURE PROCESSES
Reduplication
Deletion of final consonants
Deletion of unstressed syllables
Reduction of clusters

SUBSTITUTION PROCESSES
Stopping
Fronting
Liquid gliding

ASSIMILATION PROCESSES
Devoicing of word-final consonants
Prevocalic voicing
Labial assimilation
Alveolar assimilation
Velar assimilation

Both of these constrictions are later used as commonly occurring speech sound productions. The basic movements to and away from these constrictions involve the production of CV-like syllables as the child alternately presses the lips together and then opens the mouth. Since these movement patterns are well connected in the child's system, they likely become first approximations of the gestural control to be used in production of adult words.

Ingram (1976) cited four common error patterns that occur as children attempt to produce words with syllable structures more complex than the CV structure: reduplication, deletion of final consonants, deletion of unstressed syllables, and reduction of clusters. The terminology used to describe these processes appears to imply that the child is making active cognitive choices to "delete" consonants that occur in the adult model of a word. Within our model, deletions occur because the child has not built sufficient connection strengths to CVC or CCV syllable shapes to allow for their production. A more accurate description of what the child is doing may be to rephrase these process descriptions with wording such as "failure to approximate final consonants." However, the more traditional descriptions of these error patterns will be used at this time.

Reduplication involves the complete repetition of a syllable or partial repetition of a syllable. A child might produce the word *dog* as [dada] or [dadi]. In [dada] the first syllable of the word is repeated; in [dadi] it is partially repeated. Reduplication is more commonly seen in the preceding stage, up to about age 18 months. Many of the "baby talk" words used by adults while speaking to children use reduplication (e.g., *mama, mommy, papa, daddy, baby, doggie*). These may be cases of the adults conforming to the child's capabilities and attempting to show the child that they can use word forms that are modeled on adult speech. Reduplication may occur when children attempt multisyllabic words at a time when multisyllabic sequences are not connected well enough in the child's system. Rather than omitting a second syllable, the child repeats the syllabic-phonemic-feature pattern that has most recently been activated in his or her system.

Deletion of final consonants refers to the omission of word-final consonants occurring in adult word forms. The word *dog* may be produced as [da]. Use of this process has the effect of causing CV and CVC words to become homophonous (having the same sound representation). A child who deletes final consonants may produce both *bow* and *boat* as [bo]. A description of this error pattern that highlights the notion of "failure to approximate" a segment may be particularly useful for this error pattern. Acoustic studies of children's deleted final consonants have shown that they may be manipulating features to cue the existance of the missing consonant. Weismer, Dinnsen, and Elbert (1981) found that children who "deleted" final consonants nevertheless cued the voicing characteristic of the missing consonant by lengthening the vowel when the final consonant is voiced and shortening the vowel when the final consonant is voiceless. In other words, these children had approximated some of the features of the final consonant within a CV shape. As they approximate more of the final consonant's features, they may be able to expand on their CV shape to include CVC syllables as well.

Deletion of unstressed syllables refers to the child's production of multisyllabic words with fewer than needed syllables. The syllables remaining are typically those that are stressed in the adult model. The first unstressed syllable may be deleted from the word *banana* to produce [næne]. Within our model, learning the syllabic-phonemic-featureal aspects of a word involves stimulating a feature pattern through auditory and visual inputs. Unstressed syllables are less likely than stressed syllables to create such patterns because they are shorter in duration and not as loud. Thus, the stressed syllables in a multisyllabic utterance are probably the first to be produced because they have the strongest connection strengths.

Reduction of clusters involves the omission of one or more consonants from clusters in words. Typically, the consonant that is omitted is the one that is thought to be more difficult to produce in a motoric sense. For example, [s] + stop clusters are typically reduced to a stop consonant (e.g., *stop* [tap]). Reduction of a stop + liquid cluster typically retains the stop (e.g., *tree* [ti]). Development of consonant clusters, like development of the use of final consonants, appears to involve an interaction between the syllabic and feature levels. Some children produce single-consonant approximations of clusters in which features from the two consonants are combined (Greenlee, 1973). A common production of *swing* is [fɪn]. In the production, the child has apparently combined the fricative manner of the intended [s] with the labial place of the intended [w] to produce the consonant [f]. Acoustic studies have also shown that some children manipulate production features within their available CV syllabic frames to signal intended differences. Catts and Kahmi (1984) found a child whose productions of /s/ + stop clusters were transcribed as voiced stops (e.g., *stop* [dap]). However, acoustic analysis showed that this child distinguished this [d] from the [d]s produced in words such as *door* by voice onset time. The [d]s produced by this child for adult /d/s were prevoiced, whereas the [d]s produced for s + [t] clusters used short-lag voice onset times. Again, rather than suggesting that children actively delete consonants from clusters, within our model they have failed to produce enough of the gestural cues to approximate a production to the satisfaction of an adult listener.

Substitution Processes. Ingram (1976) described common errors in which a class of phonemes is replaced by another class of phonemes as substitutions. Each class of phonemes is describable with respect to a feature-level contrast. Voiced consonants are a class of phonemes that differ from voiceless consonants with respect to the relative timing of vocal fold movement and articulator movement. Labial consonants differ from alveolar, which differ from velar with respect to the articulator involved: lips versus front of tongue versus back of tongue. When a whole class of phonemes is approximated with a different class, a particular gesture has not been used. The *substitution processes* cited by Ingram include stopping, fronting, and gliding.

Stopping refers to the use of a stop consonant in place of another manner of articulation, usually a fricative or affricate. For example, production of the words *sue* and *chew* as [tu] would be examples of stopping. Production of the fricative aspects of the target sounds requires that a narrow articulatory constriction be held for a relatively long period of time. Such gestures require the coordination of opposing muscle forces. For example, to raise the tip of the tongue to the alveolar ridge to produce a stop [t], it may be necessary only to contract the superior longitudinal muscle of the tongue. This contraction would lift the tongue tip until its movement was halted by the alveolar ridge. On the other hand, to produce an [s], the tongue tip must be stopped a millimeter or so short of the alveolar ridge and held there for a 100 or so milliseconds. This gesture requires more muscular control inasmuch as the inferior longitudinal muscle must be contracted enough to balance the contractile force of the superior longitudinal. When children first attempt these more finely controlled gestures, they tend to produce the previously developed stop gestures.

Fronting refers to the substitution of alveolar or dental sounds for velar and palatal sounds (e.g., production of *gay* as [de]). Raising the front of the tongue to the alveolar ridge is among the most common consonantal gestures in English and other languages as well. Inasmuch as alveolar sounds are babbled more often than palatal and velar sounds, this preference may be based on the anatomical and neuromuscular structures of the vocal tract.

Liquid gliding is the common substitution of glides [w] or [j] for liquids [l] and [r]. This occurs in productions such as *lamb* [wæm] and *rim* [wɪm]. Because glides are not typically thought to occur at the ends of words, changes in [l] and [r] in this word position are referred to as *liquid vocalization* or *vowelization*. In this case, the liquid is produced as a vowel off-glide as in the production of *bar* and *bowl* as [bau]. These glide or vowellike gestures are found in children's babbling much more often than the more complex lingual articulations required for production of liquids. When attempting to replicate these more complex sounds, children use their closest available approximations.

Assimilation Processes. Whereas the substitution processes involve error approximations for whole natural classes of sounds based on articulatory gesture differences, *assimilation processes* involve feature approximations that occur in specific contexts. In a particular context, a feature that is being used elsewhere in the utterance is used inappropriately in a phoneme's representation. Ingram (1976) presented the following assimilation processes: devoicing of final consonants, prevocalic voicing of initial consonants, weakening of stops, and changes in place of articulation.

Devoicing of word final consonants involves the production of an adult voiced consonant as voiceless when it occurs at the end of the word. For example, the word *dog* would be produced as [dak]. This production may result from the child's failure to maintain an approximation of the vocal folds long enough to lengthen the vowel and produce voicing during the consonantal constriction. This failure may be related to the natural tendency to open the vocal folds at the end of an utterance to inhale.

Prevocalic voicing describes the production of unvoiced consonants as voiced when they precede vowels. This is described as an assimilation of the voicing characteristic of the vowel during production of the consonant. For example, a child may produce the words *pea* as [bi] and *sue* as [zu]. Voiceless consonants at the start of a syllable are produced by delaying the onset of vocal fold vibration for approximately 20 to 30 sec relative to release of the consonant constriction. Perhaps an easier gestural timing task is to produce the two gestures simultaneously. Such productions are categorized phonemically in English as voiced; thus an error in the phonemes signaled is produced.

Weakening of stops is seen at the ends of words and in certain clustered contexts where liquid and glide approximation gestures appear to be spread into the stop. Ingram (1976) cited the example of stops in cluster productions becoming fricatives when near liquids (e.g., *tree* [fwi]). Stops may also be expected to be approximated as a fricative at the end of a word as the vocal tract is relaxed for respiration as seen in final-consonant devoicing.

A number of assimilations are seen that involve changing place of articulation of a consonant to more closely resemble a consonant present in the word. Weiner (1979) described three types—labial assimilation, alveolar assimilation, and velar assimilation—related to the three prominent places of articulation in English. A *labial assimilation* occurs when a child produces a nonlabial sound (e.g., /t/ or /k/) as labial when preceding or following a labial consonant. For example, a child might produce the word *thumb* as [fʌm]. In this case, the dental place of articulation usually associated with production of /θ/ has been changed to a labial place of articulation because of the presence of the /m/. *Alveolar assimilation* occurs when a nonalveolar sound is produced as an alveolar because of an alveolar that precedes or follows the sound. For example, a child could produce the /g/ in *dog* as an alveolar [dɔd] because it was preceded by the /d/ at the beginning of the word. *Velar assimilation* occurs when a nonvelar sound is produced as a velar because of a velar context. For example, production of the word *dog* as [gɔg].

In summary, the common articulatory errors occurring during this time period may result from the presence of previously used connection strengths in the child's cognitive system. As the child adds new words, syllable shapes, and phonemes to his or her system, errors will tend to involve these well-used paths. Thus, the child's initial attempts at more complex utterances may be simplifications arising from previously used categorizations of features into phonemes and phonemes into syllables.

Phonemic Development

The traditional description of articulation development during this time period traces the development of adultlike phoneme production. It is generally accepted that a relatively consistent order exists in the development of consonant sounds. For example, Prather, Hedrick, and Kern (1975) asked 2- to 4-year-old children to label pictures. The picture labels included the consonants of English in word-initial and word-final positions. They calculated the percentage of children in an age group who correctly articulated each consonant sound in both word positions. Table 2-7 shows the sounds that were correctly articulated by at least 50 percent of the children in an age group.

Table 2-7. CONSONANT SOUNDS CORRECTLY PRODUCED IN SINGLE-WORD UTTERANCES BY AT LEAST 50 PERCENT OF THE CHILDREN IN AN AGE GROUP ACCORDING TO PRATHER, HEDRICK, AND KERN (1975)

Age group	*Consonant sounds correctly produced*	
2 yr	Stops	p t k b d g
	Nasals	m n ŋ
	Fricatives	h f s
	Glides	w
3 yr	Fricatives	ʃ
	Glides	j
	Liquids	l r
	Affricates	tʃ ʤ
4 yr	Fricatives	θ ð z ʒ v

As seen in this table, the consonants that are used in 2-year olds' approximations of adult words include all of the stops, the nasals, a group of fricatives including [s, f, h], and the glide [w]. With the exception of [f], these consonants are all included in the core group of sounds found by Locke (1983) in the babbling of most preverbal children. The remaining consonants need to be added to this repertoire through practice in the perception and production of words. By age 3 years, most of the children have added the use of the liquids /l/ and /r/, the glide /j/, the affricates /tʃ/ and /ʤ/, and a palatal fricative. At 4 years of age, half of the children are also producing acceptable dental and voiced fricatives.

The data from Prather and colleagues (1975) and other similar studies must be interpreted with some caution. These data are cross-sectional. Different children were studied at ages 2, 3, and 4 years. Looking at this table, we do not see the developing performance of individual children, but the average production of differing groups of children.

You would not want to conclude from this study that it takes the average child 3 years to develop production of /l/ and /r/. Studies of individual children's development have shown that large gains in percentage-correct articulation of /s/ and /r/ can be made in as little as 2 weeks (Hoffman, Schuckers, & Daniloff, 1980; Stephens, Hoffman, & Daniloff, 1986). In these studies, each child appeared to follow an s-shaped learning curve, similar to the one seen in Fig. 2-4. This learning appears to occur in three phases. We will call these experimental approximations (denoted in the figure as A), rapid development of the correct articulation (section B), and development of consistent production (section C).

Fig. 2-4. Stages in development of the correct production of a speech sound.

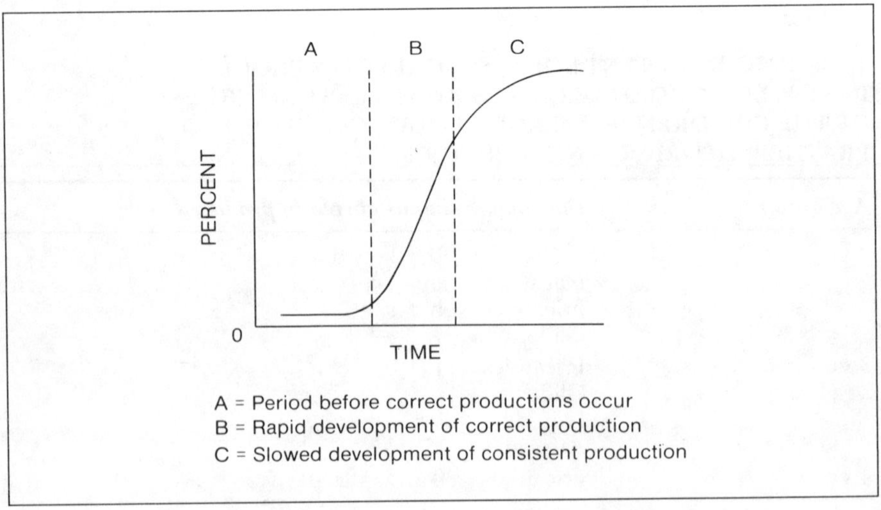

During the first period, the child maintains a relatively low percentage of correct articulations of the target consonant. At this time, the child may not have noticed that his or her speech sound approximations do not conform to the adult model. For example, the 3-year old who produces the word *thumb* as [fʌm] may find that adults understand this production and react toward the child's speech as though this production is adequate. The adults may find this production acceptable because this is "baby talk" that the child is expected to outgrow. Furthermore, no English word [fʌm] exists for the adult to be confused by in interpreting the child's meaning. Thus, there may be little communicative pressure on the child to alter this production.

In the normal course of articulation learning, children appear to be willing to experiment. Their word meanings are constantly open to revision as they learn more about the world and the way that adults make reference. Also their phonological representations must remain open for refinement as well. Stephens and colleagues (1986) observed a group of children who went through the following sequence in the development of acceptable [s] articulation. First these children produced /s/ as a dental fricative [θ]. This is the most common error substitution for [s] produced by English-learning children. It can be viewed as an approximation of [s] production that is correct in its manner, voicing, and nasality. Its only error is a small difference in the place of lingual constriction between the incisors rather than at the alveolar ridge. The sounds that are produced by these two articulations are quite similar to one another, so the child's auditory system may be telling him or her that this production is an appropriate match for the adult model. Also, few minimal pairs exist that distinguish /s/ from /θ/ in the speech of a preschool child.

This group of 5-year olds then made an adjustment in their approximation of [s]. They started to produce /s/ as [ʃ]. They have made an appropriate adjustment in the place of articulation of their dental fricative: They have moved it farther back in the vocal tract. They have just overshot their target. In a final step these children adjusted this target forward in the vocal tract to produce an acceptable alveolar constriction for [s].

Many of the phonological processes cited in the preceding section may reflect this process of approximation of the adult articulation model. Stopping involves an approximation of a fricative with a homoganic stop, a change in manner leaving the other characteristics of the target sound in place. This approximation usually allows the child to approximate an adult target using a speech sound that is already in his or her repertoire of sounds. *Fronting* can be viewed as an approximation of velar and palatal sounds with an alveolar constriction. Like the dentalized and retracted [s]s heard by Stephens and colleagues (1986), these approximations differ only in place of articulation. They also differ in the articulators used. For [t] and [d], the tip/blade articulator is used instead of the body of the tongue, which would be appropriate for [k] and [g] production. This approximation conforms to the preferences for alveolar sounds seen in preverbal speech sound production.

The child seeks to better approximate the speech sounds heard and seen being produced around him or her. During this process, the child uses well-established motor patterns. When these sounds are detected as not being adequate approximations, the child seeks to alter their production characteristics, perhaps one motor feature at a time, until the sound approximations are good enough to prove successful for the child's communicative purposes.

When sound approximations become effective in communicating with a listener, the child enters into the second stage of the s-curve development. The occurrence of acceptable productions of the sound increases rapidly. This rapid development may reflect two processes: The child will be connecting this new target configuration to appropriate words and learning to integrate this new configuration into a widening number of syllabic shapes and phonetic contexts.

The final leg of the s curve is a slow approach to completely correct articulation of the speech sound. This stage may reflect the spreading of the use of the speech sound to the less often used words in the child's lexicon, or to newly acquired words. It may also reflect continued refinement of the gestural organization of the sound.

A second way of misreading the group developmental data is to suggest that children normally misarticulate all of the speech sounds that are usually acquired at a later age. Although 50 percent of the 3-year olds do not correctly articulate /z/, /ʒ/, and /v/, this fact does not indicate that the same 50 percent misarticulate all of these sounds. A particular 3-year old may misarticulate [z] but not [ʒ] and [v].

SEMANTIC STAGE

During the *semantic stage* children develop the ability to understand aspects of language as an abstract system outside of its use. They also continue to develop the abilities to organize and execute motor programs associated with more complex propositions.

Hawkins (1984) suggested that speech production development passes through three stages that overlap the language development stages proposed by Nelson. In the first, the child's motor programs for speech production are organized primarily with respect to timing. Babbling occurs within a framework of repeating syllables whose timing is more adultlike than the particular articulatory configurations produced. The first word approximations are organized with respect to syllable shapes more than phonemic contrasts. During the second phase, children develop more accurate production of individual consonant configurations, but their timing of syllable productions does not approach adultlike performance. In the third phase, the child develops adultlike control of the temporal aspects of speech production, aspects that are based on coordination of phonemic targets within syllable trains required by the more complex propositions being expressed at this time.

Measurement of the temporal coordination of children's speech sound production has indicated that children are generally slower and more variable than adults until about puberty (Kent, 1976). Children may be slower in their articulations because they take more time to get to and away from articulatory targets. Development of speed in articulation depends at least partially on the child's development of the ability to overlap (coproduce) articulatory targets by adjusting feature-level targets of phonemes to better fit the surrounding phonemes. An experiment that demonstrates children's inability to overlap speech sounds might involve asking children to produce words containing consonant clusters and words containing the same consonants without clustering. For example, the [s] sound produced in the word *see* is typically 15 percent longer than the [s] in *ski* in the speech of adults. However, children often fail to produce the overlapping gestures necessary to produce such shortening in clusters (Hawkins, 1984).

Another indication that children are not coordinating speech sounds into larger utterances is seen in speech productions that are more stereotypical than adults (Hawkins, 1984). That is, children tend to produce particular speech segments the same way time after time, regardless of context. To speed production, it is necessary for the child to anticipate future motor targets and make changes in segments so that the transition from speech sound to speech sound will be swifter and more efficiently produced.

Children also show more variability in repeated productions of the same utterance (Hawkins, 1984). That is, when a particular word is spoken over and over again, a child will vary the durations of the individual syllables and sounds to a greater degree than adults.

Adultlike timing ability appears to be achieved at about puberty (Kent, 1976). It is not until this age that children coordinate the various levels of the verbal communication system to execute speech acts in an adult fashion.

SUGGESTED CLASSROOM ACTIVITIES

1. One class member should make an audio recording of an infant who is quietly at play. The class should transcribe utterances. What speech sounds are produced? What syllable shapes are produced? Which of Oller's sound types occur?

2. Selected class members should make recordings of a 3-year old, 4-year old, 5-year old, and 6-year old telling stories about the pictures in Appendix A. The class should decide how many of each child's utterances fall into the categories of descriptions, inferences, and interpretations. Analyze sound production errors using Ingram's phonological process categories.

CHAPTER 3

Children's Disordered Phonetic Processing

Topics in this chapter include

- Sensory Motor Aspects
  - Organic Disorders
  - Functional Misarticulation as a Sensory Motor Disorder
- Auditory Perceptual Aspects
  - Hearing Impairment
  - Speech Perception Ability
- Cognitive-Linguistic Aspects
  - General Intelligence
  - Language Ability

This chapter discusses the nature of children's disordered phonetic processing. It serves as a bridge between the discussion of normal phonetic processes and development in the preceding chapters and the assessment and treatment chapters that follow. Before speech-language pathologists decide what to assess and how to plan remediation for children's misarticulations, they should understand the factors that potentially cause and maintain misarticulation beyond the normal developmental period. They should also have an understanding of the methods employed in the theoretical study of children's misarticulation to aid in the process of keeping up with changing views in this area. Furthermore, the clinician must learn to act as a scientist does by asking questions about individual children's speech production disabilities and the manner in which the clinician goes about aiding the misarticulating child.

No universally accepted theory accounts for all of children's disordered articulation. In part this is because misarticulation has been studied within a variety of theoretical backgrounds. Individual children may misarticulate for different etiological reasons; thus attempts to define a single theoretical cause for misarticulation may always fail. Furthermore, misarticulations may be caused by different factors at different periods of development.

The earliest modern framework in which children's misarticulation was studied involved a medical orientation (Van Riper, 1939). Disorders were considered to be either *organic* or *functional.* An organic misarticulation was considered to be directly attributable to some specific anatomical or neurological deficit. Functional disorders had no such identifiable cause.

Much of the research concerning children's misarticulation conducted prior to 1970 sought organic causes in the oral sensory-motor and auditory-speech perception systems. It was found that relatively few cases of children's misarticulations could be attributed to a single organic cause. This lead some investigators to conclude that the organic causes involved in functional misarticulation were complex and subtle, but probably still there to be discovered (McDonald, 1964a). Perhaps researchers simply did not yet possess instruments capable of measuring the organic cause. Perhaps a group of subtle deficits conspires to cause an individual child to misarticulate when any one of the deficits acting alone might not. The treatment approaches that were devised to help misarticulating children during this time frame, from the 1930s through the 1960s, stressed the training of sensory motor skills and auditory perceptual skills.

As will be seen in the sections of this chapter called "Sensory-Motor Aspects" and "Auditory-Perceptual Aspects," researchers continue to study the peripheral systems of misarticulating children. The search for interactions between articulatory ability and peripheral problems is not only theoretically important, it is also of clinical importance. Although most misarticulating children may not have identifiable organic problems, some do, and the speech-language pathologist will receive referrals for such children.

Failure to discover a single underlying cause for children's misarticulations led other investigators to conclude that functional misarticulation is a problem in which physiologically normal children had mislearned the phonology of English (Winitz, 1969; Ingram, 1976). In recent years a majority of the research into children's misarticulation has focused on the child's developing conceptualization of how speech sounds are structured and used in English words. This has lead to a shift in teaching strategies away from sensory-motoric and auditory-perceptual training to training designed to help the child organize conceptual categories of words, syllable shapes, phonemes, and features in ways that approximate adult usage.

Some of this theoretical shift can be accounted for by the fact that speech-language pathologists recognized and became responsible for communication problems of younger children. Prior to this time, children were identified as misarticulating at age 7 or 8 years when normative data suggested that 90 percent of the normal population correctly produced all of the sounds of English in single words. The articulation disordered children identified at this age typically misarticulated one or two speech sounds, did not appear to have related language problems, and were expected to be able to metalinguistically understand and discuss the nature of speech sounds and their articulation. Younger children who are identified as misarticulating today typically misarticulate many speech sounds, have concomitant language problems, and are still in the stage of learning language in the context of its use. Thus, alternative methods of testing and treatment have evolved as well. However, we cannot completely dismiss the past. Children who misarticulate one or two speech sounds at age 7 still exist, and the speech-language pathologist needs to be able to efficiently deal with their problems while also being able to work with the more impaired, younger children.

This chapter presents examples of research conducted to study the nature of children's misarticulations. The scientist who seeks to understand children's misarticulations does so by conducting empirical studies. Such studies are designed to provide evidence in favor of one theory or another. Empirical evidence refers to observations that can be detected by the senses. The intent of empirical studies is to create observations on which all scientists can agree. Observations are then used to support theories. Empirical research studies can be divided into two types: descriptive and experimental.

Descriptive research in this area has detailed the relationships between misarticulation and other measurable abilities that are thought to be involved in the articulation process. One method of doing this is to describe the articulatory abilities of groups of persons who differ from one another on the supposedly related characteristic. To describe the influence of oral structure on misarticulation, a researcher could compare articulation abilities of children with cleft palates to those of children without cleft palates. Another descriptive research method compares the supposedly related abilities of misarticulating children with those of normally articulating children. Investigators have compared the sentence repetition abilities of misarticulating and normally articulating children. In a third type of descriptive study, correlations between articulation scores and other measurements are computed. Correlations are mathematical expressions of the degree to which children perform at the same level on two measures. A child whose articulation ability is below average might be found to have language skills that are also below average. If a large percentage of children performed similarly on two tasks, the tasks would be correlated.

Descriptive research has one major drawback. It cannot define the cause-effect direction of the relationships between misarticulation and these other abilities. Misarticulating children have been found to produce shorter sentences than nonmisarticulating children. This result may mean that misarticulation is caused by a language-processing problem. It may also be that children's language-processing difficulties were caused by their misarticulations. Or some third variable, such as decreased cognitive ability, may have affected both the child's articulation and language-processing abilities.

Experimental studies attempt to determine cause and effect relationships by manipulating one variable (the suspected cause) and seeing if another variable (the suspected effect) changes. For humane reasons, many of the factors associated with misarticulation cannot be studied in this manner. Hearing ability is probably related to misarticulation. However, a researcher cannot be allowed to permanently damage someone's hearing to test this relationship. In such cases, descriptive research provides all of the information that is available.

The most common experimental manipulations of children's misarticulations occur in the context of treatment studies. In these studies, experimenters wish to determine what kinds of treatment strategies change children's articulation, how the children's articulation pattern changes, and which of a variety of strategies might change children's articulation most rapidly. Since treatment strategies are often derived from particular theories of the causes of misarticulation, their success or failure is used as evidence for theories of the causes of misarticulations.

Many treatment studies use behavior modification strategies to alter children's misarticulations. These strategies seek to alter a person's behavior by manipulating the stimuli that the person responds to and the stimuli that occur after the response. These are referred to as *antecedent events* (occurring prior to the response) and *consequent events* (occurring after the response). This relationship is depicted in Table 3-1.

Antecedent events that are typically used to increase the likelihood of a correctly articulated speech sound include instructions and models. Instructions typically involve descriptions of the placement of articulators to produce the error consonant. A child who produces /s/ as [θ] is extending the tongue tip too far forward. The instruction to "Put your tongue behind your teeth" may be sufficient to allow the child to alter this typical production. Some children will alter their productions of speech sounds when they are simply given a model of the speech sound. The child who typically misarticulates /s/ may produce [s] instead of [θ] when the clinician says something like "Listen to what I say. Say [sssss]."

Table 3-1. BASIC BEHAVIORAL MODIFICATION SCHEME FOR ALTERING A CHILD'S MISARTICULATION

Stimuli	⟶ *Child* ⟶	*Response*	*Consequent event*
Instructions about sound production		Articulatory movements	Rewards
Verbal questions		Language processing	Punishments

The prompts and models used by speech clinicians to enhance a child's articulation do not typically occur in the child's day-to-day speech. During normal speech production the child is reacting to the stimuli that exist in a particular communicative setting: playing games with a friend, answering a teacher's questions, or talking to a parent. Articulation training programs typically plan to use more and more natural stimuli as therapy progresses. Part of the stimulus continuum used by Carrier (1970) is shown in Table 3-2.

In this antecedent-event progression, the child is first given a model of the sound as it occurs in a word that labels a picture. Next, the model of the word is eliminated so that the child supplies the label. The picture is paired with an object, and then the picture is removed so that the label is applied to the object. Finally, the objects are named in their usual settings (the home), in response to typical verbal statements by an adult.

Single-word–labeling responses are not typical of children's speech, so many articulation training programs seek to make the articulatory response more complex by increasing the length of utterances. For example, Hoffman (1983) taught correct production of /r/ in responses that increased through the stages shown in Table 3-3.

The first response was an isolated [ɝ] production, thought to be a good representation of the vocal tract shape involved in /r/ production. The second stage involved production of [rV] syllables such as [ri], [re], and [ru]. Third, /r/ was produced in words. Fourth, the children were required to correctly produce /r/ occurring in noun phrases. Finally, production of /r/ was required in sentences. In this case, complexity was increased by moving from meaningless responses, isolated [ɝ] and the syllables, to meaningful responses. The meaningful utterances were systematically increased in syntactic complexity. Other methods of increasing response complexity are possible and have been used by other experimenters.

To increase the percentage of correct responses made in each phase of training, the clinician manipulates the consequent events that follow the response. Consequent events that increase the frequency of a correct re-

Table 3-2. STIMULUS PROGRESSION USED BY CARRIER (1970) TO ELICIT CORRECT ARTICULATIONS OF A SPEECH SOUND

1. Model of the sound produced in a word accompanying a picture of the word.
2. Picture without a verbal model of the word.
3. Picture is presented next to the real object pictured.
4. Real object without picture or model.
5. Real objects placed around the house in their normal locations.

Table 3-3. INCREASING COMPLEXITY OF VERBAL RESPONSES UTILIZED IN TRAINING PRODUCTION OF /r/ BY HOFFMAN (1983)

1. Isolated [ɝ] productions
2. [rV] syllable productions
3. Word productions
4. Phrase productions
5. Sentence productions

sponse are called *reinforcers*. Typically, positive reinforcement (a stimulus that was chosen because it is thought to be rewarding) is used. Verbal praise such as "That was a good [s]" is often used. When positive reinforcers are witheld after a response, the clinician is trying to extinguish the response (make its rate of occurrence decrease). If the child misarticulates [s], the clinician would not use verbal praise. The lack of reinforcement for a response should cause its frequency of occurrence to lessen through a process called *extinction*. Administration of a supposedly unpleasant stimulus is used to punish a response. Like extinction, punishment is intended to decrease the rate of a response. Costello and Ferrer (1976) showed improved articulation for six children whose incorrect responses were followed by punishments including the clinician saying "No," a loud buzzer, or through the loss of reinforcers that had been previously obtained through correct responses.

In this chapter we will sample both descriptive and experimental research regarding children's misarticulations. Children's misarticulations are described using the same divisions as preceding chapters: cognitive, sensory-motor, and auditory-perceptual. However, this chapter follows a historical progression of theories of children's disordered speech production. That is, the possibility that children's misarticulations are caused by sensory-motoric problems is addressed first, followed by the possibility that children's misarticulations are due to auditory-perceptual problems, and finally, the possibility that disordered cognitive development results in misarticulations.

SENSORY-MOTOR ASPECTS

One of the first views of children's misarticulations was that it was caused by deviant anatomical structures or a lack of necessary physiological coordination. This section describes speech production effects of a variety of structural and neurological deficits. Although not responsible for the majority of disordered speech production, these problems are still encountered. Furthermore, the study of the known organic problems provides a basis for understanding the view that many cases of misarticulation require sensory-motor training. Secondly, this section will present evidence supporting the view that even children's functional misarticulations are, in large part, due to subtle sensory-motoric problems.

ORGANIC DISORDERS

A number of organic disorders may directly affect speech production processes. These are described here in two sections. "Anatomical Structure Problems" describes some of the more common physiological conditions that affect the structures that make up the vocal tract. "Neurological Disorders" describes the speech production problems encountered by persons with damaged or disordered nervous systems.

Anatomical Structure Problems

The anatomical structures of the oral and nasal cavities act to create and modify speech sounds by altering the flow of air through the vocal tract. Anatomical structures that are insufficient for this purpose can prevent adequate production of speech sounds. In Chap. 1, the speech production functions of each of the articulators were discussed. This section describes some of the more common structural deficiencies that can affect speech sound production.

Dental Structure. The teeth, especially the upper incisors, play a role in production of the fricative sounds. They provide a cutting edge for the breath stream that creates a hissing noise quality. Two dental conditions, missing incisors and misalignment of the upper and lower teeth, have been found to interact with articulatory ability.

Snow (1961) compared fricative consonant productions of children who were missing incisors and those with full dentition. She found that a higher proportion of children with missing teeth misarticulated some of these speech sounds than did the children without missing teeth. However, 75 percent of the children with missing teeth showed no misarticulation of these sounds. Thus, although missing teeth may affect the speech production abilities of some children, it does not adversely affect all children.

Dental occlusion refers to the biting relationship between the upper and lower teeth, as well as the positioning of individual teeth within the arches. In normal occlusion, the upper teeth are somewhat farther out than the lower teeth, and each tooth is opposite two teeth in the other arch (upper versus lower). The first two drawings in Fig. 3-1 show the malocclusions that result when this normal relationship between upper and lower teeth is not attained. Zemlin (1981) described Angle's (1899) classification of malocclusions as follows. Class I malocclusion involves a normal biting relationship between the upper and lower arches, but individual teeth are misaligned within the arches. In normal occlusion, the upper teeth extend out slightly over the lower teeth because the upper jaw is larger than the mandible. Class II malocclusion involves a mandible that is retruded, or too far posterior, relative to the upper jaw. This gives the person the appearance of an "overbite." Class III malocclusion involves a mandible that is positioned too far forward relative to the upper jaw.

Two other forms of malocclusion are referred to as *open bite* (shown in the last drawing of Fig. 3-1) and *closed bite*. In open bite, the upper and lower incisors fail to overlap, leaving a gap in the front of the mouth when the back teeth are closed. In closed bite, the reverse occurs: The front teeth overlap, but a gap remains between the back teeth.

Certain malocclusions, particularly open bite, have been related to *reverse swallow* patterns. In the typical swallowing motion, the tongue moves in a front to back direction. In reverse swallow, the front of the tongue is pushed forward, against or between the incisors. Reverse swallow, also known as *tongue thrust*, is a normally occurring swallow pattern that is used by fewer and fewer children from birth through puberty (Mason & Proffit, 1974). These authors suggested that its occurrence lessens as the pharyngeal cavity

Fig. 3-1. Malocclusions affecting speech production.

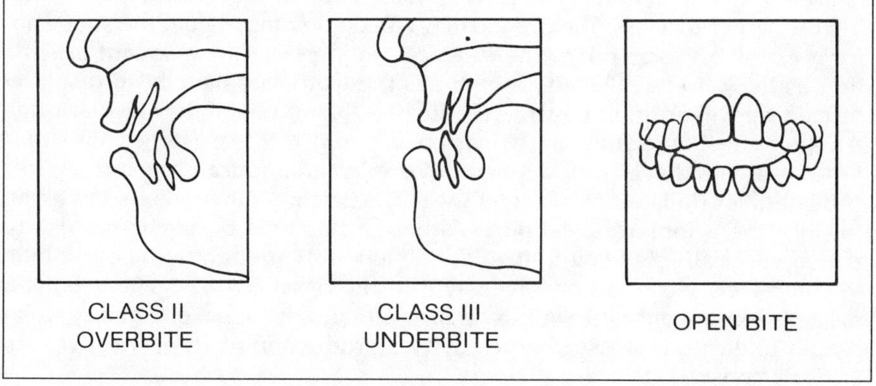

deepens and expands to allow for tongue movement in a posterior direction. This condition has also been related to thumb sucking.

Reverse swallow pattern is thought, by some, to cause both open bite and misarticulation of fricatives such as [s] and [ʃ]. However, use of this swallow pattern by much larger percentages of children than those who develop malocclusions or misarticulations speaks against its being a general causal factor in misarticulation (Mason & Proffit, 1974). In general, this statement can be applied to the other malocclusions as well. It has not been demonstrated that a particular malocclusion will invariably cause misarticulations. Children can apparently learn to adapt their speech production targets and movement patterns to a wide variety of dental structures. However, we should not rule out the possibility that a particular child may not be able to compensate for his or her particular dental differences.

Clefting. The vocal tract is formed during the first 12 weeks of embryonic development. Tissues that originate near the sides of the embryo grow together near the midline (Zemlin). In approximately 1 in 600 births in the United States, this process of fusing together components of the lip, hard palate, and soft palate is disrupted. Likely causes for this disruption include heredity, prenatal lack of oxygen, or prenatal exposure to toxic material. Figure 3-2 shows drawings of a variety of types of facial clefts. These vary in degree of involvement inasmuch as the cleft may occur on one side of the face or both (i.e, unilateral and bilateral clefts) and may be complete or incomplete (i.e., extending from lip through the velum or involving subcomponents of the lip, hard palate, and soft palate).

Clefts of the lip are often repaired surgically in the first month to aid in the child's feeding and to encourage appropriate development of the bony structures underneath. Depending on how much tissue is available, the lip may or may not be very mobile after repair. Typically, the degree of lip movement is sufficient for production of the labial consonants.

Clefting of the hard palate may occur on one side or on both sides. Wherever clefts occur they are likely to disrupt the development of the teeth nearby. When a bilateral cleft occurs, the portion of the hard palate containing the upper incisors, the premaxilla, will be floating. Thus, the shape and form of the alveolar ridge, the most common place of consonant articulation, is likely to be affected. Sometimes the teeth that have been displaced by clefting will erupt in new places, such as the middle of the alveolar ridge. Another effect of clefting on the hard palate may be the existence of fistulas. Fistulas are relatively well defined holes in an anatomical structure.

Bilateral or unilateral clefting of the soft palate impairs the person's ability to close the velopharyngeal port. Although this type of damage is also repaired surgically, the velum may not be left with enough tissue or mobility to completely close the passageway into the nasal cavities. This results in nasalization of sonorant sounds. It also impairs the speaker's ability to impound oral cavity pressure necessary for production of stop, fricative, and affricate consonants.

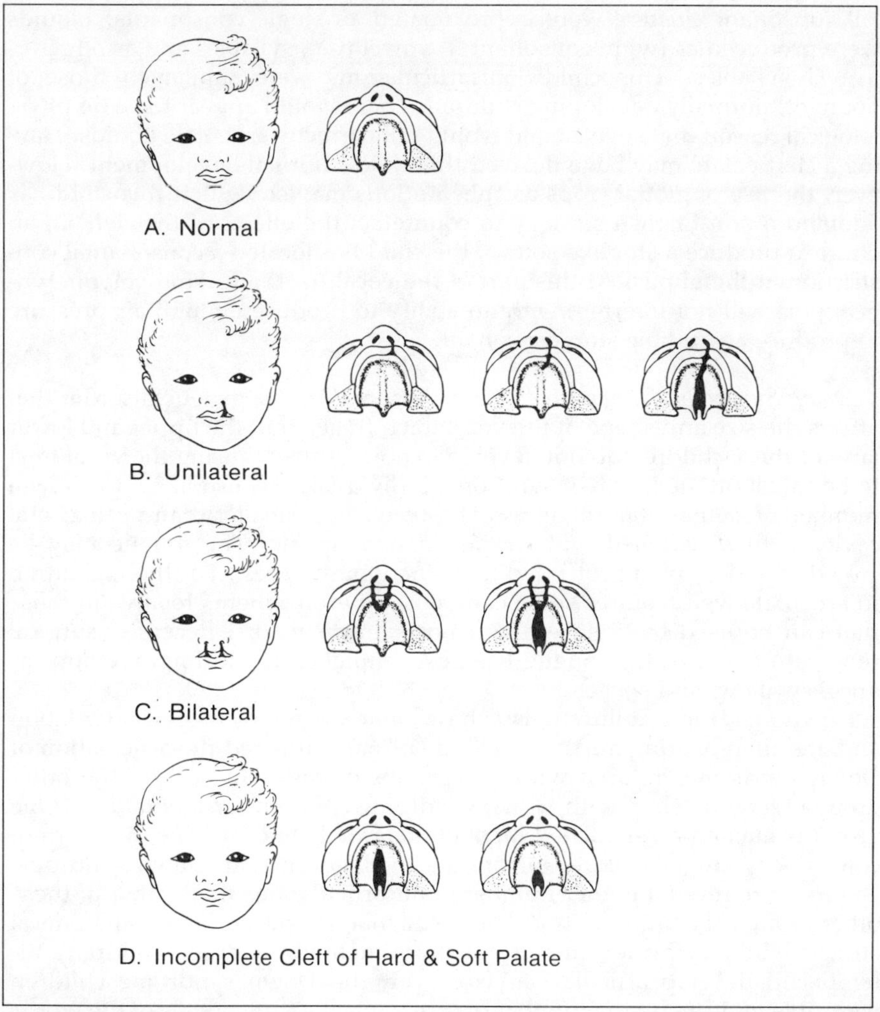

Fig. 3-2. Cleft palate types.

Hodson, Chin, Redmond, and Simpson (1983) described the misarticulations of a 5-year-old child with a repaired cleft palate. The repaired velum apparently moved well. Thus speech errors were no longer being directly caused by a lack of closure between the velum and pharyngeal wall. They found that this child produced a number of errors in production of the speech sounds, requiring increased intraoral air pressure (i.e., stops, fricatives, and affricates). Many of these sounds were omitted or produced as a glottal stop. Fricatives that were not omitted were often produced as stops.

All consonant clusters were approximated as single consonants. Liquids were produced as [w] in consonant + vowel (CV) syllables and as offglides in VC syllables. This child's misarticulations were similar to those of younger, normally developing children. There would appear to be no physiological reason that such a child would not correctly articulate liquids. Having a cleft palate may have delayed this child's normal development. However, the use of glottal stops as substitutions may show that this child has adopted a non-English strategy to counteract the effects of the cleft. In an effort to produce a stoplike sound, the child has located a consonantal constriction at the glottis. At this part of the vocal tract, a leaking velopharyngeal port will not interfere with an ability to produce enough air pressure to produce an audible stop consonant.

Down Syndrome. *Down syndrome,* or trisomy 21, is a genetic disorder that affects the size and shape of the vocal tract. In general, the upper and lower jaws of these children do not develop to normal size, causing the vocal tract to be foreshortened. Down syndrome individuals are also likely to show a number of dental abnormalities. The result is a smaller-than-normal oral cavity with a flattened and shortened hard palate. The tongue may be crowded and is often protruded from the mouth at rest. For these children to articulate well requires some compensatory movements relative to those that can be used by children with normal articulators. Recently, surgical removal of part of the tongue has been implemented to improve appearance, swallow, and speech.

Down syndrome children also show some degree of mental retardation and are often hearing impaired. Dodd (1976a) compared the articulation of Down syndrome children with two groups of children. Both of the other groups were matched with Down syndrome children for mental age. One group contained age-matched mentally retarded children. The other group contained younger children of normal intelligence. The Down syndrome children produced a higher number of misarticulations than either of these other groups of children. Thus, it appears that having a different anatomical structure added to the difficulty of these mentally retarded children's attempts to develop articulation. However, the Down syndrome children were able to decrease the number of errors when given models of the words to produce. Thus, at least for some misarticulations, the Down syndrome child's anatomy does not totally preclude appropriate speech production.

Neurological Disorders

As discussed in Chap. 1, the nervous system control mechanisms for speech production contain a variety of levels. A singularly important level of control is in the region of Broca's area of the dominant hemisphere. This area appears to prepare the final motor programs for the time course of muscular contractions needed to produce a particular speech sound sequence. Posterior to Broca's area is the portion of the motor strip that issues the actual motor commands to the muscles important for speech production. This area is the starting point for the *pyramidal tract*. The pyramidal tract is a direct pathway to the peripheral nerves of the brain stem and spinal cord. The pyramidal tract is responsible for purposeful, skilled movements. The *extra-pyramidal tract* is a less direct motor system that originates from the cortex in front of the motor strip. The extrapyramidal tract makes a number of connections on its way to innervating the peripheral nerve nuclei. The extrapyramidal system appears to be involved in the inhibition of reflexes, the maintenance of muscle tone, and posture. The *cerebellar system* appears to modulate, control, and integrate the various movements dictated by the pyramidal and extrapyramidal systems. The *cerebellum* processes information that is being fed back from the body to the cortex. This information is used to monitor intended movements and make corrections in motor plans that are failing.

Neuromotor speech disorders are generally considered to be of two types: *apraxia* and the *dysarthrias*. Apraxia is an articulation disorder that is caused by neurological damage to cortical areas responsible for selection and sequencing of the gestures associated with phonemes. The dysarthrias are a group of speech disorders caused by damage to one or more parts of the motor system including the pyramidal, extrapyramidal, cerebellar, and peripheral components.

Dysarthrias. Darley, Aronson, and Brown (1975) defined five basic types of dysarthrias: flaccid, spastic, ataxic, hypokinetic, and hyperkinetic. *Flaccid* dysarthria results from damage to the peripheral nervous system. The peripheral nervous system starts in the brain stem or spinal cord nuclei of the cranial and spinal nerves that serve speech production. The cranial and spinal nerves then connect with sensory receptors and muscles in various points in the body. Damage to this part of the nervous system results in muscular paralysis, muscular weakness, lack of muscular tone, and muscular atrophy. Basically, the affected muscles are not receiving the commands to contract. Thus, the movements controlled by contraction of a particular muscle are affected.

Respiration is controlled by a series of spinal nerves whose nuclei are in the cervical and thoracic regions of the spinal cord. The intrinsic muscles of the larynx that provide most of the control of vocal fold movement are supplied by the *vagus nerve* (tenth cranial nerve). The vagus nerve also supplies motor control of the muscles that constrict the pharynx. Muscular control of the mandible is supplied by the *trigeminal* (fifth cranial nerve). Movement of the soft palate is also controlled via part of the trigeminal nerve and the *accessory nerve* (eleventh). The intrinsic and extrinsic muscles of the tongue are largely supplied by the *hypoglossal nerve* (twelfth).

Spastic dysarthria is caused by nervous system damage to the *central nervous system* components extending from the motor strip to the peripheral nerve nuclei in the brain stem or spinal cord. Damage to the pyramidal tract results in problems in performance of discrete, skilled movements. Damage to extrapyramidal tract results in spasticity, muscular weakness, limited range of movement, and slowed movement. Basically, these are all due to the lack of muscular inhibition usually supplied by the extrapyramidal system. Muscles typically work in complementary sets. One set of muscles moves a structure in one direction, and another set moves the structure in the opposite direction. For example, the *masseter* and other muscles lift the mandible; the *geniohyoid* and other muscles lower the mandible. To smoothly lift the mandible, contraction of the geniohyoid will be decreased. When both sets of opposing muscles are allowed to compete against one another, the result is a jerky, slow movement.

Damage to the cerebellum interferes with its ability to coordinate the actions of the various muscle sets relative to a motoric goal. The results are imprecise and slowed movement and lack of muscle tone.

Damage to the extrapyramidal system can result in *hypotonic* or *hypertonic dysarthria*. Hypotonic dysarthria involves slowed movements, rigidity, and a resting tremor. Hypertonic dysarthria can be quick or slow. In its quick form, hypertonic dysarthria results in rapidly occurring involuntary movements of articulators. In its slow form, hypertonic dysarthria results in slow, writhing movements of articulators.

In general, articulatory errors associated with dysarthrias have been described as imprecise productions, including distortions or omissions of the intended speech sounds. The speech errors produced are highly related to problems in nonspeech movements. For example, flaccid paralysis resulting from damage to the trigeminal nerve will affect motion of the mandible during speech in much the same way it affects mandibular motion during chewing.

Apraxia. Apraxia is a problem of articulatory programming that has been caused by damage to the cerebral cortex. It involves inabilities to choose and sequence articulatory targets appropriate for a particular utterance. The apraxic speaker will typically have difficulty initiating an utterance and will grope for articulatory targets.

While articulatory errors of the dysarthric are typically simplifications of the movement pattern, apraxic errors often involve a degree of complication. Articulatory errors include substitution of one phoneme for another, addition of phonemes to an utterance, and repetitions of phonemes in an utterance. The substitution errors are not predictable. The same person will correctly articulate a speech sound in one utterance but not in the next. Furthermore, automatic speech such as cursing may be relatively unimpaired although more volitional speech is misarticulated. Also, as utterances become longer and more complex, the apraxic is likely to make an increasing number of errors.

Some clinicians and researchers have proposed a disorder called *developmental apraxia*. The use of this term implies that the articulation problems shown by these children are due to some form of neurological damage. However, children are sometimes labeled as *apraxic* without unequivocal evidence of neurological impairment. Rosenbek and Wertz (1972) described the speech production of a group of children who had been labeled as developmentally apraxic. They found that individual children showed some but not all of the following: (1) decreased ability to perform nonverbal oral movements, (2) more articulatory errors for the phonetically more complex speech sounds (i.e., fricatives, affricates), (3) more articulatory errors for consonant clusters, (4) more articulatory errors for longer utterances, (5) inconsistency of phoneme production, (6) transposition or misordering of sounds, and (7) errors in production of vowels. Less than 50 percent of the children studied showed clinically measurable neurological deficits.

Many of these error patterns are found in the speech of normally developing children and children whose errors are not thought to be caused by neurological damage. This overlap in performance can be interpreted in several ways. Normal articulatory development and functional misarticulation may share common mechanisms of neurological development, or, the children who are labeled as developmentally apraxic do not differ in kind from the more severely involved functionally misarticulating child.

Cerebral Palsy. Damage to the neuromuscular system that occurs before birth, at birth, or up until about the second birthday is referred to as *cerebral palsy*. As in the case of the adult, the impairment caused will depend on the areas of the nervous system that are affected. The problems of the cerebral palsied child and the adult with acquired brain damage may differ significantly. The adult has gone through normal motoric development, suppressing and mastering early reflexive behaviors. The newborn does not have the benefit of this development, and his or her nervous system impairment may prohibit normal motoric development.

Mecham, Berko, and Berko (1960) described etiologies for cerebral palsy in three time periods: prenatal, natal, and postnatal. Prenatal brain damage can be caused by anoxia (lack of oxygen supply to the fetus), maternal infections, and Rh incompatibility. Between the start of labor and birth, brain damage may result from anoxia, asphyxia (mechanical obstruction to breathing), trauma due to labor or instruments, sudden change in pressure caused by cesarean birth, or prematurity. After birth, brain damage may result from trauma, infections, anoxia, or vascular problems. These same etiologies are involved in damage to the nervous system components serving audition. The child who is at risk for cerebral palsy is also at risk for hearing impairment.

McMahon, Hodson, and Allen (1983) described the articulation errors of 10 cerebral palsied children between the ages 4 and 6 years. All of these children showed the following error patterns. Liquids were produced as glides in syllable-initial position (e.g., *lake* [wek]) and as off-glides in syllable-final position (e.g., *candle* [kændou]). Clusters were produced as single consonants (e.g., *tree* [ti]). Voiceless obstruent consonants were produced as voiced in word-initial position. Voiced obstruent consonants were produced as voiceless in word-final position. Finally, fricatives were distorted via lateralization (e.g., *sun* [lʌn]) and dentalization (e.g., *sun* [θʌn]). Again, many of these patterns of misarticulation are also seen in the articulatory approximations of normally developing children at younger ages.

FUNCTIONAL MISARTICULATION AS A SENSORY-MOTOR DISORDER

McDonald's (1964a) work exemplified the view of functional misarticulation as a motoric disorder when he defined articulation errors as "movements which are not adequate for producing the sound attempted." In McDonald's view the failure to find a particular organic cause for a child's misarticulation may result from "multiple, coexisting factors, any one of which would not result in defective articulation."

McDonald supported this view by arguing that normal articulatory development was patterned from the motorically gross to the motorically refined. He considered the vowel sounds developed relatively early to be motorically simple. These were followed in development by labials, dentals, labiodentals, "complicated tongue sounds" such as [l] and [r], and finally the sibilants. Development of production skill for these more difficult sounds necessitated the development of better sensory discrimination abilities in the tactile, proprioceptive, and auditory feedback mechanisms. McDonald also hypothesized that development of individual speech sounds proceeded from gross errors of omission to more refined errors of substitution, distortion, and finally correct production. Finally, McDonald suggested that development of an individual speech sound would progress from a time at which nearly all productions were incorrect through an increase in correct production. A major focus in this progressive development was the phonetic context in which the speech sound is produced.

The next section explores experimental evidence suggesting that functional misarticulation is at least partly a problem in learning to produce the movement patterns underlying speech production. This discussion looks at evidence regarding the changes in misarticulation of consonant sounds when phonetic context is altered, acoustic studies suggesting that misarticulating children are less coordinated speakers than nonmisarticulating children, tests of nonspeech oral-motor abilities, and the effects of training speech production as a sensory-motor task involving imitation of sounds, syllables, and words.

Phonetic Context

As seen in Chap. 1, the movement pattern required for production of a particular consonant differs with its phonetic context. Production of the [s] in the word *peace* requires little mandibular movement because the mandible is already raised for production of the [i] that precedes it. In the word *pass*, the low vowel [æ] before the [s] makes it imperative that the speaker raise the mandible as part of the [s] movement pattern. Thus, ability to produce [s] involves the ability to control these different muscular coordinations in differing phonetic contexts.

A variety of studies have shown that elementary school children who misarticulate [s] and [r] will correctly articulate these sounds in some phonetic contexts but not in others. Earlier studies noted phonetic context effects on misarticulation in single words; later investigations extended this study to contexts that crossed word boundaries.

Spriestersbach and Curtis (1951) reported data from a series of master's theses in which misarticulating school-age children were asked to name pictures that targeted /r/ or /s/. They found from 23 percent to 45 percent of these children were heard to correctly articulate [s] or [r] in consonant clusters even though they did not correctly articulate these sounds in nonclustered contexts. This is an unexpected finding given that in the normal course of development, clusters appear later than singleton consonants. As you will recall, clusters are typically first approximated as a single consonant.

Later studies have followed up on this finding. From a motoric viewpoint, misarticulation of [s] as [θ] and [r] as [w] both involve inappropriate tongue positions. If the phonetic context in which [s] or [r] is produced demands tongue positions similar to those of the error sound, then the child's tongue may be drawn through a position that approximates an appropriate articulation of the usually misarticulated [s] or [r].

Mazza, Schuckers, and Daniloff (1979) asked children who misarticulated [s] to repeat sentences in which the place of articulation of nearby consonants was altered. This occurred both within the same word and across word boundaries. Examples of these phonetic contexts and sentences are shown in Table 3-4.

It was found that these children most often correctly articulated [s] in the contexts [ps#k, p#st, ks#t, ps#p]. Each of these was correctly articulated at least 50 percent of the time. These authors described their results with respect to coproduction of place of articulation. Production of [p] requires no particular tongue position. Thus, the child is free to anticipate the alveolar tongue position involved in [s] production during production of a [p] that precedes an [s]. Production of a [t] also involves an alveolar tongue position. The child who anticipates production of [t] may correctly articulate

Table 3-4. EXAMPLES OF SENTENCE STIMULI USED BY MAZZA ET AL. (1979) TO ALTER PHONETIC CONTEXT OF [s]

Context	*Sentence*
psp	Pam keeps peeping in the window.
tst	The hot steam burned his hand.
ksk	The old man makes keys.

a nearby [s] as well by assimilation of the alveolar place from [t]. Production of [k] involves drawing the body of the tongue back in the oral cavity. Presence of a [k] may draw the usually dentalized [s] tongue position, which is too far forward, back into an appropriate position.

Hoffman, Schuckers, and Ratusnik (1977) conducted a similar study of [r] misarticulation. Children were asked to repeat sentences in which [r] was preceded by consonants of different places of articulation (e.g., [p, t, k]). These combinations occurred within words and across word boundaries (e.g., "The cat climbed a *tree*" and "Pa*t r*eads books"). These children correctly articulated [r] more often when the preceding stop consonant occurred within the same word (i.e., consonant "blends" as in the words *priest, tree, cream*), than when the preceding consonant ended one word and the [r] began the next. Furthermore, [r] was correctly articulated more often when preceded by [k] or [t] than when preceded by [p]. The authors attributed this effect to coproduction of the tongue positions involved in [t] (alveolar constriction) and [k] (velar constriction) compared to [p] (no necessary constriction). Production of [r] entails two tongue constrictions, one near the front of the mouth and one near the back. Children who produce [r] as [w] are failing to make these lingual constrictions. Perhaps having the tongue raised prior to an attempt for [r] aids in its production, especially when the preceding consonant and [r] are both part of the same word.

If functionally misarticulating children are impaired in their abilities to produce phonetic features, they may show imperceptable differences in the ability to coproduce these features in a string of speech sounds. A small number of acoustic studies have investigated this possibility.

Daniloff, Wilcox, and Stephens (1980) studied the ability of [s]-misarticulating children between the ages of 6 and 8 years to coproduce [s] with following vowels. They measured the acoustic spectrum of [s] as it was produced in [sV] syllables including different vowels. The frequencies present in the spectrum are related to the shape of the vocal tract during [s] production. Different [s] spectra in different contexts would indicate that the children were coproducing the [s] with its context. Their study indicated that children who dentalize [s] and children who lateralize [s] produce less coproduction than children whose production of [s] was acceptable.

Coproduction of a consonant with its context allows for more rapid production of the sound. Weismer and Elbert (1982) measured the durations of [s] sounds produced by 4- to six-year-old children who misarticulated [s]. They found that these children produced [s] in [sV] syllables that were longer and more variable than those of normally articulating children. Variability was measured for individual children's repetitions of the same syllables. Again, these results suggest that the functionally misarticulating child has less phonetic-level control than the normally articulating child. However, the source of this lack of control is not clear. Perhaps a misarticulating child is more variable in production of [s] because weaker connections between the /s/ phoneme and the articulatory features have been established. On the other hand, perhaps the source of the variability comes from an inability to adjust the features associated with a phoneme to become more similar to the features of the phonemes nearby in syllable contexts.

In contrast to their longer productions of [s] in [sV] syllables, Weismer and Elbert (1982) found that misarticulating children produced shorter [s] productions than normally articulating children in [sC] clusters. They attributed this shortening of [s] to an undershooting of the target configuration for [s]. In part, this shortening of [s] in the cluster context may account for the apparent facilitation of [sC] sequences seen in the studies of effects of phonetic context. Rather than facilitating [s] production, the [sC] context may affect the listener's judgment of correctness of production. In other words, the shortened [s] may make it more difficult for the listener to decide that the [s] was misarticulated.

McDonald's (1964a) treatment strategy was to locate a phonetic context in which the target [s] or [r] was correctly articulated and then train its production in a variety of other phonetic contexts. The underlying principle was that the child must learn not only an appropriate sensory-motor target for the sound but also must learn how to get to that target from a variety of preceding sounds and then must be able to move on to a variety of following speech sounds. If this sensory-motor learning were a dominant factor, then progress in speech therapy ought to be related to these phonetic context effects. A group of treatment studies have investigated this issue.

Elbert and McReynolds (1978) trained school-age–misarticulating children to correctly articulate [s] in the syllables [sʌ], [ʌs], and [ʌsʌ]. They then looked for generalization to clustered and unclustered contexts as well as to contexts involving consonants with different places of articulation. There appeared to be little difference across these factors. As children learned to produce [s] in the context of the vowel [ʌ], they generalized its production in a variety of other contexts. They did not first generalize to the consonantal contexts that were identified by Mazza and colleagues (1979) as being facilitory to correct production.

The results of these studies can be described within the parallel-processing model proposed in Chap. 1. In particular, the children in these studies were being taught to produce particular phonemes, either /s/ or /r/. Production alters the connection strengths between these phoneme categories and articulatory features within particular syllable shapes. As the children altered their featural connections to the phoneme taught, the use of the new features spread to other syllable shapes and words that also shared connections to that phoneme. The finding that learning was not completely constrained by syllable shape and phonetic context may have been caused by connections at the word level. A word that has been produced more often than others (e.g., *red* as opposed to *ray*) may have stronger connections with the old pattern involving /w/-like features. This word may not initially be correctly produced while less often used words are changed quickly. This factor may override the effect of phonetic context and syllabic shape that would predict that these two words would be learned at the same time.

Oral-Sensory and Motor Abilities

A number of studies have been conducted to determine if functionally misarticulating children have impaired oral-sensory or oral-motor abilities. All of these have been descriptive studies in which the abilities of misarticulating children are compared to those of nonmisarticulating children.

Dworkin and Culatta (1985) compared oral structures and oral-motor abilities of 24 functionally misarticulating children with nonmisarticulating children. Their measurements included diadochokinetic rate, tongue strength, and a description of oral structures. *Diadochokinetic rate* refers to how quickly a speaker can repeat a syllable (e.g., [bababab]). In this particular study, children were asked to repeat the individual syllables [pʌ], [tʌ], and [kʌ]. Tongue strength was measured by having the child press the tongue tip against a pressure sensor held between the front teeth. Oral structures were assessed for normality of appearance and nonspeech movement patterns. Results of this study showed no significant differences between groups.

In a similar study, McNutt (1977) investigated oral-sensory as well as oral-motor abilities of older misarticulating children between the ages of 12 and 15 years. Each child misarticulated either [s] or [r]. Since this group of children is older, perhaps they were more likely to show physiological problems than the typical misarticulating child seen in kindergarten or first grade. Oral-sensory ability was assessed via two tasks. In the first task, the child was to tell whether parts of the tongue were being touched by one or two points. The distance between the two points was decreased to determine the smallest distance that could be discriminated as representing two points. The second sensory task involved describing plastic shapes such as circles, squares, and stars that were placed in the child's mouth. The motor task used was a diadochokinetic task in which the disyllable [dʌgʌ] was repeated. Results of this study showed that these older misarticulating children did not perform as well as the nonmisarticulating children. Furthermore, a difference in deficit occurred among the children who misarticulated [s] and those who misarticulated [r]. Children who misarticulated [s] performed as well as normals in the sensory tasks but not the motor tasks. Children who misarticulated [r] performed more poorly on both tasks.

Conflicting results such as those cited above may be due to a number of factors, including the sampling of different populations. McNutt's results suggest that not all misarticulating children are alike and that researchers should be searching for subgroups of misarticulating children. In a later study, McNutt and Hamayan (1984) divided misarticulating children into subgroups using a variety of nonarticulation tasks having to do with language ability, auditory perception, and other skills. They measured the articulatory and nonarticulatory abilities of 60 misarticulating children between the ages of 8 and 12 years. They used the nonarticulatory measures to subgroup children. That is, the children in a particular subgroup would show a similar pattern of performance (e.g., high on tests of auditory perception and low on gross motor skills). The children in many of these groups also showed similar patterns of misarticulation. For example, one group of children was found to perform most poorly in language tasks and memory tasks. This same group evidenced a larger number of misarticulation patterns similar to those of younger children than any other group. Their misarticulations included production of velar consonants as alveolars, producing fricatives as stops, producing liquids as glides, and producing clusters as CV syllables. This subgroup of children may typify the children discussed in the third section of this chapter whose misarticulations appear to be related to problems in cognitive categorization of linguistic symbols. A second group of children had the poorest scores in oral-sensory abilities. These children also showed the largest number of fricative errors. This group may typify children who are thought to have oral-sensory motor problems. In all, 12 subgroups were defined. Results of this study should remind us that we should not easily talk about "functionally misarticulating children" as a single group.

Training Syllabic Production

Studies of the sensory-motoric characteristics of functional misarticulation have also looked for syllabic-level effects in rates of misarticulation and in the effects of therapy. Misarticulating children typically misarticulate consonant speech sounds as opposed to vowel sounds. Consonants and consonant clusters act to initiate syllables (e.g., *see, ski,* and *scree*). They also act to close syllables (e.g., *at, act,* and *acts*). Consonants also act to bind two syllables together as in the intervocalic consonants in *writing* and *reading*.

From a motoric viewpoint, articulation therapy has as its first goal the teaching of an appropriate articulatory target for the speech sound. A second goal is teaching the child to use this newly acquired target in a variety of syllabic positions. This approach to articulation therapy is exemplified by the training sequence outlined in Table 3-5.

Syllable-based goals for articulation therapy may be accomplished using both meaningless utterances (e.g., [isi asa usu]) and meaningful utterances

Table 3-5. SYLLABLE-BASED TRAINING GOALS FOR [s] PRODUCTION

1. Correct production of isolated [s]
2. Correct production of [sV] syllables
3. Correct production of [Vs] syllables
4. Correct production of [VsV] syllables
5. Correct production of [sCV] syllables
6. Correct production of [VCs] syllables

(e.g., "He sees me," "You sued him"). It has been suggested that practice in production of nonmeaningful syllabic sequences be used prior to practice in production of meaningful utterances (Winitz, 1975). In essence, the 6-year-old child who produced the word *sun* as [θʌn] has had 3 or 4 years' practice in this production. The connection strengths between the word *sun* and inappropriate phoneme and feature level classifications are very strong. By using nonmeaningful syllables (e.g., [sɪ, sæ, sʌ]), the child can practice manipulation of appropriate features without interference from the already formed word-level patterns.

One question that arises from this viewpoint is whether or not training children to correctly articulate a speech sound in non symbolic syllables will directly affect their production of the speech sound in words. Powell and McReynolds (1969) trained four misarticulating children to correctly produce [s] in isolation, and in the syllables [sa], [as], and [asa]. After these children learned to reliably produce isolated [s], their ability to articulate [s] in a set of untrained words was assessed. Two of the subjects had begun to use correct [s] productions in some of the untrained words. The remaining children did not start to use correct articulation of [s] in words. Thus, training in just the correct articulator positions for this consonant does not appear to cause the child to use correct articulation in a wide variety of words. Training in correct production of the [sV] context resulted in almost equal amounts of generalization to the different syllabic positions in words. That is, no tendency existed for children, having been taught [sV] production to articulate better in similarly shaped words (e.g., *see* and *sigh*) than other syllabic shapes (e.g., *ice*).

Similar results were demonstrated for /r/ training by Hoffman (1983). In the initial stages of this study, misarticulating children were taught to correctly articulate an isolated [ɝ] production. Next, individual subjects were taught production of one syllabic type—either [rV] (e.g., [ri]); [CrV] (e.g., [gra]); [CɝC] (e.g., [tɝt]); or [VCɚ] (e.g., [atɚ]). As was seen during [s] training, training in the isolated production of [ɝ] did not result in extensive generalization of learning to words in which the various forms of /r/ were included. Training in any of the syllabic forms resulted in equivalent amounts of transfer to production of meaningful utterances. Little tendency existed for training of one syllable type to be reflected only in words of particular syllable types.

Results of these studies indicate that learning of the motor pattern associated with isolated production of a particular consonant sound is not sufficient training for the misarticulating child. Training of correct articulation in a syllable or group of syllables does produce some improvement in correct production of words, but the generalization is incomplete. Furthermore, the generalization does not appear to be strictly related to the syllabic shape taught. Thus, syllable motor production factors are not the only, or perhaps not even the major influence in determining treatment outcomes.

Training Phonetic Feature Production

The verbal communication model presented in Chap. 1 included a level of organization for articulatory features. These features describe the vocal tract constriction place and type as well as laryngeal activity involved in production of the speech sound. Descriptive studies have shown that functionally misarticulating children, like normally developing children, tend to make errors in production of particular phonetic features more than others. Training studies have demonstrated that learning to produce a phonetic feature in one phoneme may also result in its use in others. Within our model, this would occur as a particular articulatory gesture incorporated into the feature level and is related to the various phonemes in which it occurs. Restrictions on the spread of this new gesture may be caused by prior connections to other phonemes, connections at the syllable level, and connections for particular words. Learning a particular gesture in a particular phoneme in a particular syllable shape may start the process of altering the child's system but is not likely to cause a complete transformation.

An early indication that phonetic feature production was learned during articulation training was found by Elbert, Shelton, and Arndt (1967). These authors trained children who misarticulated [s] and [r] to produce [s] in syllables and words. After training they found improvement not only in [s] production but also in [z] production. They found no improvement in [r] production ability. They argued that the children had learned to produce an appropriate place of articulation for [s], which they also applied to [z] production.

Compton (1970) was one of the first researchers to study children's misarticulations using articulatory features. He found that a child's misarticulation of a number of phonemes could be described using a smaller number of feature changes. This was due to the fact that features define natural classes of phonemes that are treated similarly in the child's substitutions. For example, Compton found that one of the children he studied produced word-initial /p/ as [b], word-initial /t/ as [d], and word-initial /k/ as [g]. These three errors share a common property. In each approximation, a voiceless stop has been produced as voiced. Compton argued that the child had mislearned the use of the voicing feature for stop consonants. An alternative explanation is that the child had some difficulty in producing a particular gesture, which led to misproduction of all phonemes incorporating that gesture.

Following this line of argument, McReynolds and Huston (1971) analyzed the speech sound substitution errors of 10 children between the ages of 4 and 6 years whose speech contained numerous articulation errors. They did this by looking for consistencies in the use of distinctive features such as +voice and −voice or +continuant and −continuant. They found that the most often misarticulated feature specifications for misarticulating children were fricative manner (continuant, strident). Furthermore, children misused features in one of two ways. A particular feature might not be produced by a child. For example, five of their subjects never produced sounds that were characterized as +strident (i.e., the lingual fricatives s, z, ʃ, ʒ). This error pattern was called *phonetic,* suggesting an inability to produce a particular motor pattern. The second error pattern was called *phonological.* It involved the misuse of a feature specification that was produced in some context. For example, they found that some of their children produced sounds that were +voice and some that were −voice. However, the children's misarticulations included a misproduction of voicing in some speech sounds. This type of error is discussed in more detail in the final section of this chapter entitled "Cognitive-Linguistic Aspects."

The discovery that multiple phoneme misarticulation could be described via a relatively small number of feature errors led Compton (1970) to state the "generalization hypothesis." He argued that if a child were taught to correctly produce the misarticulated features in one phoneme, all other phonemes would be correctly articulated. A child who produced all fricatives as stops would be taught to correctly produce one fricative in the hope that the features learned in this one exemplar would then be used in the other fricatives.

Costello and Onstine (1976) tested this hypothesis with two preschool children who produced fricatives as stops. In general, these children produced /θ/, /s/, and /ʃ/ as [t]; /ð/, /z/, and /ʒ/ as [d]. To teach these children that frication is an important feature of these phonemes, they were simultaneously taught to correctly articulate [s], [θ], and [t]. Of course, these children already correctly articulated [t], but it was used in the program as a contrast to the two fricatives. In essence, Costello and Onstine (1976) chose examples of the children's stopping patterns. They taught the children to correctly articulate these sounds in syllables, words, phrases, sentences, story telling, and conversation. They then measured the children's success in production of the trained sounds and the other fricatives that were also stopped.

Costello and Onstine (1976) reported good improvement in production of [θ] and [s] as seen in a set of syllables, words, and phrases that the children were asked to repeat. Before training, the two children correctly articulated less than 5 percent of these [s] and [θ] items; after training they correctly produced [s] (93% and 97%) and [θ] (80% and 57%) at much higher rates than they had before treatment. More important for assessing the generalization hypothesis, they also improved in production of fricatives that were untrained. The two children correctly produced [ð] (47%, 50%), [z] (95%, 85%), and [ʃ] (90%, 70%). Thus, these authors found support for the generalization hypothesis.

In summary, studies of children's learning during articulation treatment based on repetition activities show that articulatory gestures may be taught in a particular phoneme, and their use will occur in other phonemes. However, learning to produce a feature in a particular phoneme does not necessarily ensure its use in others. Furthermore, practice of production of a phoneme in one syllabic context does not ensure that it will be produced in all words containing that syllable structure.

AUDITORY-PERCEPTUAL ASPECTS

The primary pathway through which children learn the articulation of their language is auditory in nature. Recall from the last chapter that the infant's auditory nervous system appears to be tuned to discriminate the important auditory characteristics representing speech sounds prior to development of speech sound production capabilities. Impairment of this processing capability would have drastic effects on children's ability to learn the phonemic classes, syllabic shapes, and words of the parent language. In this section we present studies of the relationship between articulation, learning, and impairment that have been associated with hearing impairment, impairment of acoustic cue detection and storage, and perceptual phonemic categorization abilities.

HEARING IMPAIRMENT

Hearing impaired children should logically have difficulties learning the relationship between acoustic aspects of the speech signal and the expression of meaning. Children with sensory-neural hearing losses receive an acoustic input that is degraded by frequency distortion and filtering. Often such children do not hear the higher frequencies where much of the information in stop and fricative consonants is contained. Children who suffer from repeated bouts of middle-ear infections must learn to cope with acoustic representations of sounds that change depending on whether their ears are affected or not at any particular time.

One of the earliest studies of hearing impaired children's articulation ability was conducted by Hudgins and Numbers (1942). These investigators recorded the speech of 192 students enrolled in residential schools for the deaf. Speech samples were gathered by asking the students to read 10 sentences. Subjects in this study were categorized by degree of hearing loss: hearing impaired, partially deaf, and profoundly deaf. In general, a correlation existed between the degree of hearing impairment and impairment of articulation. The mean number of articulation errors increased as the children's hearing ability decreased.

Hudgins and Numbers described the children's errors with respect to their place manner and voicing characteristics. The largest group of errors involved the voicing distinction. Voiced consonants such as /b, d, g/ were produced as voiceless (i.e., [p, t, k]. The reverse was also found with voiceless sounds being produced as voiced. Another common misarticulation pattern of the hearing impaired involved misproduction of nasality. Nasal consonants were produced as oral stops, and oral stops were produced as nasals. Consonant clusters were often reduced to single consonants and fricatives produced as stops. These children also produced vowel misarticulations that typically involved use of a neutralized vowel for more extreme point vowels.

Two characteristics of the hearing impaired population's misarticulations appear to be noteworthy. First, misarticulations appear to be related to characteristics of articulation that are not visible. The hearing impaired child can see some differences in the place of articulation of certain consonants (e.g., the labials and dentals). No such visual cue exists for the position of the velum (responsible for nasality differences) or the action of the vocal folds (responsible for voicing differences). Second, misarticulations that occur are reversible in nature. That is, a child may substitute a voiced sound for a voiceless sound in one production and then do the opposite in another production. This bidirectionality of substitutions is not typical of children whose misarticulations are caused by motoric or structural problems. Recall that children who are normally learning articulation and those who have organic involvements typically simplify the phonetic task (e.g., producing fricatives as stops, rather than producing bidirectional errors in which fricatives may be produced for stop consonants).

In support of these general conclusions, Nober (1967) found that hearing impaired children most often correctly articulated visible sounds (i.e., the bilabials, labiodentals, and dentals). The least well articulated consonants were palatal and velar. Another characteristic of a speech sound that affects its production by hearing impaired children is its acoustic frequency. Nober (1967) found that among the most often misarticulated sounds were the fricatives that generally contain higher-frequency acoustic information. Since sensory-neural hearing loss typically affects hearing for the higher frequencies, these sounds are less likely to be heard by hearing impaired children.

SPEECH PERCEPTION ABILITY

Few areas of misarticulation research have sparked as much interest as the ability of misarticulating children to perceive speech sound differences. Following the model of speech perception presented in Chap. 1, we will look at the speech perception abilities of misarticulating children at two levels: the extraction of phonetic cues and phonemic categorization.

Perception of Phonetic Cues

One hypothesis about the origin of children's misarticulations is that these children cannot easily extract the important acoustic phonetic cues that signal the differences between phonemes. Children with such a difficulty would obviously be impaired in the ability to learn about speech sound differences, thus forming inappropriate phonemic classes. They might also be impaired in their ability to separate the acoustic speech stream into words, morphemes, or other higher-level syntactic units. Thus, a low-level acoustic cue perceptual deficit might account not only for misarticulation but also for the development of language problems at higher linguistic levels. Such a theory is appealing because it would also account for the relationship between misarticulation and language deficits to be discussed in the final section of this chapter.

Researchers have tested misarticulating children's abilities to detect acoustic features of speech sounds by using discrimination tasks in which pairs of syllables or words that differ by one phoneme are presented and the child's task is to say whether the pair is "same" or "different." Half of the pairs contain two productions of the same syllable, so there is a 50 percent chance that a particular pair is the same.

Some of the earliest studies of misarticulating children investigated the relationship between ability to discriminate speech sounds and the ability to produce speech sounds. Travis and Rasmus (1931) administered a discrimination test in which a large number of speech sound contrasts were tested in syllable productions. This test was administered to misarticulating children from first through fifth grades. These children performed poorly compared to their nonmisarticulating age mates. Sherman and Geith (1967) reversed the logic of this experiment by choosing groups of children based on their speech sound perception performance. They then compared the articulation performance of these groups and found that the children who discriminated speech sounds better also correctly articulated more often. From these and similar studies, one can conclude that children who make many speech sound production errors are likely to make many speech sound discrimination errors and vice versa.

One explanation for this finding is that children who misarticulate many speech sounds have reduced ability to detect the acoustic cues underlying speech sound categorization. Tallal and Stark (1981) conducted a study that asked which kinds of acoustic cues to speech perception misarticulating children might be misperceiving. They studied the abilities of language impaired children, many who misarticulated as well, to discriminate syllable pairs representing a variety of acoustic cues. Compared to age mates with normal articulation and language abilities, the language impaired children made more errors in discrimination of /ba/-/da/, /da/-/ta/, and /sa/-/ʃa/. The misarticulating children did not make more errors in discrimination of the following syllable pairs: /e/-/æ/, /dab/-/dæb/, and /sa/-/sta/. These results suggest that language impaired children have some difficulty in processing the acoustic cues that are rapidly changing (i.e., those that occur in the consonant transitions of stops such as /ba/, /da/, and /ta/. They also may show some difficulty in discrimination of frequency components of fricative consonants as in the /sa/-/ʃa/ contrast. These children showed normal abilities for discrimination of vowel contrasts /e/-/æ/ and /dab/-/dæb/, which are represented by relatively stable formant patterns for a relatively long period of time.

In another study, these authors analyzed the articulation errors of the language impaired children and found that the acoustic characteristics that were more likely to be misperceived were the same characteristics that were likely to be misproduced (Stark & Tallal, 1978). In particular, they found that language impaired children showed less precise control of voice onset time production in the transitions of stop consonants than did their normally developing age mates. The language impaired children with less ability to perceive acoustic cues showed more errors in their consonant productions.

Phonemic Categorization

An alternative explanation for the finding of a relationship between number of misarticulations and number of misperceptions is that children misperceive those sounds that they misproduce. As one type of error includes more phoneme contrasts, so will the other. Monnin and Huntington (1974) provided evidence that misarticulation and misperception are tied to one another. They selected groups of children: kindergarten children who correctly produce [r], kindergarten children who produce [r] as [w], and preschool children who produce [r] as [w]. The first and third groups were chosen to represent normal development; the second group was thought to be disordered inasmuch as most children correctly articulate [r] by this age. These children were tested in ability to identify phonemes in word pairs (e.g., the words *tub* and *cub* were presented in randomized order, and the child was asked to point to one of two pictures representing these words). A variety of phonemes was contrasted in this manner. It was found that the children classified as disordered made more errors than the other children in identification of /r/ and /w/. They did not differ in their ability to identify other phonemes. Thus, their misperception appears to be directly related to their phonemic classification of /r/ and /w/ as a single phoneme. The preschool children, many of whom misarticulated /r/ as [w], also performed better than the misarticulating children. This suggests that their classification of the phonemes /r/ and /w/ was better than those of the disordered group.

To probe this possible difference in more detail, Hoffman, Daniloff, Bengoa, and Schuckers (1984) tested misarticulating first-grade children's abilities to identify and discriminate synthetic stimuli representing the difference between /r/ and /w/. The synthetic stimuli varied the onset frequencies of the first three formants. The normally articulating children identified nearly all of the first two stimuli as /w/. Almost all of the last three stimuli were judged to be /r/. By contrast, the misarticulating children did not identify these stimuli as well. Although all of the normally articulating children consistently heard some of the stimuli as /w/ and others as /r/, most of the misarticulating children were unable to reliably identify two phonemes in this acoustic continuum. That is, an individual child may identify some of the stimuli as /w/ and none as /r/, or some as /r/ but none as /w/. Many of the misarticulating children appeared to be guessing throughout the task.

The ability of these two groups of children to discriminate pairs of stimuli showed that both groups behaved in a categorical fashion. That is, if a child identified one stimulus as /w/ and another as /r/, he or she would be able to say that the two were "different" when presented together in a discrimination task. Thus the misarticulating children did not perform this task as well as the normal subjects, apparently because their phonemic categorization was not as good.

Broen, Strange, Doyle, and Heller (1983) found somewhat different results for a group of younger children, ages 3 to 4 years. The children who were judged by standard articulation tests to be normal could reliably identify contrasts among /w/, /r/, and /l/, regardless of how they articulated the /r/ and /l/. For these children, ability to perform perceptual tasks preceded ability to produce the speech sounds. Some but not all of the misarticulating children made perceptual errors. Perceptual errors were usually related to speech sounds that were misproduced.

Locke (1980) has gone further in specifying a relationship between misarticulation and misperception by suggesting that misarticulating children may misperceive an error in phonemic contrast only in certain contexts. To test this hypothesis, he designed a special perceptual task. In this task, a child would misarticulate a word (e.g., *lake* produced as [wek]). The examiner would question the child about the label of a picture of a *lake* by saying, "Is this a [lek]?" (the correct form), "Is this a [wek]?" (the child's error form), and "Is this a [jek]?" (an incorrect form that is similar to the other two). Testing of a large number of misarticulating children between the ages of 3 and 6 years indicated that approximately 30 percent of the contrasts misproduced were misperceived. Most of the contrasts that were misperceived involved voiceless fricatives.

The phonemic identification abilities of misarticulating children may be related to the types of misarticulations used. Smit and Bernthal (1983) compared the abilities of normally articulating children with children who substituted target phonemes or deleted phonemes in their productions. Both of these groups were comparable in their ability to identify phonemes perceptually in two tasks: identifying word-final consonant voicing (e.g., *cup-cub* and *beet-beed*) and identifying initial-consonant clusters (e.g., *steer, tear, deer*). Both groups performed as well as normally articulating children in perception of final-consonant voicing, and both performed below normal levels in identification of the consonant clusters. These misarticulating children also demonstrated misarticulation of the voicing characteristic of the initial consonants of these words, so the direct linkage between perceptual categorization and productive differentiation appears to have held true.

Training Speech Perception

It has long been logically argued that misarticulating children should be trained to perceptually discriminate and categorize their error sounds from others. Van Riper (1939) argued that "ear training" should precede production training so that the misarticulating children will learn the characteristics of the sound they are going to learn. When children can easily identify the characteristics of their error sound and their production of that sound, they will be able to use this ability to monitor correctness of their productions. Winitz (1975) has argued that auditory discrimination training should make articulation training faster, more efficient, and better retained. Unfortunately, not much data exist detailing the effectiveness of this auditory-perceptual training.

Williams and McReynolds (1975) taught an artificial phonemic contrast to four children. The contrast taught involved speech sounds that were misarticulated by the children (e.g., [k, t]) in syllables that were used as labels for nonsense drawings. A particular child was taught two contrasts. One contrast was taught perceptually and the other was taught productively. When a child was taught to perceptually discriminate two drawings using two labels, he learned to perceive the difference but not to produce it. When a child learned to produce contrasting labels, he also learned to perceive the auditory differences. Thus, production practice appears to provide the child with strengthening relationships between words, phonemes, and both auditory and gestural features. Perceptual practice does not appear to enhance the use of appropriate gestures in representing a word or phoneme. However, systematic investigation has not been conducted to test the short- or long-term effectiveness of including aspects of auditory-perceptual categorization training in articulation treatment.

COGNITIVE-LINGUISTIC ASPECTS

The cognitive-linguistic characteristics of misarticulation can be described in a number of ways. In this section we will first look at the relationship between general intelligence and articulatory ability. This is followed by a discussion of the relationship between language ability and articulatory ability, and finally, the theoretical view that misarticulation is a manifestation of a language problem occurring in the organization of syllables, phonemes, and features.

GENERAL INTELLIGENCE

When the study of articulation disorders began in earnest in the 1930s, one of the first factors investigated was the relationship between articulation ability and measures of intelligence. Winitz (1969) reviewed studies in which the children serving as subjects had IQ scores in the normal range. In these studies, researchers looked for a correlation between IQ scores and articulation test scores. Winitz' (1969) review of studies that correlated articulation scores and IQ scores showed only small correlations between these two variables, ranging from 0.05 to 0.48. Thus, there appears to be little relationship between general intelligence and articulation ability *when normal children are studied. This is an important point.* These studies all involved children whose IQ scores placed them in the normal range. When children with lower-than-normal IQs are studied, a relationship between these two variables emerges. In particular, children with lower-than-normal IQs show a higher percentage of articulation errors, that is, more of these children have articulation problems than seen in the normal population.

Bangs (1942) described the articulation errors of mentally retarded children. Many of the errors produced by these children were similar to those of younger, normally developing children. These errors were described in Chap. 2 as resulting from the application of phonological processes. The most common misarticulations were approximations of [w] for /r/, [f] and [t] for /θ/, and [d] for /ð/. Bangs (1942) noted that omission of consonants was a characteristic that might distinguish errors of the mentally retarded from those of normally developing children.

Dodd (1976b) compared the articulation errors of a group of mentally retarded children and normal children who were matched for mental age. The average chronological and mental ages of the normal children was 3.6. The mental age of the retarded subjects was also 3.6, but their average chronological age was 10.7. Dodd found that the retarded children did not differ in the number or types of errors produced. Thus, she concluded that articulation errors of the mentally retarded are similar to articulation errors made by normal children whose chronological age matches the mental age of the mentally retarded subjects.

In summary, it appears that articulation ability is only related to general intelligence for those at the lower end of the intelligence range. For these individuals, the articulation errors are similar to those made by younger children. Error approximations appear to be appropriate for the individual's mental age.

LANGUAGE ABILITY

Inasmuch as cognitive abilities measured in IQ tests depend on language coding, a strong relationship exists between IQ and language abilities. Thus, it is not surprising to find that articulation ability would be related to language ability. Furthermore, since articulation ability is directed by a portion of the cognitive linguistic system (i.e., the feature, phoneme, syllable, and word levels), disordered articulation may result from disordered organization of the units and relationships within these levels. The following sections describe relationships between children's misarticulation and organization of the language system.

Misarticulation Related to Language Impairment

One way of looking at the relationship between articulatory performance and other levels of language performance is to see if misarticulating children also show deficits in language processing. Paul and Shriberg (1982) studied the use of grammatical morphemes by a group of children who demonstrated impaired articulation ability. They found four subgroups of misarticulating children, which they labelled pattern I, II, III, and IV.

Pattern I children showed a general impairment in use of grammatical morphemes and an even greater deficit for morphemes that were expressed with a phonologically complex production. An example of a phonologically complex morpheme is the plural marker [s], which forms a word-final consonant cluster in the word *cats*. Thirty percent of their misarticulating children showed this pattern. For this group of children, impaired morphological ability is reduced by impaired articulatory ability. Twenty percent of their subjects fell into pattern II. In this pattern, the children showed age-appropriate use of all grammatical morphemes except those that are realized in a phonologically complex production. For these children, an articulation problem may be the root cause of their morphological errors. Pattern III children showed generally poor syntactic ability that was not made worse in phonologically complex utterances. Thirty-six percent of the children fell into this category. The remaining 14 percent showed no syntactic problems in spite of their faulty articulatory performance.

Himmelwright-Gross, St. Louis, Ruscello, and Hull (1985) suggested that two groups of misarticulating school-age children exist: those with multiple phoneme errors and those with residual errors. Children in the residual-error group typically misarticulate one or two of the commonly misarticulated /r/, /l/, and /s/ phonemes. The multiple phoneme–misarticulating children produce numerous articulation errors that can be described via such devices as phonological process rules. Their assessment of language performance indicated that the multiple-phoneme error group produced more syntactic errors than did a group of normal children. The residual error group did not differ in syntactic performance from the normal children. Articulation errors of the multiple-phoneme–misarticulating group also contained more omissions of speech sounds than in the residual group.

Smit and Bernthal (1983) found similar subgroups of misarticulating children. They divided a group of 5-year-old misarticulating children into two groups: syllable reducers and substituters. The syllable reducers were children who deleted consonants either at the ends of words or in clusters. The substituters maintained the shape of syllables in their productions but used some of the substitution processes such as stopping or gliding to alter articulations. They found differences in the expressive syntactic abilities of these children in comparison to a group of language-normal children. The syllable-reducing children scored worse in expressive syntax measures than did the other two groups. The children whose misarticulations consisted of substitutions were more like a normal control group than were the children who deleted segments.

Articulation Interacting with Processing at Other Levels

Shriner, Holloway, and Daniloff (1969) compared the syntactic performance of a group of school-age children described as having "severe" articulation problems with their normally articulating age mates. They found that the misarticulating children's spontaneous speech was comprised of syntactically simpler sentences than the normal children's. Production of shorter, less complex sentences may be a strategy used by the misarticulating children to maximize their intelligibility. Shorter sentences will leave the most important noun and verb components. To avoid this effect in measuring syntactic abilities of misarticulating children, Panagos, Quine, and Klich (1978) asked children to repeat sentences. The sentences were systematically increased in syntactic complexity from noun phrase ("the boy") to active declarative ("The boy thanked the man") to passive declarative ("The book was read by the boy"). The children produced more articulation errors as the utterances increased in syntactic complexity.

Panagos and colleagues (1978) concluded that children have a finite amount of cognitive-processing ability. When more of that ability is devoted to processing syntactic complexity, less remains for articulatory processing, and more articulatory errors are made. To provide further support for this theory, Panagos and Prelock (1982) measured the syntactic errors that resulted as phonological complexity was increased. Sentences were constructed to be either phonologically simple or phonologically complex. The phonologically complex sentences contained more multisyllabic words and more consonant clusters than the phonologically simple sentences. For example, "The kid pushed the car in the room" was considered to be phonologically simple, whereas "The customer smeared the chocolate in the napkin" was considered to be complex. The language impaired children who repeated these sentences made more syntactic errors in recall of the complex than simple sentences; thus, the authors concluded that the relationship between phonological and syntactic processing is reciprocal (i.e., increases in complexity of one can cause errors in processing the other).

Syntactic processing is not the only language level that interacts with articulation ability. Leonard, Schwartz, Chapman, Rowan, Prelock, Terrell, Weiss, and Messick (1982) exposed language impaired children to a novel set of words and measured the children's learning of those words. The language impaired children ranged in age from 2.5 to 4.0 years of age, yet they were still functioning at a single-word utterance level. Like normal children who are in this phase of learning the first 50 words, these children were better at learning object words than action words. They also learned more words that conformed to already established syllable shape and phoneme connections within the child's system.

Articulation ability also interacts with processing of pragmatic demands. Campbell and Shriberg (1982) described misarticulating children's articulation errors as a function of pragmatic context. Pragmatic context was defined with reference to discussion topic and comments. Essentially, the *discussion topic* is the common thread that holds together a portion of a conversation. For example, you might introduce a discussion topic by saying, "Hey, did you go to the ball game Saturday?" Later references to the game in the conversation will be repetitions of the topic. The other portions of the conversation will be comments about this topic. For example, a reply to the above question might be "Yeah, we really played well." Since the topic is understood by both the speakers, it is not as important to the conversation as the new information added by each comment. Campbell and Shriberg (1982) found that misarticulating children apparently understand this distinction. They produced fewer misarticulations in production of the comments than the topics.

In summary, children's articulatory ability is related to their linguistic ability. Syntactic, semantic, and pragmatic demands affect articulatory ability. Children who misarticulate a large number of phonemes are also likely to suffer from language problems as well.

Knowledge of this relationship has a number of clinical implications. The diagnostician is alerted to the possibility that young children referred for misproduction of speech sounds may have pervasive language problems as well. This is particularly true for children who delete consonants and syllables in their speech productions.

Training for articulation skills should be included in treatment strategies that improve the child's overall language ability when necessary. Training of articulation skills should be integrated as rapidly as possible into pragmatically useful utterances so that they will become part of the overall communication network.

Misarticulation as Disordered Conceptual Organization

Younger children who misarticulate many phonemes do so in patterned ways. The regularities in children's misarticulations can be described with respect to the communication model at the following levels: syllabic, phonemic, and featural. Clinical intervention for such misarticulations has taken these patterns into account in structuring remediation approaches.

Syllabic Level Organization. As discussed above, misarticulating children have been subdivided according to whether or not they "reduce syllables." Children who do not approximate complete shapes of syllables are more likely to present disordered language at other levels. Two studies have confirmed this relationship by describing the misarticulations of children whose speech is described as being "unintelligible."

Hodson and Paden (1981) tested the articulation abilities of 4-year-old children whose speech was described as unintelligible because of multiple phoneme misarticulations. They compared the test results from this group of children with 60 other 4-year olds whose speech was regarded as normal. The single-word responses of these children were analyzed for the occurrence of a variety of error patterns common in the speech of younger normally articulating children. These investigators found that over 50 percent of the disordered group produced errors in which syllable-final consonants were not produced, unstressed syllables were not produced, and consonant clusters were produced as single consonants. Fewer than 10 percent of the normally articulating children produced similar errors.

In a similar study, McReynolds and Elbert (1981a) studied the spontaneous speech articulation abilities of misarticulating children between the ages of 3.7 and 13.0 years. They also found that over 50 percent of these children produced these three errors of syllabic shape. This list of error types might be an exaggeration of misarticulating children's use of these patterns if each were found only occasionally in the speech of an individual child who was counted as producing the error. To account for this possibility, McReynolds and Elbert applied the following criteria. First, an error pattern must have had an opportunity to occur in at least four utterances. For example, if a child never attempted a multisyllabic word, he or she would not have an opportunity to delete unstressed syllables. Second, the error patterns counted must occur in at least 20 percent of possible occurrences. For example if a child produced 10 words with final consonants, the final consonant must have been deleted in at least two of these before he or she would be described as using an error pattern of approximating CVC syllables as CV syllables. Given these minimal criteria, a drastic reduction occurred in the number of misarticulating children who appeared to use many of the error patterns. In fact only one error pattern was still attributed to at least half of the children: deletion of final consonants.

Having found that misarticulating children tend to organize complex syllables (i.e., syllables with final consonants and consonant clusters) as simple CV syllables, researchers have sought to teach children to expand their syllable structures.

Weiner (1981) taught two misarticulating children to use final consonants in words. His teaching strategy was to demonstrate to these children that their misarticulations were causing their word productions to be misunderstood. To show the importance of producing final consonants, four pairs of words were chosen. One word of each pair was a CV word (e.g., *bee, pie, no, tea*). The other word of each pair contained these CV sequences but included a final consonant (e.g., *bead, pipe, nose, teeth*). The clinician would display five pictures of each member of a pair (e.g., five pictures of bows and five pictures of boats). The children were instructed to name pictures that the clinician would then remove. The object of the game was to get the clinician to remove all of the pictures. To get the clinician to pick up the picture of the boat, the children were required to mark the existence of a final consonant. Any final consonant was accepted: It did not have to be /t/ in the case of *boat*.

Having taught the children to distinguish this particular set of minimal pairs, the major question was whether or not the children would generalize the use of CVC-syllable structure to other words that had not been taught. This was assessed by asking the children to name pictures using words that contained final consonants. Both children showed an increase in the percentage of production of CVC syllables in these untaught words. Thus, it can be argued that teaching children to produce a small set of words with a particular syllable structure pattern will improve production of other words with similar syllable patterns.

Weiner's (1981) experimental results showed that children could learn to mark the existence of word-final consonants, but they would not automatically learn the production of the correct final consonants for nontaught words. The children in Weiner's study did tend to learn correct production of the final consonants in the words that were trained, but not necessarily in the words to which they generalized production of final consonants. This is probably due to the practice in strengthening connnections between the words taught, their syllable structures, and the phonemes involved.

Dinnsen and Elbert (1984) reported a study in which four children who deleted final consonants were taught production of final consonants in syllables and then tested for generalization to production of words. These children were first taught either production of syllable-final stop consonants or word-final fricative consonants. Generalization was measured to production of word-final stop and fricative consonants. It was found that generalization was limited to the natural class of phonemes trained. That is, if children were taught to produce syllable-final stop consonants, they may show generalization to word-final stops, but they would not show generalization to word-final fricatives. Similarly, if children were taught syllable-final fricatives, they may generalize to word-final fricatives but not to word-final stops.

A similar result has been seen in training of cluster reduction. McReynolds and Elbert (1981b) taught four children who reduced consonant clusters to produce either [s] + stop clusters or stop + liquid clusters. Training and generalization probe items in this study were limited to meaningless syllables. In general it was found that these children generalized only to the class of clusters that had been trained. Children who received training on a liquid cluster would generalize to other liquid clusters but not to [s] clusters. Children taught to produce [s] clusters did not generalize to liquid clusters.

The children in the studies cited above did not correctly articulate the [s] or liquid segments that made up the clusters being reduced prior to training. Powell and Elbert (1984) studied generalization across cluster types when the children were able to produce the [s] or liquid segments when they occurred as singletons. Their results showed that children who learned to produce fricative + liquid clusters or stop + liquid clusters did show generalization to the other type of cluster. Thus, training at the syllabic-shape level involves interactions with the phonemic level as well.

Results of these various training studies show the importance of the syllabic level of organization. However, they also show the importance of the interrelatedness of this syllabic level to the phonemic, feature, and word levels. We probably cannot expect to show a child how to produce a particular syllable shape without considering the words that include those shapes and the phoneme and feature units that are being taught as well.

Phonemic Level Organization. Misarticulating children have been shown to manipulate phonemic levels that do not contain the full set of English phonemes. This results in what appears to be a variety of speech sound errors when the children's productions are compared to those of adults.

Camarata and Gandour (1984) analyzed the initial-consonant productions of a 3-year-old misarticulating child. A variety of these productions are shown in Table 3-6.

Assuming that these productions are typical of this child's speech, his productions can be described fairly well by saying which consonant and vowel sounds the child produces and which are used phonemically to distinguish words. This child produces voiced stops [b], [d], and [g]. By looking for minimal pairs, it can be shown that /b/ and /d/ contrast phonemically

Table 3-6. WORD FORMS SPOKEN BY A THREE-YEAR-OLD CHILD FROM CAMARATA AND GANDOUR (1984)

bee	[bi]	tea	[di]	kite	[gæ]
bath	[bæ]	key	[di]	tie	[gæ]
bus	[bʌ]	kick	[di]	clown	[gæn]
boot	[bu]	two	[du]	train	[gæn]
book	[bu]	cook	[du]	cup	[gʌ]
boat	[bo]			duck	[gʌ]
ball	[ba]			goat	[go]
pan	[bæn]			toe	[go]
				car	[ga]
				dog	[ga]

in this child's system (e.g., *bee* [bi] versus *tea* [di]). However, [d] and [g] never contrast in a minimal pair. Instead, these consonants occur in different contexts: [d] appears before high vowels, and [g] appears before low or mid vowels.

The child studied by Camarata and Gandour had developed a very restricted set of phonemic classes that might have resulted from stopping normal development at a very early stage. Other children show disordered phonemic organization that is not typical of early development. Weiner (1981) described a 4-year-old child who used [θ] and [ð] in production of words whose adult forms contained a variety of fricatives, affricates, and liquids; and a 5-year-old who used [l] in production of words whose adult forms contained stops. In both of these cases, the sounds produced by the child, and presumably the phonemic classes underlying them, were out of developmental order with relatively late-appearing sounds being used rather than relatively early appearing sounds.

The phonemic level interacts with the syllable structure level as seen in the results of a treatment study by Powell and Elbert (1984). They trained a group of six cluster-reducing children to produce either stop + liquid clusters (e.g., /bl tr gr/) or fricative + liquid clusters (e.g., /fr sl sr/). Training in one class of clusters did result in improvement in articulation of the other class. This is contrary to the evidence found by McReynolds and Elbert (1981b) who saw little generalization across cluster types. The primary difference between these two studies was that the children in Powell and Elbert's study were able to correctly articulate the fricatives, stops, and liquids involved in the clusters prior to training. That is, the individual speech sounds in the clusters were present in the children's phonetic and phonemic inventories prior to training in cluster production. The children in the previous study, in which generalization did not occur across cluster types, did not correctly articulate all of the speech sounds as singletons prior to cluster training.

Feature Level Organization. As seen in the sensory-motor section, misarticulating children may not develop the use of a particular gesture that limits the sounds used phonemically. Hodson and Paden (1981) found that over half of the misarticulating 4-year olds studied produced such errors. Errors included the following: stopping (i.e., production of stop manner rather fricative manner); gliding (i.e., production of a glide rather than a liquid); fronting (i.e., production of velars as alveolars); and backing (i.e., production of alveolars as velars). Furthermore, when children are taught to produce these gestures within particular speech sounds, some spread of the use of those features to other phonemes occurs, but this spread is not complete.

Another variety of error patterns shows that misarticulating children are organizing features within phonemes, syllables, and words. These errors are often called *assimilations* because features that are associated with one phoneme are produced during the positional slot associated with another phoneme. Hodson and Paden's study of misarticulating 4-year olds revealed that over half of the children made such errors. Examples of such errors include assimilations of place of articulation (e.g., *dog* produced as [gog] [the velar feature of /g/ appears in the time slot associated with /d/] or [dod] [the alveolar feature of /d/ appears in the positional slot associated with /g/]. These children also produced prevocalic voicing in which a voiceless consonant appears to be affected by the voicing of the vowel that follows it (e.g., *pat* produced as [bæt]).

Studies of the acoustic characteristics of misarticulating children's syllabic shape errors also show organization of features. Weismer, Dinnsen, and Elbert (1981) analyzed the vowel lengths produced by misarticulating children in approximations of CVC words that contained only a CV syllabic shape. In adult speech, the length of the vowel in CVC syllables varies with the voicing of the final consonant: It is longer preceding a voiced consonant and shorter preceding a voiceless consonant. These children were heard to "delete final consonants" (i.e., transcriptions of the words *beat* and *bead* were likely to both be [bi]). However, these children were producing the appropriate vowel durations associated with the missing final consonant. That is, the vowels produced in the [bi] meaning *bead* were longer than the vowels in the [bi] meaning *beat*. It appears that these children were approximating the features of the final consonant without yet producing enough of those features to trigger the perception of a final consonant in the adult listener.

Similar organization of features can be seen in misarticulating children's productions of consonant clusters. Assimilations of the features of both adult phonemes into a single phoneme have been reported in the normally developing child (Greenlee, 1973). For example, a production of the word *swing* as [fi] apparently combines the fricative manner and voicelessness of [s] with the labial place of [w]. Similar error patterns have been shown in the cluster reductions of misarticulating children as well (Hoffman & Damico, 1988).

We have expressed the view that verbal communication depends on a synergystic cognitive system that includes levels of cognition and language knowledge. The fundamental entities of this system are perceptible, gestural features that are related to visual, auditory, and kinesthetic sensations. All higher cognitive levels represent more elaborate organizations of these sensations for use in the perception and production of speech. These perceptions are organized into phonemic, syllabic, and word units.

The misarticulating child is also organizing language concepts with respect to these sensations. However, the quality and quantity of organization that have occurred have not yet become adultlike or they significantly trail the development that has typically been achieved by a particular age. The misarticulating child's organization may have been arrested or slowed by faulty feature-sensing systems—either auditory or motoric. On the other hand, organizational shortcomings may be caused by impoverished environmental inputs in the form of models of speech organization or the need to socially interact using speech and language.

The ultimate answer to the question "Why do children misarticulate?" may never be known. Some of us have become intrigued with the chase, even if the fox is never found. Some of you may one day be similarly moved and you are welcome. Others of you will be satisfied to know that the problem can be described and remediated. These are the topics of the concluding chapters.

SUGGESTED CLASSROOM ACTIVITIES

1. Make recordings of a variety of patients within your department's clinic as they tell stories about the pictures in the Appendix. Choose patients who (1) are preschool age with many misarticulations, (2) are school age with one or two misarticulations, (3) are hearing impaired, and (4) demonstrate a known physiological problem related to speech production. Analyze their productions for the error patterns described by Ingram's phonological processes (listed in Chap. 2). Describe the complexity of their propositions using the categories of descriptions, interpretations, and inferences (described in Chap. 1). Compare their performance in these tasks to the normally developing children you recorded for the last chapter.

2. Assess the speech sound discrimination abilities of a school-age child who misarticulates one or two phonemes. Contrast his error sound with his usual production in word pairs, e.g., *ring* and *wing*. Draw pictures of these two words and ask him to point to the appropriate picture when you name them one at a time. Ask him to point to one of the pictures five times and the other five times. Then test his judgment of his own productions of these words. Have him name pictures whose labels use the error sound, e.g, /r/ in *ring*. Then ask one of the following types of question for each production: "Did you say [rɪŋ]? (use the correct form of the word), or "Did you say [wɪŋ]?" (use the child's error production of the word), or "Did you say [lɪŋ]?" (use an error form that is different from that produced by the child).

CHAPTER 4

Assessment of Children's Phonetic Ability

Topics in this chapter include

- Gathering Data
  - Background Information
  - Assessing Children's Articulation
- Asking Clinical Questions
  - Is This Child's Articulatory Ability Normal?
  - How Does This Child's Articulation Differ From Normal?
  - Does This Child Have the Necessary Structural and Physiologic Movement Patterns?
- Reporting Results

Each time a speech-language pathologist assesses a child's articulatory skills, he or she conducts an empirical study like the research projects discussed in the last chapter. Table 4-1 portrays the parallels between these two endeavors.

Both researcher and clinician first review what is already known about their topics. For the researcher, this involves reading research reports related to a specific area of knowledge. Researchers interested in children's development of speech perception review what is known about this area by reading studies like those cited in Chap. 2 and would summarize this literature search in the beginning of their articles. For example, Hillenbrand (1983) reviewed the studies demonstrating that infants are able to discriminate the acoustic cues to stop consonant place of articulation and also studies of the distinction between oral and nasal stop consonants as an introduction to his experimental questions. Clinicians read information available on particular children and will often have referrals regarding their problems. At many clinics, the patient referred for evaluation, or the patient's parents, will fill out a case history information form prior to being seen. These forms provide a wealth of information to the clinician attempting to synthesize the factors important to an explanation for the communication problem.

Having read research literature, an investigator will ask questions that are intended to extend the scientific community's knowledge of the topic area in some specific way (Silverman, 1977). Hillenbrand's (1983) review of literature led him to ask if infants categorize speech sounds into natural classes of stops and nasals using the acoustic cue differences they had been shown to discriminate. An answer to this question fills in a piece of the puzzle concerning infants' speech perception abilities and the manner in which these develop. Prior to meeting a child who is referred for speech-language problems, the clinician asks questions about the child that are

Table 4-1. STEPS IN THE PROCESS OF ARTICULATORY ASSESSMENT COMPARED TO CONDUCT OF A RESEARCH STUDY

Researcher	*Clinician*
Reads previous studies in a topic area	Reads intake information about client
Formulates research questions	Formulates clinical questions
Designs an experiment	Chooses tests and procedures
Runs experiment	Gives tests and procedures
Analyzes data with respect to particular questions	Analyzes data with respect to particular questions
Reports findings	Reports findings

based on the clinician's knowledge of normal and disordered articulation and their interactions with other levels of processing within the child's verbal communication system.

With respect to articulatory ability, the clinician wants to answer three basic questions. The first asks whether a child exhibits normally developing speech sound production. If the answer to the first question is "no," the clinician will then want to describe the child's articulatory performance. Thus, the second question is "How does this child misarticulate?" The third and final question is whether other related factors of communication processes or the physiological mechanism underlying speech production and development contribute to the problem. As seen in Chap. 3, a number of factors are related to children's misarticulation. A child's disordered articulation may be related to hearing loss (Nober, 1967), deficits in speech perception (Broen, Strange, Doyle, & Heller, 1983) or deficits in orofacial structure or muscular coordination (Dworkin & Culatta, 1985). Children who misarticulate many phonemes are likely to have disordered language processing as well (Himmelwright-Gross et al. 1985). The clinician will want to question the child's abilities in each of these areas so that his or her communicative needs can be fully addressed in the most efficient manner through treatment.

The researcher and clinician gather data using appropriate observational techniques for each question. Observable behaviors constitute evidence for description of a child's cognitive or physiological abilities.

Hillenbrand (1983) trained infants to turn toward an animated toy by activating the toy (an interesting event) as a reward for correct perceptions of the distinction between oral and nasal stops. A series of syllables was presented in which oral stops were followed by nasal stops or vice versa, e.g., [ba]..[da]..[ga]..[ma]..[na]..[ŋa]. The correct response in this series was to turn toward the toy when the first nasal consonant, [m], was heard. The head turn was an observable behavior that could be tallied as evidence regarding the child's speech discrimination abilities. Similarly, it is impossible to directly view a child's phonemic organization or understanding of syllable structure. The clinician seeking to describe a child's articulatory ability must elicit behaviors useful as inferential evidence regarding cognitive organization and physiologic abilities. As will be seen, a variety of speech sound elicitation procedures have been used for this purpose, including picture naming, speech imitation, reading, and storytelling.

Having designed an experiment to answer specific questions, the researcher conducts the experiment by observing subjects under controlled conditions. The observer scores the child's responses. For example, Hillenbrand's observers simply noted whether or not an infant looked toward the toy during the presentation of the fourth syllable in the series. The clinician elicits articulatory responses from a child using chosen test materials and then scales these responses with respect to some coding scheme that is intended to represent the child's behavior. An often overlooked, but always crucial, aspect of articulation assessment is the clinician's role as response scorer. The child's speech act is fleeting in time. It is observed by the clinician who records on paper his or her impression of the child's sound production. These impressions constitute the data for making decisions about the child's speech development.

Next, experimenters and clinicians organize their observations with respect to the questions asked. Both make assertions about their topic that must be supported by empirical data. The researcher reports an analysis of data in the results section of a research report that clearly shows the relationship between the research questions and the data used to answer each. Hillenbrand (1983) found that infants' learning was faster when the sound classes compared were similar in phonetic features (e.g., nasals versus orals) than when two random assortments of nasal and oral stops were compared. The clinician reports findings to clinical questions in diagnostic reports and treatment summaries. If a clinician concludes that a child's articulation is abnormal, the statement is accompanied by data derived from observations of the child. These typically include summary statements of the results from the test procedures that were chosen.

The remainder of this chapter discusses the process of articulatory assessment within this framework. The first section discusses commonly used procedures for gathering data, including background information used to formulate questions and articulatory assessment procedures. The second section discusses the questions that are typically asked regarding misarticulating children and the types of procedures used to provide data for each. The procedures and analyses are derived from two major viewpoints of children's misarticulations (i.e., (1) they represent a phonetic production problem and (2) they represent a cognitive organization problem). These processes are described with respect to two children who are typical of the populations these two differing views of misarticulation were developed to describe. The first child is a 7-year old with few misarticulations; the second is a 4-year old with many misarticulations.

GATHERING DATA

Data gathering for diagnosis of children's misarticulations presents distinct activities: gathering background information and interaction with the child. The gathering of background information may occur as the clinician is preparing to see the child and may then be used to guide direct observations that the clinician will make. Direct observation of the child's behaviors occurs in an interaction between clinician and child that has been orchestrated by the clinician to provide appropriate data.

BACKGROUND INFORMATION

The speech-language pathologist uses two basic sources of background information to decide what form of articulatory assessment is likely to be necessary for an individual child or patient: the referral and case history information. This information is used to guide the asking of appropriate questions.

Referral

Referrals come from a variety of persons who have differing kinds and depths of knowledge about speech and language disorders (e.g., parents, pediatricians, teachers, audiologists, and other speech-language pathologists). Referrer's knowledge of normal and disordered communication development often dictates how specific their request for diagnostic information will be.

Children are often referred to the speech-language pathologist by their parents. Parents often ask whether their child's communication skills are age-appropriate. They worry whether or not their child may require treatment. Most parents will not easily distinguish between speech and language production. The descriptions of a problem received in a referral are likely to be general in nature (e.g., "J. is hard to understand").

If the referral is for a first or an only child, the parents may not know much about normal speech and language development. In such cases, the speech-language pathologist assesses the child's speech and language abilities. If the child's development does not appear to be progressing normally, the clinician will seek to determine an appropriate course of action. If the child appears to be progressing normally, the clinician's role becomes that of counselor. Basically the clinician will seek to convince the parents that their child's misarticulations are not of concern at that time; to aid in that process, follow-up screening or diagnostic rechecks for the child may be scheduled.

An experienced teacher or pediatrician will have seen a number of children and may have a good feel for what normal communication skills are like. If the referral comes directly from one of these, the speech-language pathologist must determine if the child's speech is disordered and may have to convince the parents that something needs to be done.

Sometimes referrals from other professionals are made for specific reasons. The pediatrician may have detected an organic problem that is usually related to impaired speech development. The pediatrician or audiologist may refer a child because of impaired hearing ability, either permanent or fluctuating. This information will be used by the clinician to help structure the specific questions to be asked. The clinician might suspect that a child's hearing impairment has led to a lack of phonemic distinctions among speech sounds with high-frequency acoustic representations. A referral for a child with a repaired cleft or cerebral palsy will lead the clinician to ask questions related to the child's ability to produce various motor gestures crucial to speech production.

Case History

Speech-language pathologists often use a case history information form to gather information prior to seeing a child. Such forms offer a time-efficient way of gathering a large amount of information. However, the answers are only as good as the parents' understanding of the questions. These forms typically ask questions related to the child's health and physiological development. Such questions seek information about possible organic problems that could affect speech and language development. The questions also seek information regarding a child's environment that might affect speech and language development. Areas of questioning typically used are shown in Table 4-2.

Identifying information is primarily intended for record keeping purposes. Accurate information about a child's parents' names and home and work addresses is necessary for keeping appointments, sending reports, and billing. The child's date of birth is used to calculate chronological age, a necessary step in using standardized test procedures.

The second section should allow parents to make as full a statement of their concerns as possible. This is typically done with open-ended questions such as "Describe your child's communication problem." "When was the problem first noticed?" "How has it changed over time?" Typical responses indicative of an articulation problem include references to the child's not being understood when talking or not producing particular sounds or letters correctly.

Questions about a child's speech and language history are intended to help the clinician define what kind of communication problem the child is exhibiting. Specific characteristics of the child's speech and language use are addressed in the following sample questions. "At what ages did your child first babble, say the first word, use two-word phrases, use sentences?" "What is your child's preferred form of communication now?" "How well

Table 4-2. AREAS OF QUESTIONING TYPICALLY INCLUDED IN CASE HISTORY INFORMATION FORM

Identifying information
Description of problem
Speech and language history
Developmental/medical history
Social/educational history
Family history

is your child understood by the parents, siblings, others?" Does your child understand and follow directions?" "Do you question your child's ability to hear?"

The child's current level of language use and the ability of others to understand the child are of concern in choosing articulation-oriented measurement procedures. If listeners have a great deal of difficulty understanding what the child says, it is possible that the child is language disordered including misorganized syllabic shapes and phonemic classes. On the other hand, if the child is well understood and the parent supplies a short list of speech sounds that are misproduced, it is likely the articulation problem is limited to later-developing speech sounds.

The developmental/medical history section serves to alert the clinician to potential etiologies for the speech and language disorders. Table 4-3 displays developmental milestones that are normally attained in an orderly fashion and some of the conditions that may cause or indicate the possibility of neurological or oral structural problems (King & Berger, 1974). These conditions are divided into three time periods: prenatal, natal, and postnatal.

The *prenatal* section refers to activities of the mother (e.g., smoking), conditions of the mother (e.g., viral infections), and conditions of the fetus (e.g., Rh incompatibility) that may affect the fetus' development.

The *natal* period refers to the time of labor and delivery. Again, this refers to conditions that may affect the child's nervous system (e.g., long labor period), medical procedures that are used when the delivery is difficult (e.g., use of oxygen), and characteristics of the child that indicate the infant was stressed by the birth process (e.g., jaundice).

The *postnatal* list also refers to indications that something might be wrong with the child's nervous system (e.g., sleeping problems) or oral development (e.g., feeding problems). It also includes disease processes (e.g., convulsions, high temperature) that cause nervous system damage and medical procedures (e.g., tonsillectomy) related to vocal tract structure and function. The developmental milestones section gives an indication of the child's general neuromuscular development. On average, children sit at about 6 months, feed themselves with utensils and walk at 12 months, and are toilet trained at about 2.5 years. Each of these ages represents the lower age of development of these abilities.

The social and educational section seeks to describe aspects of the child's environment that are important for development of normal speech and language: opportunities to interact with others using language and appropriate models of normal speech and language. In general, the clinician wants to know who the child interacts with verbally, how often verbal interaction occurs, and what kinds of interactions these are.

From a description of the immediate family, the clinician can get a view of who is likely to be interacting with the child. One parent may be at home with the child and other siblings, or both parents may work. Having siblings who are close in age offers the possibility that the child will be interacting with others of similar or slightly better verbal ability. This situation may

Table 4-3. SPECIFIC INFORMATION SOUGHT IN CASE HISTORY FORMS RELATED TO EARLY PHYSIOLOGICAL DEVELOPMENT AND PRESENT ENVIRONMENT

PRENATAL	
Length of pregnancy	Viral infection
Bleeding	German measles
Swelling	Diabetes
High blood pressure	Heart condition
Low blood pressure	Asthma
Convulsions	Thyroid condition
Excessive weight changes	Vomiting
Toxemia	Kidney disease
Medications	Accidents
Anesthetics	Surgeries
Drinking alcohol	Smoking
NATAL	
Length of labor	Anesthetics
Type of delivery	Anoxia
Birth weight	Jaundice
Oxygen used	Complications
Incubator	Head shape
POSTNATAL	
Convulsions	High fever
Infections	Hospitalizations
Traumas	Sleeping problems
Feeding problems	Fussiness
Tonsillectomy	Adenoidectomy
Ear surgery	Transfusions
Breathing difficulty	Intravenous fluids
DEVELOPMENTAL MILESTONES	
Sit without support	
Walk independently	
Feed self with spoon	
Toilet trained	
Solid foods	

offer the child opportunities to use speech and usable models of appropriate language forms. If both parents are working and there are no siblings, perhaps the child is in a situation in which there is little time available for close interactions with others. In either case, the clinician will want the informant to supply a description of the child's typical day to help determine to whom and for what purposes the child is likely to be talking.

Other questions seek to ascertain how well a child socializes with others. In large part, social skills depend on the concurrent development of linguistic skills. Questions such as "How does your child get along with adults . . . siblings . . . other children . . . at school?" attempt to describe how well a child is communicating in each of these situations. Parents and siblings are more likely to be able to interpret the child's intentions than are other adults or playmates. Ability to get along at school involves being able to internalize rules of school behavior, most of which are imparted through teacher language. The child who is described as hyperactive in such formal situations may be one whose language system is not sufficiently developed to understand what is expected of his or her behavior.

Although a form containing check-off lists and simple questions provides a rapid acquisition of information, the clinician will probably also want to interview a parent. This allows the clinician to ask for information that was not clear in the parent's responses to the form. It allows the clinician to expand on questions that may provide useful information. A parent may check the box regarding high fevers, and the clinician will want to inquire as to when such fevers occurred, how often, and what medications were given as a result. The personal interview also gives the parent an opportunity to ask questions of the clinician. The parent will be much more likely to be open and share information with the clinician if the clinician appears to be genuinely concerned about the well-being of the child. As such it is important that the parent's concerns be given an open forum and that the clinician really listen to these.

ASSESSING CHILDREN'S ARTICULATION

Having used the background information to formulate particular questions, the clinician can then contrive a situation in which he or she will be able to elicit verbal responses from the child. The responses are then evaluated by the clinician who assigns a scale value to each response. These scalar values become the data for answering questions about the child's articulatory ability.

Eliciting Articulatory Responses

Every articulation assessment procedure has at its core an interaction between the child and examiner, each taking specified roles with respect to particular materials at hand. The examiner brings a set of stimuli to the situation. These stimuli have been organized to elicit verbal responses from the child. Organization of stimuli attempts to accomplish particular test purposes that are directed by the test maker's and user's theoretical viewpoint regarding what an articulation disorder is, how it should be measured, and how it should be remediated.

The child is prompted to produce speech in a number of different ways. The manner in which stimuli are used determines the level of processing that the child must use to accomplish the task. Although the verbal communication model indicates that all levels are engaged simultaneously during speech and language production, it is possible that the child can focus attention on different levels and perform differently under different speaking conditions. A variety of these are shown in Table 4-4.

Picture Naming. Perhaps the most recognized format for eliciting articulation responses is the picture articulation test format in which a child is shown a series of pictures and requested to name the picture or describe some aspect of the picture. The response is usually intended to be a single word.

The *Templin-Darley Tests of Articulation* (2nd ed.) (Templin & Darley, 1969) will be used as an example of a picture articulation test. This test offers a series of colored line drawings that are to be used as stimuli. The first drawing depicts a robin sitting on a tree branch. The targeted response is *bird.* The examiner prompts this response by saying "This is a . . ." However, a child does not necessarily have to respond with the desired response. The astute child may respond by saying *robin.* This leaves the clinician with the option of trying to elicit the response with reference to some other knowledge (e.g., "That's right. This is a robin, and a robin is a type of . . ."). The problem with this strategy is that these verbal prompts are quite different with respect to the cognitive processing they demand. The first allows for a simple labeling; the second demands that the child take a specific animal (robin) and infer an appropriate supraordinate category (bird).

Table 4-4. CHILD SPEECH TASKS USED TO EVALUATE ARTICULATION PERFORMANCE

Picture naming
Syllable repetition
Single-word repetition
Repetition of multiword utterances
Description of pictures
Reading
Story retelling
Conversational speech

Furthermore, it is easier to picture objects than actions, so the intended responses in picture articulation tests are usually nouns. Recall from the normal developmental literature that very young children tend to produce object names before actions. It may also be the case that misarticulating children correctly articulate nouns before verbs or adjectives. Again, the level of processing required may vary with the type of word. For example, the Templin-Darley test attempts to elicit the response *red* using a drawing of three red blocks. The examiner's prompt is "What color are these?" From the discussion of normal development in Chap. 2, you should recognize that this response is a level II response on Blank and colleagues' (1978) scale of complexity compared to the level I response to "What is this?"

Speech Repetition Tasks. Researchers and clinician's have used repetition of sample utterances for a number of reasons. To gather data for her developmental study, Templin (1957) decided to use a word imitation if the child failed to spontaneously produce the desired word. This decision was based on an earlier study (Templin, 1947) in which it was found that *normally developing children's overall articulation test scores* did not differ when single words were repeated rather than named spontaneously. There are some important assumptions in this choice. First, Templin's data showed no differences in the performance of normally developing children, but the clinician is usually testing the child with disordered articulation. Second, overall scores did not change. It is often not an overall score, but responses to particular speech sounds that concern the clinician. Later studies have shown that misarticulating children's imitations of words are produced with fewer speech production errors than naming responses (Snow & Milisen, 1954; Carter & Buck, 1958). Thus, the difference between imitative and spontaneous elicitation is a parameter the clinician must take into account when planning testing procedures.

This finding can be explained with respect to the verbal communication model. In a spontaneous naming task, the child is activating connections to the motor, auditory, and visual feature system from internal stimulation related to the concept and meaning level connections associated with the picture shown. This stimulation may prove to be *weaker* for *less well learned* patterns than when speech production is stimulated by a strong auditory and visual input from another speaker. In the case of a repetition response, the child's system has been patterned by the auditory and visual inputs. This priming of the speech feature systems may lead to a better than usual speech sound production.

The use of single-word responses in the picture naming task has been criticized from a motoric viewpoint of children's misarticulations because utterance of single words overemphasizes the beginning and end of the word. A word may be produced differently when embedded in a larger utterance than when standing alone. Evidence for such differences was found by Faircloth and Faircloth (1970), who made spectrographic measures of words produced by children in conversations and when repeated as single words. The single-word repetitions were longer and contained better approximations of the consonants and syllable structures of the words. However, Bankson and Bernthal (1982) found that misarticulating children did not produce more errors or different kinds of errors when they repeated sentences compared with repetitions of single words. Furthermore Haynes and Steed (1987) found that a sentence repetition task designed to sample all speech sounds in a variety of word positions was reliably related to percentage of consonants correctly produced in spontaneous speech.

Table 4-5 contains a sentence repetition task that should be suitable for overviewing a young child's articulatory performance. Each of the consonants is assessed in syllable-initial and syllable-final position. The sentences are all at a descriptive level, and the targeted words are all nouns, verbs, or

Table 4-5. SENTENCE REPETITION SURVEY

/p/	The pig was fat.	The cup is full.
/b/	My ball is red.	The cab is yellow.
/t/	My toe hurts.	The cat meowed.
/d/	The dog barked.	My bed is soft.
/k/	I kiss mommy.	You look happy.
/g/	I go fast.	The bag is full.
/m/	Daddy is a man.	The lamb is white.
/n/	I know the alphabet.	I won the race.
/ŋ/		The ring is yellow.
/f/	My face is clean.	The knife is sharp.
/v/	I broke a vase.	The cave is dark.
/θ/	My thumb hurts.	The bath is hot.
/ð/	I saw them.	I bathe at night.
/s/	My soup is hot.	The ice is cold.
/z/	The zoo is fun.	The cheese is yellow.
/ʃ/	My shoe is brown.	The fish is wet.
/h/	I help daddy.	
/w/	I won the game.	
/j/	I saw you.	
/l/	The lion roars.	The ball is red.
/r/	I ran fast.	My car is blue.
/tʃ/	I chew gum.	The witch is flying.
/ʤ/	I jump rope.	The badge is shiny.
/sp/	The spoon is silver.	The clasp broke.
/st/	The step is high	Run fast!
/sk	The sky is blue.	I'll ask mommy.
/pr/	Thorns can prick you.	
/tr/	The train is fast.	
/kr/	The baby cries.	
/pl/	Please say yes.	
/gl/	The glass is full.	

adjectives. The organization of sentences follows the manner of articulation of the target sound, and finally a number of allowable consonant clusters is included.

Some studies have shown that misarticulating children will produce fewer misarticulations if they repeat nonmeaningful syllables rather than meaningful words (Carter & Buck, 1958). One explanation for this is that meaningful words have been heard and produced often enough to create strong connection strengths at the phoneme and feature levels that determine that an error will be produced. For example, the 7-year old who misarticulates /r/ as [w] has had a lot of practice connecting [w] gestures to the word *red*. He is more likely to produce an acceptable [r] in a novel utterance in which a clinician provides visual and auditory features not associated with a known word (e.g., [ɛrɛ]).

In summary, imitative responses have been used because they rapidly provide the clinician with speech productions representing a variety of phonemes that might otherwise take a long time to collect. They have also been used to control the syllabic context and phonetic context of a target sound. However, the clinician should be aware that the child's articulatory performance is likely to be better when a production is elicited through imitation rather than through more spontaneous speech productions.

Storytelling. Another task used to target production of a particular set of words involves telling stories about a picture or series of pictures chosen to elicit particular words. This can be done either with a clinician modeling a particular story or without modeling. This procedure allows for the sampling of a child's articulation in connected speech utterances that are motorically more like the child's day-to-day speech and also allows for the influences of higher-level processing as the child seeks to organize and tell the story. Dubois and Bernthal (1978) compared the number of misarticulations produced by children when they named pictures, repeated a modeled story, or produced their own story. They found that picture naming produced the smallest number of articulation errors. Apparently, as the child must coordinate more information, articulation deteriorates. As further evidence of this relationship, children also produced fewer errors when the story had been modeled for them.

Conversational Speech. In conversational speech with a clinician, a child must cope with following an adult's conversation, often about actions and things that are distant in time and space. This added communication burden appears to affect the child's articulation ability. Both Klein (1984) and Andrews and Fey (1986) found that children's misarticulations increased from picture naming to conversational speech tasks

In summary, picture naming appears to underestimate a child's misarticulations compared to other speaking situations. All of the parameters affecting this relationship have yet to be mapped, but no one would accept single-word–naming responses as typical examples of a child's articulatory ability. Furthermore, as the clinician adds information to the child regarding an utterance by providing models of the utterance, articulation ability improves. As we will see, this relationship has been used in attempts to predict a child's chances of improvement and is also a key element in basic therapy techniques.

Scaling Articulatory Responses

Once the clinician has prompted a child to produce an utterance, the response must be scaled to produce data for answering questions. Using a personal speech perception system, the clinician attempts to interpret how the child has moved the articulators. The clinician then writes down on paper some scale value that reflects his or her interpretation. The following section presents some of the scales that have been used.

Correct-Incorrect. The *correct-incorrect* scale is the simplest of the scales used in judging children's articulation. When a speech production has been judged to be correct, the clinician is stating that the production is an acceptable representation of the intended phoneme in the intended word or utterance.

This scale obviously hinges on the judge's communication system. A midwestern clinician would judge the utterance [ka] for *car* to be unacceptable inasmuch as it lacks a final [r] consonant, or [r] coloring of the vowel. However, the clinician in Boston is likely to find this an appropriate representation within a local dialect. The clinician using this scale must be attuned to the phonetic variations that are possible for the child's dialect and judge accordingly.

A correct-incorrect scale is probably most useful when the form of a particular child's phonetic errors is relatively stable and known to the clinician. A child whose only error is production of /s/ as [θ] may be judged using a correct-incorrect scale for purposes such as tracking improvement over therapy time. The clinician can calculate a percentage correct production of /s/ or other target phoneme relatively easily using a tally of correct and incorrect scores.

Another positive aspect of this simple scale is that it is the most reliable of scales. Reliability of judgments has always been a concern in research regarding children's misarticulation. Virtually every article measuring children's articulation reports indices of interjudge and intrajudge agreement. These are calculated by measuring the number of times a second judge agrees with the first or the number of times a judge reviewing a tape recording agrees with him- or herself. Judgment reliability becomes a major clinical concern if errors in judgment are many compared to the degree of change a child is supposed to exhibit during treatment. For example, if you give an articulation test to a child on one day and the child scores 30 percent correct, and then you rejudge the tape recording and find that the score is

40 percent correct, the error is 10 percent. The child would have to improve over the course of therapy by more than 10 percent for you to be confident that he or she has indeed improved.

Correct-Omission-Substitution-Distortion. Another traditionally used scale elaborates on the more simple category of responses called "incorrect." In this scale, the most severe error is omission of a speech sound, followed by substitution of another English speech sound, followed by a distortion of the intended speech sound. Each of these errors will be discussed with respect to the *verbal communication model* below.

Omission of a speech sound relates to the syllabic level of the verbal communication model. As seen in the preceding chapter, typical syllabic-level errors involve a tendency to produce consonant vowel (CV) syllables instead of syllables with final consonants or syllables including consonant clusters. Other syllabic-level errors involve failure to produce all of the syllables in a word. Either of these cases would result in omission of speech sounds.

As seen in the last chapter, misarticulating children may be approximating the features associated with a missing consonant, (i.e., producing changes in vowel duration associated with the voicing characteristic of a missing final consonant) (Weismer et al., 1981). Some of these feature changes may be subphonemic and therefore not recognized by the judge. Recall that normal speech perception is often categorical in nature; a change in features that does not cue a phonemic distinction may well go undetected by the listener.

Many children who misarticulate a number of speech sounds appear to approximate consonant productions by using a glottal stop consonant (e.g., "Sally saw Suzie" produced as [ʔæʔi ʔɔ ʔuʔi]). In such cases the child appears to have marked the appropriate syllable boundaries of the utterance but needs to elaborate the consonants involved at the phonemic level by including more gestural features (e.g., appropriate place manner and voicing characteristics). Such productions are likely to be recorded by the clinician as "omitted." One of the reasons for describing a [ʔ] as omitted is that this sound is not phonemic in English. Therefore, its use cannot be described as a substitution.

Substitutions involve use of a speech sound that is identifiable as a member of a phonemic class other than the one included in an adult version of an utterance. An English-speaking scorer would classify the use of a dental fricative for an adult word containing /s/ as a case of a substitution because English uses a dental fricative phoneme. However, use of a lateralized fricative for an /s/ would be classified as a *distortion* because no phonemic class of lateral fricatives exists that contrasts with /s/. The distortion category has drawn the greatest amount of criticism in the use of this scale because it is ambiguous. A sound is distorted if either an inappropriate allophone of a phoneme is used in its production or a non-English sound is produced. Use of the category *distortion* does not clarify which of these possibilities has occurred. Both cases involve inappropriate gestures associated with a phoneme in a particular utterance.

Phonetic Transcription. Transcription of a child's utterance provides a clearer description of what a child has produced. The scale values in phonetic transcription are the individual symbols. Each symbol characterizes the articulatory configuration inferred to underlie a speech production. Use of the symbol [p] means the transcriber has inferred that the speaker produced a complete constriction of the vocal tract at the lips, the vocal folds were apart, and the velum was raised.

A phonetic transcription of what a child says provides a great deal of information regarding the child's production of particular speech sounds. However, it must be recalled that much of what the listener transcribes has been inferred by the listener. The listener cannot see velar movement and thus must infer that the velum is raised appropriately or not. Furthermore, phonetic transcription is often highly variable from listener to listener.

The clinician will have to deal with two types of children: younger children with multiple phonemic errors and older children with errors involving one or two phonemes. In the former case, a phonemic-level transcription is often adequate because measurement will revolve around describing the child's syllabic and phonemic organization. For the older child, the primary task is description of the phonetic characteristics of a few errors, which may be accomplished using phonetic diacritic marks or even a verbal description of the child's production inasmuch as a number of diacritic systems are available. After the initial description is made, the clinician will primarily want to describe how often the child is using a typical pattern and how often he or she is using an adultlike pattern. This type of measurement can be accomplished with the more basic correct-incorrect scale.

ASKING CLINICAL QUESTIONS

When a child is referred to the speech-langauge pathologist because his or her speech is difficult to understand, one of the questions asked is whether a child's articulation ability is normal or disordered. Because articulation ability is a developmental skill, answering this question requires that the clinician compare the individual child to age mates using normative data. If a child's articulation development is not appropriate for his or her age, the clinician asks how the child's articulation ability is disordered. Answering this question requires the use of some theoretical model of articulation ability, for it is the components of such a model that the clinician will seek to assess.

IS THIS CHILD'S ARTICULATORY ABILITY NORMAL?

Two methods are typically used to compare a child's articulatory ability to what would be expected in normal development. In the first method the child's articulation errors are compared with normative data provided by studies such as those reviewed in Chap. 2 or by norm-referenced tests, which supply data from a study of responses of normally developing children.

Comparison to Normal Developmental Literature

Chapter 2 provided a description of speech sound production and perception development. Figure 4-1 reiterates the major phases of speech production development. These may be used as a rough guide to a child's development of speech sound production.

The first portion of Fig. 4-1 lists the common preverbal sound productions at approximately the time they occur (Oller et al., 1975; Irwin, 1947a, 1947b). It should be kept in mind that studies that identified these sound production types have often found that not all normal infants produce all types. It is highly likely that in the short period of time one has available for interacting with a child for testing purposes, a normal child would not produce the full repertoire of preverbal sound types.

The second portion of Fig. 4-1 lists the consonants of English in the order in which they are typically successfully used by a majority of children in an age group in simple word forms (Prather et al., 1975). It also includes the consonant clusters that occur in English words. Most of these are adequately produced by age 4 years. From a sample of the child's speech, the clinician transcribes the child's representations of these sounds or clusters.

These checklists could be used to judge the adequacy of a child's speech with respect to age. Particular attention should be paid to the child's production of clusters and word-final consonants. Failure to produce segments in these contexts is not typical of normally developing children at age 4 years (Hodson & Paden, 1981). Errors in which segments are not produced in word-final position are also an indication that the child may have failed to organize his or her language system at other levels as well (Panagos, 1974; Smit & Bernthal, 1983). Such children should receive further diagnostic attention for both articulation and other levels of language processing.

Table 4-6 shows part of a 4-year-old boy's version of the *Three Bears* story as told using a picture book. In most cases each utterance is in response to a particular picture. Although we will not attempt to analyze this child's language ability, it should be noted that his utterances stay at a fairly low level of description. For example, referring to Goldilocks' breaking the baby bear's chair, this child says, "Then sat on baby's chair." The adult prompts for more, and the child says, "Chair breaked." The first portion of this ut-

Fig. 4-1. Stages of speech sound production acquisition.

Prelexical Stage

Age	*Speech sound production*	
6 mon	Quasi resonant nucleus	_____
	Fully resonant nucleus	_____
	Raspberry	_____
	Yell	_____
	Squeal	_____
	Growl	_____
10 mon	Canonical babbling	_____
12 mon		

SYLLABIC SHAPES PRODUCED

	Meaningful	*Nonmeaningful*
CV	_____	_____
CVCV	_____	_____
VC	_____	_____
CVC	_____	_____

PHONETIC PRODUCTIONS

		Meaningful utterances	*Nonmeaningful utterances*
Labials			
	[p]	_____	_____
	[b]	_____	_____
	[m]	_____	_____
	[w]	_____	_____
Alveolars			
	[t]	_____	_____
	[d]	_____	_____
	[n]	_____	_____
	[s]	_____	_____
	[z]	_____	_____
Velars			
	[k]	_____	_____
	[g]	_____	_____
Glottals			
	[h]	_____	_____
	[ʔ]	_____	_____

Fig. 4-1 (continued)

Conceptual Phase

APPROXIMATIONS OF ADULT PHONEMIC TARGETS

Age	*Consonants*				
2;0	p ______	m ______	h ______	w ______	
	b ______	n ______	f ______		
	t ______	ŋ ______	s ______		
	d ______				
	k ______				
	g ______				
3;0			ʃ ______	j ______	tʃ ______
				l ______	ʤ ______
				r ______	
4;0			θ ______		
			ð ______		
			ʒ ______		
			v ______		

APPROXIMATIONS OF ADULT CLUSTERS (AGE 4;0)

Word-initial

sp ______	st ______	sk ______	sm ______	sn ______	
sw ______	sl ______				
fr ______	fl ______	θr ______	ʃr ______		
pr ______	br ______	tr ______	dr ______	kr ______	gr ______
pl ______	bl ______	kl ______	gl ______		
tw ______	kw ______				
spl ______	spr ______	str ______	skr ______		

Word-final

kt ______			
ft ______			
sp ______	st ______	sk ______	
lp ______	lt ______	lk ______	lf ______
mp ______	nt ______	nd ______	ŋk ______

Table 4-6. FOUR-YEAR-OLD BOY'S TELLING OF THE *THREE BEARS* STORY

də papə be sɛt mai powiʤ iz tu hat.
The papa bear said, "My porridge is too hot."

dɛn dɛ mami sɛt mai powiʤ iz tu koud.
Then the mommy said, "My porridge is too cold."

dɛn dɛ bebi sɛt mai powitʃ iz tu doun nou.
Then the baby said, "My porridge is too . . . don't know."

goudilaks kem.
Goldilocks came.

dɛn hɪm sɛd dæt powitʃ iz tu hat.
Then him said, "That porridge is too hot."

dɛn kem tu də ədə powɪtʃ æn sɛd dæt dɪs powitʃ iz tu kat.
Then came to the other porridge and said, "That . . . this porridge is too cold.

dɛn hɪm et təm əf bebɪz powiʤ
Then him ate some of baby's porridge.

dɛn hɪm dɛd da wəz dʌs wait.
Then him said, "That was just right."

dɛn sæʔ an bebiz se.
Then sat on baby's chair.

tʃe wekt.
Chair breaked.

terance failed to include the agent of this action (Goldilocks). The child also did not supply the causal linkage between these two propositions (i.e., that the chair broke because Goldilocks sat on it). Furthermore this child produced syntactic errors when attempting to use pronouns and when referring to time relationships. Both of these attributes would cue the clinician to further investigate this child's language organization.

Table 4-7 compares this child's data to normal development of consonants and consonant clusters. He produces a number of consonant errors for speech sounds that a majority of children at age 4 years are able to appropriately produce: /t/, /d/, /s/, /z/, /r/, /tʃ/, and /ʤ/. He also fails to produce some word-final consonants as well as consonant clusters, both cues that this child's articulation ability may be disordered.

This technique of screening has a number of flaws. As seen in this sample, a number of English consonants were not attempted, so no data exist on this child's use of these consonants. A very large number of possible consonant clusters also did not appear in the sample. A second problem is that this process offers no quantitative basis for making the decision that this child's speech is disordered. A related problem is that using the ages at which 50 percent of the children correctly produce some speech sound as a

Table 4-7. ANALYSIS OF A 4-YEAR-OLD CHILD'S SPEECH SAMPLE FROM TABLE 4-6 IN THE CONCEPTUAL PHASE

Approximations of adult phonemic targets

Age	Consonants										
2 yr	p	[p]		m	[m]	h	[h]	w			
	b	[b]		n	[n]	f					
	t	[t]	[ʔ]	ŋ		s	[s]	[t]	[d]		
	d	[d]	[t]								
	k	[k]									
	g										
3 yr	ʃ	[s]	[t]	[d]	j				tʃ	[s]	[tʃ]
	l				ʤ	[ʤ]	[tʃ]	[d]			
	r	[w]									
4 yr	θ										
	ð	[d]	[ʔ]								
	z	[z]	[s]								
	v	[f]									

Approximations of adult clusters (age 4 yr)

Word-initial							
sp	st	sk	sm	sn			
sw	sl						
fr	fl	θr	sr				
pl	bl	kl	gl				
tw	kw						
spl	spr	str	skr				
Word-final							
kt							
ft							
sp	st		sk				
lp	lt		ld	[d]	[t]	lk	lf
mp	nt	[n]	nd	[n]		ŋk	

criterion opens the possibility of deciding that half of the children in an age group are speech disordered. Each of these concerns is addressed by using more formal approaches.

To overcome some of these problems, clinicians often use a picture-naming task to elicit responses. The pictures are chosen to elicit all of the speech sounds of English in various word contexts such as word-initial, word-medial, and word-final. They then apply a more stringent age criterion. In particular, traditional practice for the older child who misarticulates speech

Table 4-8. AGES AT WHICH 90 PERCENT OF THE CHILD POPULATION IS EXPECTED TO CORRECTLY ARTICULATE CONSONANT SOUNDS IN SINGLE-WORD–NAMING RESPONSES ACCORDING TO SANDER (1972)

Age	*Sounds*					
3 yr	p	m	h	n	w	
4 yr	b	d	k	g	f	j
6 yr	t	ŋ	r	l		
7 yr	s	tʃ	θ	ʤ		
8 yr	ʃ	ʒ	v	z		

sounds is to use the age at which 90 percent of the children correctly articulate a speech sound as a cutoff. Sander (1972) estimated "ages of mastery" for the consonant sounds of English as shown in Table 4-8.

Use of these more stringent age boundaries suggests that this child's productions are normal inasmuch as error sounds are not expected to be appropriately articulated until age 6 years. Although normative data are currently lacking for such a measure, Shriberg and Kwiatkowski (1982) have proposed using the "percentage of consonants" correctly articulated as a metric for children's articulation errors. The consonants that occur in the adult form of a word are taken as the base number in calculating this metric. For example, the word *cold* contains three consonants: [k], [l], and [d]. This child's production of this word as [koud] would give him two-thirds of the consonants correctly articulated or 66.6 percent of the consonants correct. Overall, this child correctly articulated 88 in 138 consonants in this sample for a correct articulation of 64 percent.

Table 4-9 shows the responses of a 7-year-old boy to the *Goldman-Fristoe Sounds in Words Subtest* (Goldman & Fristoe, 1969). This boy made errors in production of the consonants /r/ and /ð/. According to the studies of normal development, both of these sounds should be correctly articulated at this age. Treatment for this child's articulation of these two sounds would be considered justified, and further testing would be used to better define the child's ability and perhaps to make decisions about the particular approach to treatment that would be used.

Standardized Tests

A standardized test has been given to a sample of persons from a target population to find out what scores would be expected from a person in that population. The test manual presents typical articulation scores for children at different ages. The test performance of an individual child can be compared to those of this normative group to see if the child fits within the group. For example, a 5-year-old child entering school might be given an

Table 4-9. RESPONSES OF A 7-YEAR-OLD CHILD TO THE SOUNDS IN WORDS SUBTEST OF THE GOLDMAN-FRISTOE ARTICULATION TEST WITH CONSONANT TARGETS UNDERLINED

house	haus	carrot	kɛwət
telephone	tɛləfoun	orange	owənʤ
cup	kʌp	bathtub	bæθtəb
gun	gʌn	bath	bæθ
knife	naɪf	thumb	θʌm
window	wɪndoʊ	finger	fɪŋgə
wagon	wægən	ring	wiŋ
wheel	wil	jumping	dʒʌmpɪŋ
chicken	tʃɪkən	pajamas	pəʤæməʒ
zipper	zɪpə	plane	plen
scissors	sɪzəz	blue	blu
duck	dʌk	brush	bwʌʃ
vacuum	vækjum	drum	drʌm
lamp	læmp	flag	flæg
matches	mætʃɪz	Santa	sæntə
shovel	ʃʌvəl	Claus	klɔz
car	kar	Christmas	kwisməs
rabbit	wæbɪt	tree	tri
fishing	fɪʃɪŋ	squirrel	skwoul
church	tʃoutʃ	sleeping	slipɪŋ
feather	fɛðə	bed	bɛd
pencils	pɛnsɪlz	stove	stouv
this	dɪs		

articulation test so that his or her total score can be compared to age mates. If his or her score is low relative to those of age mates, further assessment is indicated, or a program of articulation therapy may begin. Perhaps the most important precaution about standardized tests is that they be used only with persons who are from the target population. It would obviously be unfair to administer a French articulation test to a native speaker of English from Chicago. Less obvious, but equally unfair, is the administration of a test normed on a group of speakers of standard American English to a speaker of black vernacular English. Table 4-10 displays the names, publishers, and age ranges for commonly used standardized articulation tests.

The articulatory responses of the 4-year-old child while producing the words from the Templin-Darley screening Test of Articulation are shown in Table 4-11. The screening portion of the Templin-Darley test is an example of a measurement tool that supplies normative data for children. In this test,

Table 4-10. TEST INSTRUMENTS THAT SUPPLY AGE-REFERENCED NORMATIVE SCORES

Arizona Articulation Proficiency Scale
Western Psychological Services
12031 Wilshire Blvd.
Los Angeles, CA 90025
Age range: 3:0–11:11

Coarticulation Assessment in Meaningful Language
Communication Skill Builders
3130 Dodge Blvd.
Tucson, AZ 85733
Age range: 2:6–5:6

Denver Articulation Screening Examination
Ladoca Project and Publishing Foundation
East 51st Avenue and Lincoln
Denver, CO 80216
Age range: 2:5–6:0

Goldman-Fristoe Test of Articulation
American Guidance Services, Inc.
Publishers Building
Circle Pines, MN 55014
Age range: 6:0–12:0

Photo Articulation Test
Interstate Printers and Publishers, Inc.
19–27 North Jackson St.
Danville, IL 61832
Age range: 3:0–8:0

Predictive Screening Test of Articulation
Continuing Education Office
Western Michigan University
Kalamazoo, MI 49001
Age range: 6:0–7:0

Screening Deep Test of Articulation
Stanwix House
3020 Chartiers Ave.
Pittsburgh, PA 15204
Age range: 5:0–8:0

Templin-Darley Tests of Articulation
Bureau of Educational Research and Service
University of Iowa
Iowa City, IA 52242
Age range: 3:0–8:0

Table 4-10. (continued)

Weiss Comprehensive Articulation Test
Teaching Resources
50 Pond Park Rd.
Hingham, MA 02043
Age range: 3:0–8:0

Table 4-11. A 4-YEAR-OLD BOY'S RESPONSES TO THE TEMPLIN-DARLEY SCREENING TEST

Word	*Target*	*Response*	*Score*
bird	ɝ	bud	0
music	ju	muzək	0
red	r	wɛd	0
arrow	r	ɛwou	0
leaf	l	lif	1
valentines	v	vælətaims	1
thumb	θ	təm	0
toothbrush	θ	tufbwʌs	0
teeth	θ	tif	0
feathers	ð	fɛvəs	0
there	ð	deə	0
smoothe	ð	smuf	0
zipper	z	dipə	0
shoe	ʃ	ʃu	1
fish	ʃ	fɪʃ	1
dishes	ʃ	dɪsəz	0
television	v	tɛləvɛʃən	1
yellow	j	jɛlou	1
onions	j	ʌnjəns	1
chair	tʃ	seə	0
matches	tʃ	mætsəz	0
watch	tʃ	wats	0
jump	ʤ	dʌmp	0
engine	ʤ	ɛnʤən	1
presents	pr	wɛzənt	0
bread	br	wɛd	0
tree	tr	wi	0
drum	dr	rʌm	0

Table 4-11. (continued)

Word	*Target*	*Response*	*Score*
crayons	kr	weans	0
grass	gr	wæs	0
frog	fr	fwok	0
three	θr	fwi	0
shredded	ʃr	ɛtʌd	0
planting	pl	plænt	1
clown	kl	laun	0
glasses	gl	læsəs	0
flower	fl	slawe	0
smoke	sm	ʃmok	0
snowman	sn	nomæ	0
spoon	sp	pun	0
steps	st	dɛps	0
skates	sk	kets	0
sled	sl	slɛt	1
swing	sw	wɪŋgz	0
twins	tw	twɪns	1
queen	kw	kwin	1
splash	spl	plas	0
sprinkler	spr	wɪŋkələ	0
string	str	wɪŋ	0
scratch	skr	ʃræt	0
		Total	12

children are asked to name 50 pictures. Each labeling response contains a particular targeted speech sound or consonant cluster. The examiner observes the child's production of that speech sound or cluster and decides whether it is "correct" or "incorrect." For each correct response, the child receives one point; thus a child's score may vary from 0 to 50 points. This particular child produced the word *bird* as [bud], which was judged to be an inappropriate production of the vowel /ɝ/ by the midwestern test administrator. Thus, his response was scored incorrect and was assigned a numerical value of 0.

The items appearing in the screening portion of the Templin-Darley test were those 50 responses from the total test that best distinguished the top performing 27 percent of the children in the normal sample from the bottom 27 percent. Analysis of the items tested shows a high proportion of liquids, fricatives, and consonant clusters containing fricatives and liquids. In essence, this approach maintains that children who can correctly articulate the later-developing speech sounds are those who will develop appropriate articulation.

The authors of this test instrument assessed the articulation of a sample of children to find out what an average score would be for a particular age group. The test was given to 30 boys and 30 girls in each of 8 age groups: 3 years, 3.5 years, 4 years, 4.5 years, 5 years, 6 years, 7 years, and 8 years. The average scores for children in an age group are shown in the first row of Table 4-12. As expected, the average score increases as the age of the children tested increases. The average 3-year old correctly articulates 21 of the target sounds; the average 8-year old correctly articulates 48.

For purposes of calculating a score for this particular child, the last column showing whether a production was correct (1) or incorrect (0) would suffice. A response is counted as correct if the targeted speech sound is acceptable to the examiner. The remainder of the word may contain misarticulations without causing the production to be marked as incorrect. For example, his production of *sled* as [slɛt] is scored as correct because the targeted portion of this word is the [sl] cluster not the final [d]. This child's score of 12 places him two standard deviations (one standard deviation = 11) below the average score (average = 34) for 4-year olds.

Now the clinician must decide at what point a child's articulation ability is considered to be normal. In psychological fields it is usually assumed that scores related to an ability are normally distributed. This is a statistical concept that indicates that the underlying population of scores is bell shaped. That is, most of the people in a population will score near the mean of the score scale. As the score either increases or decreases from the mean, fewer and fewer persons obtain these scores.

The mean score of the population is the fiftieth percentile of the distribution. That is, 50 percent of the population are expected to receive scores below this score. For example, according to Table 4-12, 50 percent of the 4-year olds should score below 34 on the Templin-Darley test.

Table 4-12. AVERAGE SCORES WITH STANDARD DEVIATIONS FOR THE TEMPLIN-DARLEY SCREENING TEST

Age	*Mean*	*Standard deviation*
3.0	21	13
3.5	28	14
4.0	34	11
4.5	36	12
5.0	38	13
6.0	41	11
7.0	46	6
8.0	48	4

Also, within normal distributions there is a standard percentage of persons in the population within each standard deviation range. Approximately 16 percent of the population will score below one standard deviation below the mean. Therefore, 50 percent of the 4-year olds score below 34 on the Templin-Darley test, and 16 percent score below 23. The score 23 was derived by subtracting one standard deviation (11) from the mean (34). Furthermore, approximately 2 percent of a population is expected to score below two standard deviations below the mean. In this case, 2 percent of the 4-year olds would be expected to score below 12.

Many state school systems require that a child score two standard deviations away from (usually below) the age-group mean on a standardized test to be included in a treatment program. The 4-year old in our example would be judged to be articulation disordered using this criterion because his score of 12 is two standard deviations below his age group's average. Nothing is magic or predictive about this second percentile. Unfortunately, even the articulation tests that have been normed either do not supply the necessary information to compute this cutoff score or have not used large enough sample sizes to avoid having standard deviations that are too large to be useful. For example, look at the average score for a 3-year old: the mean is 21, and the standard deviation is 13. To be two standard deviations below the mean, a child would have to score -5. Obviously this is impossible.

This commonly used cutoff, like many governmental decisions, is at least partly based on economic considerations. School systems cannot afford to supply speech-language pathology services to children who may not need it. Many parents will be concerned about the economics of hiring a private practice–based speech-language pathologist for children who will not require a service as well. No simple test instrument–based answers to such problems exist at the present time.

Since the Goldman-Fristoe Test of Articulation (Goldman & Fristoe, 1969) has been normed for a population of 7-year olds, it is possible to compute a total error score for the child whose productions are shown in Table 4-9. His misarticulation of /r/ in the words *rabbit, carrot, brush,* and *Christmas* and his misarticulation of /ð/ results a total error score of 5. The manual for this test shows that this number of errors is produced by 35 percent of the children in this child's age group. This percentile would often be called normal. Notice that the decision to call this child's misarticulations normal differs from the decision to call them disordered, which occurred when his errors were compared to the normal developmental literature. Testing and prediction of human performance is often an inexact science with different answers being obtained when different methods are being used. In this case, the child's errors are not sufficient to cause him to be identified as misarticulating because his errors are inconsistent (i.e., he does not misarticulate all occurrences of /r/ and /ŋ/).

Other test instruments have been normed with scores that are derived from the raw number of errors rather than just the error score itself. For example, the *Arizona Articulation Proficiency Scale* (Fudala, 1974) computes an estimated percentage of speech sounds produced in error rather than simply counting the number of errors. This percentage is based on the relative frequency of occurrence of a speech sound in a particular word position. For example, a word-final [t] is the most often occurring consonant, so it is given a weight of 4.0. A word-final [ʒ] occurs less often, so it is given a weight of 0.5. Each error is multiplied by its weight so that a child who misarticulates the more frequently occurring sounds receives a higher error score and therefore a lower percent correct score. The basic rationale is that misarticulation of the more frequently occurring speech sounds is more damaging to a child's intelligibility than misarticulation of those sounds that do not occur so often.

This test supplies average, weighted percent correct scores for a variety of ages of children. Each of the weighted scores is related to a verbal description of intelligibility. For example, a score of 70 is described as "Speech is intelligible with careful listening." However, the normative data do not readily convert into percentile scores or standard deviation scores that might be used to meet governmental criteria.

A comparison of three standardized screening tests by Everleigh and Warr-Leeper (1983) showed that the three tests used identified to a high degree the same children as requiring attention. Children in this study ranged in age from 3 to 5 years. Furthermore, 95 percent of the children identified as needing attention by the formal screening tests were also identified as needing attention by experienced speech-language pathologists who made decisions based on a short sample of the child's conversational speech. The 5 percent disagreements occurred for 3-year olds, suggesting that the judgment of a trained individual is as accurate as the use of standardized test procedures for children entering kindergarten. These clinical judgments were most likely made with reference to the normal developmental literature as described in the preceding section.

Although a standardized test allows you to compare a child's performance to that of peers, it does not tell you whose articulation is disordered and whose is not. The choice of a standardized cutoff for screening purposes should be based on research that shows that receiving a particular score at one age will predict how well a child will do at a later age. Such data are generally lacking in our field.

Studies have shown that children who can correctly imitate their error sounds are more likely to improve their articulation without therapy. Snow and Milisen (1954) gave a group of children an articulation test in two manners: by asking children to name pictures and by asking the same children to imitate the words. They found that children who could correctly imitate words that were misarticulated when named were more likely to correctly articulate the sounds involved 6 months later. Carter and Buck (1958) found that children who could correctly imitate error sounds in nonmeaningful syllable repetitions were more likely to develop correct articulation with or without therapy. This ability would appear to indicate that the child has the anatomical and neuromuscular abilities necessary for articulation.

The *Goldman-Fristoe Test of Articulation* (Goldman & Fristoe, 1969) has formalized this relationship in its testing procedures. Each error sound is recorded during picture naming. Then, each error is assessed during imitation of the word and imitation of the sound in a nonsense syllable. The 7-year old whose misarticulation of /r/ was not consistent enough to be deemed disordered in the picture-naming portion of the Goldman-Fristoe was able to correctly produce /r/ in single words when given a verbal model of the word. This evidence supports the decision not to enroll this child in therapy inasmuch as it is an indication that he may develop appropriate production of /r/ without remedial help.

The Predictive Screening Test of Articulation (Van Riper & Erickson, 1969) combines a number of these indicators of articulatory ability. Children's articulations of sounds is scored, as in most screening tests. Ability to modify an incorrect production given instruction is assessed. Also included are nonspeech tasks, such as rhythmic finger tapping, that are theoretically indicative of motor control. Unlike other screening tests, the Predictive Screening Test of Articulation is based on a longitudinal study that suggests the probability that a child obtaining a particular score will have improved his or her articulation by the end of the school year.

HOW DOES THIS CHILD'S ARTICULATION DIFFER FROM NORMAL?

The manner in which a clinician seeks to describe a child's ability varies with the clinician's theoretical model of articulation ability. The earliest descriptive tests were designed to assess articulation of each consonant sound of English in the initial, medial, and final positions of words as well as allowable consonant clusters. This test format was developed within a theoretical view that misarticulation is an inability to produce speech sounds, primarily consonants that are learned in word frames.

When studies of children's misarticulations indicated that phonetic context affected speech sound production, other tests were developed to assess production of a speech sound in a wider variety of phonetic contexts than was being assessed in single-word–naming responses. Phonetic context testing was used as a follow-up procedure for each sound identified as being misarticulated. When research suggested that misarticulating children produced articulatory feature errors, tests were designed to assess if a particular feature was being produced in error across phonemes. Such procedures became relatively lengthy and would show that a child was misarticulating a relatively abstract feature such as "stridency" in some percentage of its occurrences.

Speech sounds distribute themselves into natural classes (e.g., all stop, all alveolars, all voiceless sounds) that share the key features such as named above. Error patterns may invade part or all of a natural class in a particular case, and the error production may produce a systematic shift into another natural class. For example, one error pattern involves stopping (making stops from) all fricatives. The use of such patterned error processes as a way to evaluate phonetic disorders has great theoretical power.

Most recently, test instruments have been designed around commonly occurring patterns of misarticulation such as cluster reduction and final-consonant deletion. These typical patterns include the feature-based errors as well as errors that involved failure to approximate the syllabic shapes of adult utterances.

The following discussion describes three types of analysis in order of their historical development. The first describes production of individual speech sounds in word position. In the second, speech sound errors are described with respect to syllable boundaries. In the final analysis, common error patterns are described with respect to levels of the verbal communication model, in particular, the syllabic shape level and the articulatory feature level. For each type of analysis, particular test procedures are presented as well as examples taken regarding the articulation data of the two misarticulating children referred to in this chapter.

Sound-in-Word Position

The traditional analysis of articulation ability is based on testing the production of particular speech sounds in particular word positions. For example, the Goldman-Fristoe test assesses production of /s/ in word-initial (*scissors*), word-medial (*pencil*), word-final (*house*), and consonant clusters (*sleeping, stove, squirrel*). This organization is common to many of the earlier articulation tests.

Table 4-13 shows an analysis of the errors produced by the 7-year-old misarticulating child while producing the words from the Goldman Fristoe test. Only those sounds produced in error are shown.

This analysis shows that the child misarticulates two sounds: /r/ and /ð/. Both are inconsistently misarticulated, that is, each error sound is correctly articulated in some word positions but not in all. /r/ is correctly produced in word-final position and in /tr/ and /dr/ clusters. /ð/ is produced as [d] in word-initial position and is correctly produced in word-medial position.

This organizational scheme makes a number of assumptions about the nature of children's misarticulations. First of all, it assumes that a child learns articulation one phoneme at a time. For example, learning to produce

Table 4-13. ANALYSIS OF ERRORS SHOWN IN TABLE 4-8

Sound	*Initial*	*Medial*	*Final*	*Clusters*
r	w	w	r	tr, dr, bw
ð	d	ð		

an /s/ is thought to be distinct from learning a /z/. For children who are nearing the final stages of articulatory development, this may not be a critical assumption. This 7-year old does appear to be misarticulating two speech sounds that are unrelated to one another at the articulatory feature level.

Second, this format assumes that production of a sound is meaningfully described with respect to word boundaries. That is, it is expected that children may have an easier or more difficult time producing a speech sound in word-initial, word-final, or word-medial positions.

A classic problem arises when word-medial position is considered. For example, the Goldman-Fristoe test uses the following words to assess word-medial productions: tele*ph*one, win*d*ow, and Sa*n*ta. When considered at a syllabic level, these word-medial positions appear to be different. The [f] in *telephone* occurs between two vowels and seems to be the first consonant of the last syllable of the word. The [d] in *window* also starts the final syllable of a word but is bordered by one consonant and one vowel rather than two vowels. The [n] in *Santa* also connects to a consonant and a vowel but appears to end the first syllable of the word rather than starting the final syllable. The question can be raised regarding the effect of these differing contexts on the production of these sounds. For example, is production of [f] the same in an intervocalic, word-medial position like *telephone* as it is in other word-medial positions such as *infant*?

Furthermore, to the extent that the articulators remain in motion from one word to the next, a sound's production may be affected by contexts that extend across word boundaries due to the process of coproduction. It has been argued that only the beginning of an utterance and the end of an utterance are really in "initial" or "final" position; everything else is "medial."

Objections such as these led McDonald (1964) to propose that children's misarticulations were better analyzed with respect to syllable position rather than word position. He also proposed that phonetic context (i.e., the speech sounds that precede and follow a particular consonant) will affect its articulation. Analysis of articulation errors from this perspective is discussed in the next section.

Although such a traditional analysis is relatively straightforward for the 7-year old who exhibits few misarticulations, it becomes somewhat unwieldy for the 4-year old. Table 4-14 shows an analysis of the errors produced by the 4-year old's responses to the words in the Templin-Darley test shown in Table 4-11.

The errors have been listed in order of intended consonant manner of articulation. The first error is for the nasal consonant /n/. It was produced as [m] in the word *valentines.* /r/ is often misarticulated as [w] but is sometimes appropriately articulated in consonant clusters. /f/ is misarticulated in the cluster /fl/. The dental fricatives /θ/ and /ð/ are consistently misarticulated. Usually, the dentals are produced as labials [f] and [v]. /z/ is produced as a [d] in word-initial position and as [s] in word-final position. /s/ is misarticulated in consonant clusters. Consonant clusters are sometimes pro-

Table 4-14. ANALYSIS OF THE 4-YEAR OLD'S ERRORS IN THE TEMPLIN-DARLEY SCREENING TEST

Sound	*Initial*	*Medial*	*Final*	*Clusters*
n		m		
r	w	w	ə	w
f				s
ð	d	v	f	
θ	t	f	f	f
z	d		s	
s				ʃ, –, s
ʃ		s		
tʃ		ts	ts	
ʤ	d			

duced as single consonants. Such an organization of this child's data does not easily lead to a coherent description of how this child misarticulates, and this state of affairs led to the practice of analyzing young children's misarticulations for common error patterns.

Sound-in-Syllable Position

McDonald's (1964a) discussion of motor aspects of children's misarticulations led to the use of syllabic position rather than word position as a descriptive device in articulatory assessment. He chose two functions for consonant sounds. A consonant could either release a syllable (*see*) or arrest a syllable (*ice*). At other times a consonant could be "ambisyllabic" in that it could be considered to arrest one syllable and begin the next as in *icy*. This latter syllabic context could also occur in an utterance between words (*I see*).

This type of analysis stands apart from the word position analysis because it does not consider word boundaries to be important determinants of misarticulation. In some respects it offers useful divisions. For example, it allows a means of distinguishing different types of word-medial positions. The word-medial contexts for [s] in the following words involve quite different syllabic contexts: *icy, pest, pester*. The [s] in *icy* is ambisyllabic; the [s] in *pest* is part of a consonant cluster occurring within one syllable; the [s] in *pester* probably ends a syllable while the [t] begins the next. Like the word-position analysis scheme shown above, this analysis involves an appeal to logic. Only data from children's misarticulations will ultimately show if their systems have organized articulation according to word boundaries or syllabic boundaries. For example, data from Hoffman, Schuckers, and Ratusnik (1977) suggest that both syllable and word boundaries are important in some respect. Children who misarticulated [r] were asked to produce [tr] clusters when the two consonants were part of the same word *tree* and when they were separated by word boundaries such as "Pat reads." Fewer misarticulations occurred when the consonants were in the same syllable.

This type of detailed phonetic-level analysis is typically used with the older child who misarticulates one or two speech sounds. To further quantify a child's production of a particular consonant and to search for phonetic contexts in which it may be correctly produced, McDonald developed a procedure called *deep testing*. In the *McDonald Deep Test of Articulation*, (McDonald 1964b), a child is asked to rapidly name two pictures. One of the pictures is used to elicit production of the target consonant in either syllable-releasing or syllable-arresting position. For example, the word *sun* contains a syllable-releasing [s], and the word *bus* contains a syllable-arresting [s]. The consonant preceding the [s] in *sun* is altered in the deep test by changing the first picture (e.g., a [g] would precede the [s] if the first picture is of a dog; a [t] would precede the [s] if the first picture is of a cat).

Some children find the task of naming the two pictures rapidly somewhat difficult. Furthermore, some clinicians object to the lack of a meaningful relationship between the two words in the standard deep test. McDonald (1964c) also published a form of the deep test in which the two-word combinations are embedded in sentences. Table 4-15 shows some of the responses of the 7-year-old child who misarticulates /r/ to the syllable-releasing /r/ contexts. His production of syllable-arresting contexts showed all appropriate [r] productions.

One use of this form of testing is to gain a measurement of the consistency with which a sound is misarticulated. In this case, it could be said that the child correctly articulates [r] in syllable-releasing position in 6 in 30 utterances or 20 percent of the time. The responses to the McDonald Deep Test would also be analyzed for phonetic contexts in which correct productions occur. In this case, the child correctly articulates [r] when it is preceded by labial stops [p, b], alveolar stops [t, d], one velar stop [k], and [ɝʃ]. One or more of these contexts might be used in therapy to help elicit appropriately articulated /r/ productions. A number of sentence sets called *sound-in-context surveys* for speech sounds commonly misarticulated by older children are listed in Appendix B.

Another test instrument using this syllabic-based logic is the *Coarticulation Assessment in Meaningful Language Test* (Kenney & Prather, 1984). This test uses a two-word production task like the McDonald Deep Test (1964b) but seeks to improve on the deep test by using two-word combinations that are meaningful. The task used is picture naming after a model of the desired response has been given. Commonly misarticulated phonemes /r, l, s, f, c, k, t/ are targeted in syllable-releasing and syllable-arresting positions. For example, the 7-year-old boy who misarticulated /r/ produced the responses to /r/ productions in this test shown in Table 4-16.

The items used in this test are hoped to be meaningful to the child in a way that the items in the McDonald picture test are often not. For example,

Table 4-15. RESPONSES OF A 7-YEAR-OLD /r/-MISARTICULATING CHILD TO SOME OF THE SYLLABLE-RELEASING [r] CONTEXTS IN THE McDONALD DEEP TEST, SENTENCE FORM

Context	*Syllable-releasing sentence*	*Production*
pr	The sheep ran up the hill.	r
br	Bob read a book.	r
tr	The cat ran after the dog.	r
dr	I did read the book.	r
kr	I like red apples.	w
gr	We saw a big red house.	w
mr	We saw him run to school.	w
nr	He can run fast.	w
fr	Ask if red is the right color.	w
vr	I have red shoes.	w
θr	Make the mouth red.	w
sr	The class rode on the bus.	w
zr	Eat these ripe apples.	w
ʃr	Is that dish red?	w
tʃr	Which rope is mine?	w
ʤr	Paint the cage red.	w
lr	Watch the ball roll.	w
ɝr	That is her red shoe.	r
ŋr	We had a long ride.	w
ir	She read the book.	w
ur	Did you read the book?	w
ɔr	We saw red shoes.	w

Table 4-16. PRODUCTIONS OF THE /r/ ITEMS FROM THE COARTICULATION ASSESSMENT IN MEANINGFUL LANGUAGE (KENNEY & PRATHER, 1984)

Syllable releasing		*Syllable arresting*	
bus ride	[r]	fire man	[r]
keep right	[w]	car door	[r]
bed room	[r]	four kids	[r]
park road	[w]	her shoe	[ɝ]

one of the two-word combinations in the picture form of the deep test is "cup sun." It is also hoped that the pictorial reference will make these utterances more meaningful to the child than simple sentence repetition tasks.

Common Error Patterns

Failure of the traditional sound-by-sound approach to coherently describe the errors of multiple phoneme–misarticulating children leads to the use of linguistic descriptive devices by speech-language pathologists. Since the early 1970s linguistic notation has been used by speech-language pathology researchers, and later clinicians, to describe error patterns occurring across phonemes. The devices used have included distinctive features (McReynolds & Engmann, 1975), phonological processes (Weiner, 1979), phonotactic constraints, and phonological rules (Elbert & Geirut, 1986).

Descriptions of children's misarticulations using distinctive features are capable of summarizing a child's misarticulation of a natural class of phonemes. Consider a child who produces the misarticulations such as the following: [di tup tud be ʔat]. ("The soup should be hot"). This child consistently produces stop consonants in words that adults produce as containing fricatives. Linguistic feature systems have been devised to describe such natural class differences. For example, Chomsky and Halle (1968) used a single two-level feature to describe the difference between stops and fricatives. The feature is called *continuant*. The two levels of this feature are + and −. A sound is +continuant if it does not involve a complete articulatory constriction (e.g., fricatives are +continuant). A sound is −continuant if it does involve a complete closure of the vocal tract (e.g., the affricates and stops are −continuant). Using this feature, the child who produces all fricatives as stops has apparently failed to distinguish +continuant from −continuant sounds.

Following Ingram's (1976) publication of *Phonological Disability in Children*, researchers and clinicians have investigated errors using phonological process notation. The processes include the errors that can be described by feature errors. For example, the production of fricatives as stops is typically called *stopping*. Processes also describe misarticulations in which sounds are not produced (e.g., cluster reduction would be used to describe the production of *stew* as [tu], and final-consonant deletion would be used to describe the production of *cat* as [kæ]). Processes were also used to describe feature errors occurring only in some contexts, called *assimilations*. A child who produces *Coke* as [kok] and *coat* as [tot] would be exhibiting an assimilation in which the place of articulation features of the [k] sound assimilate or become like those of [t] because [t] is in the word.

Although phonological process notation provides a description of children's misarticulations relative to the adult model, it may not describe the psychological processing that is involved in production of these errors. An alternative phonological description has suggested that a single phonological process may result from different forms of phonological knowledge

(Dinnsen & Elbert, 1984; Elbert & Gierut, 1986). For example, a final-consonant deletion may result from one of two kinds of errors. In the first, the child has not learned that words may have final consonants. This is described as a phonotactic constraint against word-final consonants. In the second, the child knows that the words affected contain final consonants but is deleting those consonants by using a rule.

To assess a child's articulation ability Elbert and Gierut (1986) wished to define a number of phonologically defined products of the child's organization: a phonetic inventory, a phonemic inventory, sequential constraints, and the underlying forms of certain morphemes. The phonetic inventory represents the speech sounds that the child produces but does not necessarily contrast at a phonemic level. Consider the fairly typical speech productions shown in Table 4-17. This child would be said to have misarticulated the adult phoneme /θ/ but is producing [θ] phones. This child certainly can physically produce [θ] because it appears regularly where adults would use an [s]. This child can also physiologically produce an [s] although it is inconsistently produced correctly.

The child's phonemic inventory represents contrasts that the child produces among speech sounds. The productions in Table 4-17 show that this child has both an [s] and a [θ] in his phonetic inventory, but he does not contrast these phonemically. Rather they appear to be interchangeable in some word forms.

In their typology of types of misarticulation Elbert and Gierut (1986) allowed for a category of errors in which a particular word or morpheme is produced with a syllable shape or phoneme error although others are not. They refer to such cases as *fossilized forms.* For example, if the child were to start to correctly produce other word-initial [s] words but maintained the error productions for *soap,* the form of this word would be described as fossilized.

A number of tests and analysis manuals have been constructed to measure commonly occurring error patterns. A list of these is included in Table 4-18.

The *Compton-Hutton Phonological Assessment* (Compton & Hutton, 1978) and *Phonological Process Analysis* (Weiner, 1979) tests provide picture stimuli to be used in gaining specific utterances. These utterances were chosen to test particular error patterns. For example, the Phonological Process Analysis elicits productions of the following words to measure "weak syllable deletion": *giraffe, elephant, telephone, umbrella, envelope,* and *pajamas.* The child's productions are scored as correct if all of the syllables are produced.

Table 4-17. EXAMPLE PRODUCTIONS OF FRICATIVES BY A CHILD

soap	[θoup], [soup]	bus	[bʌθ], [bʌs]
thumb	[fʌm]	bath	[bæf]
shoe	[θu]	bash	[bæθ]

Table 4-18. ARTICULATION TESTS THAT MEASURE OCCURRENCE OF COMMON ERROR PATTERNS INCLUDING SYLLABLE STRUCTURE ERRORS

Assessment of Phonological Processes Interstate Printers and Publishers Danville, IL
Compton-Hutton Phonological Assessment Carousel House San Francisco, CA
Elicited Articulatory System Evaluation Pro-Ed Austin, TX
Handbook of Clinical Phonology Taylor & Francis, Ltd. London, England
Natural Process Analysis John Wiley & Sons New York, NY
Phonological Process Analysis University Park Press Baltimore, MD
Procedures for the Phonological Analysis of Children's Language University Park Press Baltimore, MD

The authors of the *Handbook of Clinical Phonology* (Elbert & Gierut, 1986) and the *Assessment of Phonological Processes* (Hodson, 1980) provide lists of words to be elicited. Elbert and Gierut's words are elicited in single-word repetition responses, and the Hodson words are elicited through naming of objects that are assembled by the clinician.

The authors of *Natural Process Analysis* (Shriberg & Kwiatkowski, 1980) and *Procedures for the Phonological Analysis of Children's Language* (Ingram, 1981) provide instructions and forms for the analysis of children's spontaneous speech. Lowe (1986) provides forms for the Goldman-Fristoe Test of Articulation and the screening portion of the Templin-Darley test.

In the discussion that follows we will describe common error forms from a somewhat different perspective, using the lower levels of the verbal communication model from Chap. 1. In particular, error patterns will be described using a syllabic shape level, a phonemic level, and a production feature level.

Syllabic Shape Level. The infant's primary oral gestures to be organized into speech productions involve moving from a closed to open vocal tract. These primitive gestures are best suited to rhythmical production of repeated CV syllables (e.g., [dadada]). Children's development of articulation involves adding consonant clusters and syllable-final consonants to these more basic syllable shapes. The child must also develop the ability to produce controlled multisyllabic utterances.

Common errors occurring in this developmental process are described in Table 4-19. The transcribed words in this table are taken from the 4-year old's telling of the *Three Bears* story. This child approximates all of the syllables contained in the utterances produced. He also produced final consonants where appropriate. However, he did not always produce consonant clusters.

A similar pattern of syllable production errors is seen by reviewing this child's single-word productions from the Templin-Darley in Table 4-11. He approximated all of the syllables in the words. He did produce one error by adding a syllable (i.e., *sprinkler* [wɪŋkəlɚ]). However, this error is more likely to be related to the production of the three consonants in the middle of this word. He has added the vowel [ə], which breaks up this string of consonants. As in the spontaneous speech sample, he fails to produce all of the consonants in consonant clusters, especially clusters involving three consonants (e.g., *string* [wɪn] and *skates* [kets]).

Misarticulating children do not often produce only CV syllable shapes in monosyllabic words. More often failures to produce final consonants, clusters, or syllables interact with the levels of phonemes and meaningful linguistic units. For example, the 4-year old generally produces consonant clusters with a reduced number of consonants. However, he produces two-consonant clusters in which one of the consonants is a glide (e.g., [kwin] and [twɪns]). He also produces two consonants in clusters in which his [w] approximation of an /r/ is being used (e.g., [fwok] and [fwi]). A number of cases have been cited in the literature in which children will produce a particular class of word-final consonants such as stops, nasals, or fricatives before producing the other consonant types in word-final position. Such differences in development show the interaction of the syllable shape level with the other levels of the model (i.e., meaningful linguistic units, phonemes, and features)

Table 4-19. SYLLABIC ERROR ANALYSIS FOR THE 4-YEAR-OLD'S SPONTANEOUS SPEECH SAMPLE

Failure to produce all syllables
Failure to produce all syllable-final consonants
Failure to produce consonant clusters
  cold [koud] [kat]
  breaked [wek] [wekt]

Phonemic Level. As a child organizes a phonemic level to conform to that of the adult's usage, he or she will have a system that is incomplete in the phonemes and their contrasts with one another. Consider the productions listed in Table 4-17. Among the fricatives that this child produces, he does contrast [θ] and [f] productions as seen in the use of word-initial and word-final [θ] and [f], with no cases in which these sounds are used in the same position in the same words. However, even though he produces an [s] sound, he does not contrast it with [θ]. Multiple productions of a particular word that show differences in production of a particular consonant are one form of evidence that a child has not distinguished the speech sounds that are substitutable for one another in a word as different phonemes.

Analysis of the data in Table 4-11 shows that the 4-year old makes a number of these phonemic-level errors. /r/ is produced as [w], suggesting that this child does not distinguish /r/ and /w/ at a phonemic level. /θ/ is produced as [t] or [f], suggesting that /θ/, /t/, and /f/ are not separate phonemic categories for this child. Similarly, /ŋ/ is apparently not distinct from /d/, /f/, and /v/ in this child's organization of phonemes. Errors in production of /z/ suggest that this is not a separate phoneme distinguishable from /s/ (*feathers* [fɛvəs) and /d/ (*zipper* [dɪpə]). Furthermore, repetitions of a single word in different forms provide evidence that some contrasts are not complete. The 4-year old's productions show a number of cases in which contrasts between phonemes are incomplete. For example, adult /d/ is produced both as [d] in *cold, don't,* and *said* and as [t] in *said* and *cold.*

Providing a more complete description of a child's phonemic contrasts involves describing whether contrasts occur in all possible syllable structures or word positions. For example, the 4-year old does produce some appropriate [z]s (e.g., *music* [muzək]). Perhaps his failure to distinguish /z/ from other phonemes is bound to a particular set of word positions (e.g., word-initial). The analysis procedures provided by Elbert and Gierut (1986) seek to make such an analysis by assessing production of each consonant in each word position in minimal pairs of words. For example, the contrast between /p/ and /b/ can be heard in the words *pig* and *big;* the contrast between /k/ and /g/ is assessed in the word pairs *coat* and *goat.* Essentially, these authors suggested extending the "sound-in-word position" test construction to include (1) more than one example of each phoneme in each word position, and (2) words in each word position that provide for near-minimal pair contrasts of each phoneme.

An alternative strategy for analysis of a child's phonemic categorization is to measure the child's speech perception abilities. Although not often used clinically, such procedures can provide information about the child's phonemic categorization.

One procedure would be to assess the child's ability to point to the appropriate picture when given two choices that represent the phonemic contrast in question (Oller and Eilers, 1983). For example, a child who misarticulates /r/ as [w] might be asked to point to pictures of *wing* and *ring.* To produce a reliable assessment of this ability, the child must be observed in a number of repeated trials of this task. If the child is guessing, he or she will get the first trial correct 50 percent of the time. Each consecutively correct response reduces the probability that a child is only guessing. A child would have to make at least five consecutive correct responses so that the probability that he or she was guessing would be below the 5 percent level. Other possibilities that allow for one error include seven correct out of eight, eight out of nine, and nine out of ten. An alternative is to use Locke's (1980) procedure in which the child is asked to compare his own production to that of the clinician. For example, a child is asked to name pictures containing word-initial /r/s. The clinician follows each response with a question such as "Did you say [rɪŋ]?" or "Did you say [wɪŋ]?" The clinician scores these with respect to their correctness (i.e., whether the child recognized the comparison between his production and that of the clinician). Since these can be scored as correct/incorrect, the probability of guessing the correct answer is the same as in the preceding procedure.

Feature Level. When a child does not produce a particular articulatory gesture during speech production, a whole class of phonemes will be produced in error. For example, a child who does not lift the tip of the tongue toward the alveolar ridge will misarticulate all of the alveolar phonemes. An alternative for such a child would be to approximate alveolar consonants with velar articulations. Thus, /t/ would be produced as [k], /d/ would be produced as [g], and so forth. Common patterns of feature errors are listed in Table 4-20, with examples from the 4-year old's Templin-Darley productions.

Although each of these error patterns is seen in this child's productions, they are certainly not universal to all phonemes or word positions. For example, his gliding of liquids is restricted to /r/ not /l/ and is not even present in all productions of /r/. When such feature errors are consistent, a number of phonemic contrasts would be impossible at the phoneme level.

A number of authors have suggested measuring what is possible for an individual child at the feature level by listing the sounds that are produced (Shriberg & Kwiatkowski, 1980; Elbert & Gierut, 1986). This listing is called

Table 4-20. COMMON FEATURE PRODUCTION ERRORS EXEMPLIFIED BY THE 4-YEAR-OLD'S SPONTANEOUS SPEECH SAMPLE

Fricatives or affricates produced as stops thumb [tʌm], there [deə], zipper [dɪpə]
Liquids produced as syllable-initial glides or syllable-final vowel off-glides red [wɛd], arrow [ɛwou]
Palatals and velars produced as alveolars chair [se]
Linguals produced as labials teeth [tif]

a *phonetic inventory*. A phonetic inventory of the sounds produced by the 4-year old is shown in Table 4-21.

From this list, we see that this child produced all of the consonants except /ŋ/, /θ/, /ŋ/, and /ʒ/. Inasmuch as each of these sounds should have occurred in the sample, it can be concluded that these sounds are not part of this child's phonetic inventory. That is, he does not appear to use these sounds to represent words. It is possible that some low-level physiological inability is present in this child's failure to move the tongue to the front teeth. The other sounds do appear in the child's speech output so we can conclude that the child has the physiological capability to associate the required articulatory gestures for each of these.

Feature organization interacts with the phonemic and syllabic levels of organization within words and even within whole utterances. Children's production of a particular gesture within a phoneme may be affected by the gestures, or features, in nearby phonemes. This type of error is most often called an *assimilation,* in which some of the feature characteristics of neighboring speech sounds are produced within the target sound. Some common assimilations in children's speech are shown in Table 4-22, with examples from the 4-year old's Templin-Darley.

Table 4-21. CONSONANT SOUNDS PRODUCED BY THE 4-YEAR-OLD IN THE TEMPLIN-DARLEY SCREENING TEST INDICATED BY AN x

Stops						*Nasals*			*Fricatives*								*Affricates*		*Glides*		*Liquids*	
p	b	t	d	k	g	m	n	ŋ	f	v	θ	ð	s	z	ʃ	ʒ	tʃ	ʤ	w	j	l	r
x	x	x	x	x	x	x	x		x	x			x	x	x		x	x	x	x	x	x

Table 4-22. COMMON ASSIMILATIONS PRODUCED BY CHILDREN

Palatals and velars produced as alveolars or dentals when produced near alveolars or dentals

Alveolars and dentals produced as palatals or velars when produced near palatals or velars

Linguals produced as labials when produced near labials, e.g., valentines [væl taims] (/n/ affected by /v/)

Stops and affricates produced as fricatives when produced near fricatives or glides

Voiceless word-initial consonants produced as voiced

Voiced word-final consonants produced as voiceless, e.g., sled [slɛt]

DOES THIS CHILD HAVE THE NECESSARY STRUCTURAL AND PHYSIOLOGICAL MOVEMENT PATTERNS?

When a child does not produce a whole class of speech sounds at the phonetic level, a logical question is whether or not the child has a subtle neuromotor or anatomical structure deficit that impairs articulatory ability. A time-honored procedure in the speech-language pathologist's repertoire has been the oral-peripheral mechanism examination. In large part, this procedure was developed because of the earlier theoretical view that children misarticulate because of subtle organic problems. The oral-peripheral mechanism examination attempts to assess whether or not a child has the anatomical structures and neuromotor coordinations necessary for production of all articulatory gestures.

Table 4-23 provides a checklist of structures and gestures that are typically assessed in such an examination. The clinician should be quite wary of making claims about the organicity of a child's misarticulation based on results of such an evaluation. Many of the gestures that are asked for in such an exam are embedded in speech sounds (e.g., tongue-tip raising is assessed in [t] production). Children who misarticulate a particular sound have not organized its connections with the gestural system to the same degree as nonmisarticulating children. Thus, the clinician may conclude that the gesture is at fault when it is really the phonemic organization that is lacking. You can demonstrate this effect in your own speech by repeating the syllables [ŋu ŋu ŋu] and [nu nu nu] as rapidly as possible. Your rate is probably better and your productions smoother in [nu], a combination of gestures that is often used by English speakers in which the phoneme /n/ occurs frequently in CV syllables. You will probably produce [ŋu] more clumsily because you are not used to producing a syllable-initial [ŋ], which does not occur in English words.

On the other hand, when a clinician asks a child to "Smile or spread your lips," the child may not understand that the clinician is looking for a maximal lip-spreading gesture, or that he or she is expected to execute such a gesture as rapidly as possible. Since we are mostly interested in the child's ability to coordinate auditory, visual, and motor features, most of the tasks suggested below can be executed as imitations of the clinician's modeling of each gesture or sound production and thus are a use of sound or syllable imitation procedures as described earlier.

Lips

The examiner looks at the lips for any obvious clefting or surgical repair of a cleft. Of primary structural interest is whether or not enough tissue is present to make a complete closure of the lips. A drooping of the corners of the lips may indicate damage to the facial nerve. This nerve also supplies

Table 4-23. ORAL-PERIPHERAL MECHANISM EXAMINATION CHECKLIST

LIPS	
Describe appearance:	
Rounding	"Pucker your lips" "Show me a kiss" "Say [u]"
Spreading	"Spread your lips" "Smile" "Say [i]"
Closure	"Close your lips and don't let me open them" "Say [ip]" "Say [ip ip ip]"
Opening	"Say [pi]" "Say [pi pi pi]"
TEETH	
Missing teeth	
Occlusion	
MANDIBLE	
Describe resting position:	
Lowering	"Open your mouth slowly as wide as you can" "Say [pa]" "Say [pa pa pa]
Raising	"Open your mouth wide. Now close it" "Say [ap]" "Say [ap ap ap]"
HARD PALATE	
Description	
VELUM	
Describe resting position:	
Raising	"Say [a]" "Say [ab]"
Lowering	"Open your mouth and breathe through your nose" "Say [a]" "Say [am]"
TONGUE TIP	
Appearance	
Forward-backward	"Touch tip of tongue to teeth then behind teeth" "Say [θ]"
Up-down	"Touch tongue tip behind teeth" "Say [iti]" "Say [ata]"

Table 4-23. (continued)

Groove	"Blow air straight ahead with tongue tip extended" "Say [isi]"
TONGUE BODY	
Appearance	
Forward-backward	"Say [i]" "Say [u]"
Up-down	"Say [ki]" "Say [ku]"

the area around the eyes, and these may also look droopy. The basic movements to be assessed are those of *rounding-spreading* and *opening-closing*. Keep in mind while watching these movements that the mandible may aid in the opening-closing gesture. Movement of the lips can be isolated to a certain degree by holding down the child's mandible and requesting that lip closure be made. In assessing these basic movements, the clinician is looking for the speed and smoothness of the movements.

Teeth

The teeth are described while the examiner asks the child to open the mouth. Of particular interest are missing incisors that may affect the hissing quality of strident sounds or teeth that are displaced into unusual locations that interfere with movement of the tongue. Malocclusions, particularly open bite, are noted as possibly affecting fricative production. Occlusion is observed by asking the child to bite down on the back teeth. The examiner moves the lips away using a tongue depressor to look at the biting relationship between the upper and lower first molars. If the upper molar is approximately one-half tooth ahead of the lower, the occlusion is normal. If the upper molar is behind the lower, it is referred to as a class II malocclusion; if the upper molar is more than one-half tooth ahead, it is called a class III malocclusion.

Mandible

The resting position of the mandible should be up so that the mouth is closed. However, the presence of a lowered mandible may have more to do with an inability to breathe through the nose than with any neuromotor problem of mandibular movement. Movements of the mandible should be symmetrical, not favoring movement to one side or the other.

Hard Palate

The primary concern regarding the hard palate is the presence of clefts or holes (fistulae). The relative size of the palatal vault is judged with respect to the size of the tongue. Palatal vaults may range from relatively flat to relatively peaked.

Velum

A structural description of the velum should note if it appears to be symmetrical or if it appears to hang to one side. The relative arch of the faucial pillars may be described if they are apparently too tight or angular. It is quite difficult to judge the length of the velum with respect to the depth of the pharynx. The movement of the velum is typically described with respect to speed and symmetry. Some indirect measures are often used. Clinicians will hold a mirror under the nose of the child while asking for production of vowel and fricative sounds. If the mirror fogs, then there is an apparent leak at the velopharyngeal port.

Tongue

The tongue is described with respect to size relative to the oral cavity. Clinicians also look for small rapid movements (fasciculations) while the tongue is at rest. Symmetry and speed of movements are judged. Strength can also be judged by asking the child to push against a tongue depressor placed on the outside of the right and left cheek.

REPORTING RESULTS

Researchers ultimately seek to tell others about the results of their studies by writing papers for journals or by presenting reports to technical or poster sessions at association meetings. These reports take a standardized form that presents specific questions asked in a study, observations that are related to each question, and a discussion of how these results should change the study of a particular topic area. Clinicians write reports about patients that should address clinical questions asked, observations made, and recommendations about what should be done on behalf of that patient.

Clinical writing, like research writing, should make as clear as possible the relationship between the clinical questions asked, the data supplied by test administration, and the recommendations. One way of achieving this purpose is to organize the report with respect to the clinical questions. In this section a report regarding the 4-year old's articulation performance is presented as a demonstration.

The first section describes the child's articulatory performance by first answering the question of age-appropriateness of his ability. The claim is made that his articulation ability is not normally developing, and this is backed by the observation that Joe's performance on the Templin-Darley was more than two standard deviations below his age group's average score.

Joe's articulation ability is below that expected of a child his age as seen by his raw score of 12 on the Templin Darley, which places him below the second percentile for four year olds.

The next paragraph describes his inappropriate approximations of adult articulation performance. This section is organized from syllable level to phonemic level to feature level. Errors at the syllable level are described with respect to affected phonemes. Phonemic errors are described with respect to features involved.

In single-word productions, he produced single consonant approximations of consonant clusters in 14 in 25 words (e.g., *spoon* [pun]). Correctly approximated clusters included [tw, kw, sl]. He produced stop and labial approximations of dental fricatives that were never produced (e.g., *thumb* [tʌm] and *teeth* [tif]). He produced inconsistent fricative and stop approximations for the affricates (e.g., *chair* [se] and *watch* [wats] and alveolar approximations of palatals (e.g., *dishes* [disəz]). Similar approximations were produced in a story telling task in which his overall score of consonants correct was 64 percent.

Each statement is accompanied by an example utterance that is used as evidence. The type of speaking task, single-word naming versus storytelling, is also made clear. Numerical indices are provided where possible.

The report will ultimately conclude with statements about clinical goals and a rationale for these.

Due to Joe's restricted abilities to express propositions beyond the descriptive level, treatment will focus on expanding his abilities to organize concepts in storytelling tasks. Modeling and feedback regarding articulatory ability will be included in this process. Percentage correct syllables and percentage of cluster approximations will be tracked for improvements.

In this case, as in many in which the child misarticulates many phonemes, a concomitant problem exists regarding the child's ability to organize propositions, concepts, and higher-level language symbols. As a result, the articulation goals of improving this child's syllabic shape and phonemic organizations will be approached within an overall program to improve language organizational abilities.

SUMMARY

In this chapter we sought to show similarities between the clinical process and the conduct of empirical studies. We exemplified this process using data from two children's responses to a group of articulation tests. New tests are published constantly, but the process remains essentially the same. In the following chapter we look at what the clinician does in an attempt to improve children's phonetic organization within their communication attempts. One of the characteristics of the treatment process is that the clinician continues to measure changes—improvements, it is hoped—in a child's articulation ability over time. The questions asked by the clinician during the first diagnostic meeting with a child were only the first questions: Clinicians continue to pose and answer questions regarding their patients

CLASSROOM ACTIVITIES

1. Record an interview with a friend about the development of their normally developing preschool child. Frame your questions so that you ask them directly, in a logical order. As a class, take notes and organize the information into a report.
2. Give an oral-peripheral mechanism examination to a classmate, then to a child. Note how you have to change your instructions and models for the child and how their responses differ.
3. Divide the class into small groups. Make the groups responsible for presenting information about a commercial test of articulation. Demonstrate its use for the class, and discuss its scoring, normative data, and underlying view of misarticulation.
4. Analyze the performance of the children you recorded for the last chapter using the syllable level, phoneme level, and feature level tables provided in this chapter.

CHAPTER 5

Treating Children's Phonetic Ability

Topics in this chapter include

- Treatment Components
  - Goals
  - Procedures
- Treatment Programs
  - Treatment Program Review
  - Suggested Treatment Strategies

This chapter discusses approaches to treatment of children's sound production errors. At its conclusion we will present two approaches to articulation treatment that we believe to be most useful for children at different stages of language development: those in the conceptual phase and those in the semantic phase. Like all treatment programs that have been developed prior to these, and those that will follow, our programs were developed with knowledge of work done by others who preceded us. Thus, the procedures we use are never completely novel. Often they are rearrangements of procedures used by others. To understand our approach, and those of others, it is necessary to be able to dissect the therapy process into components that can be contrasted and compared. We seek to present such a dissection in the first section of this chapter.

Once we acknowledge basic components, we can study the makeup of various approaches to articulation treatment that have been developed in the past. In the second section of this chapter, entitled "Treatment Program Review," we analyze some of the better known treatment approaches in an historical overview of their development.

The final section, entitled "Suggested Treatment Strategies," reflects our current views on structuring articulation therapy. We advocate use of two general approaches to accommodate the child's ability to view language as an abstract system. The intent of these approaches is to alter the child's verbal communication system by adding missing information to the child's syllabic, phonemic, and featural levels of knowledge organization. These organizational levels are altered by the child as he or she constructs speech acts to communicate with the clinician. The clinician uses speech acts to help the child organize his or her next speech production attempt. Following a child's speech production, the clinician provides feedback regarding the child's speech production errors in an attempt to improve the child's organization. Finally, the clinician provides another opportunity for the child to organize information in production of another speech act, and the cycle is repeated. Each time the child prepares a speech act, he or he is using and reinforcing the pattern of connections that represent the organization of the utterance produced. The clinician provides information regarding how the child's organization differs from others around him or her and how that organization helps or hinders communication attempts. The clinician helps the child reformulate utterances so that their production will reshape the child's system.

For the child in the *semantic phase* of language development, this process takes place fairly directly in the context of "working on the child's speech." For the child in the *conceptual phase* of development, the process is embedded within activities in which the child is communicating about some topic, usually a story that is constructed, acted out, or read. The younger child's focus is not on "working on speech" but on "telling a story." The clinician's focus remains the same.

TREATMENT COMPONENTS

Ideally, treatment is based on a carefully designed plan that incorporates knowledge of normal and disordered articulation processes. Much like the researcher, the clinician plans activities in a scientifically based manner. As illustrated in Table 5-1 the overall method of planning treatment is similar to the researcher's planning of an experiment. All too often, clinicians labor under the illusion that their work is inferior to or less "scientific" than their fellow professionals whose major responsibility is research. This should not be the case.

The researcher starts with a question about the nature of human communication processes. The clinician seeks to alter some aspect of the patient's communication processing that is judged to be less than optimal. The researcher designs and executes an experiment in which subjects experience particular stimulus inputs that are thought to require the communication processes under question. The clinician plans and implements a treatment strategy in which patients experience planned sensory inputs that are thought to lead to changes in communication processing. Both researcher and clinician must plan for subject and patient behavioral responses to make results of their work observable. The researcher uses these observed behaviors to evaluate questions asked; the clinician uses them to evaluate effectiveness of treatment. The sections that follow elaborate on each of these phases of the treatment process. The first section discusses the goals that clinicians set for their patients. The second discusses basic procedures used by the clinician. The third discusses measurement strategies.

GOALS

Any treatment plan can be described as a series of goals to be attained. In many clinical settings, particularly the public schools, goals for an individual child are mandated by law and must be written in behavioral responses that the child is expected to produce at the end of some therapy period. In plan-

Table 5-1. COMPARISON OF A RESEARCHER'S ACTIVITIES AND THOSE OF A CLINICIAN IN THERAPY

Research design	*Treatment plan*
Statement of a question	Statement of goals
Methods of a study	Treatment activities
Results of the study performance	Measurement of patient performance

ning treatment, clinicians typically deal with two levels of goals: generalized goals and behavioral objectives.

Generalized Goals

As implied by their title, *generalized goals* refer to long-range expectations of patient performance. Such goals are like expectations we set for ourselves when we enter college and our generalized goal is to obtain a degree. Similarly, at the start of each semester we establish general goals for the successful completion of various courses we have either selected or were required to take. In either case, successful completion of these goals depends on day-to-day performance, analogous to the more discrete behavioral obectives discussed next.

Not only are generalized goals long-range, they tend to be relatively nonspecific. The general's order to advance an army 20 miles one day takes on many different characteristics depending on existing conditions. It is one thing to move a national guard unit via truck convoy up Interstate 75 from Detroit to Pontiac in 1988 and another to move 20 miles via landing craft and against armed opposition at Omaha beach on D-day. The most general goals for articulatory performance might be stated as "to improve speech production" or "to increase articulation ability." But the particulars of achieving these goals may be quite different for individual children.

Generalized goals will differ in composition according to components of the model of articulation processes used by a clinician. Generalized goals for articulation treatment based on our verbal communication model could be stated as follows: increase the complexity of the child's system at the syllabic structure level, phonemic level, and feature level. These statements imply our view that development of articulation is an additive process, one in which the child is continually refining his or her productions to improve communicative efficiency. Other clinicians, using a phonological process model, as described in Chap. 2, would write goals to "eliminate the use of stopping of fricatives, or final-consonant deletion," or other error patterns.

Table 5-2 shows some more specific goal statements at the various levels of the verbal communication model with respect to common patterns of misarticulation. Since misarticulating children's general tendency at the syllabic level is to produce single CV syllables, general goals for improvement include expanding the child's system to include multisyllabic meaningful units, consonant clusters, and meaningful unit final consonants. Common error patterns at the phonemic and feature levels interact to such a degree that they are presented together and organized by feature. Typical patterns of development with respect to manner of articulation involve failures to develop phonemic contrasts between stops and fricatives, stops and affricates, stops and glides, and liquids and glides. Differentiation of place of articulation commonly involves failures to differentiate labial from lingual consonants and front from back lingual consonants, and failure to differ-

Table 5-2. GENERALIZED TREATMENT GOALS RELATED TO LEVELS OF THE VERBAL COMMUNICATION MODEL AND COMMON MISARTICULATION PATTERNS

Syllable level
- Increase production of unstressed syllables
- Increase production of final consonants
- Increase production of consonant clusters

Phoneme and feature levels
- Manner of articulation contrasts
  - Increase contrast between stops and fricatives
  - Increase contrast between stops and affricates
  - Increase contrast between stops and nasals
  - Increase contrast between liquids and glides
- Place of articulation contrasts
  - Increase contrast between labial and lingual consonants
  - Increase contrast between front and back consonants
  - Increase place contrasts within words
- Voicing contrasts
  - Increase contrast between voiced and voiceless consonants
- Nasality contrasts
  - Increase contrast between stops and nasals

entiate place of articulation among consonants within a word (assimilations). Voicing errors are common and involve tendencies to produce voiced prevocalic consonants and voiceless postvocalic consonants. Failure to produce nasality appropriately results in lack of contrasts between stops and nasals.

Generalized goals may serve as the basis for a treatment plan when dealing with the young child who produces many misarticulations. As seen in Chap. 3, such children are likely to have disordered processing of language at all levels. Our approach to such children is to seek improvements in *all levels of language processing simultaneously*. The 4-year old referred to in Chap. 4 who misarticulated many phonemes was treated in this fashion. Generalized articulation goals that were suitable for him included the following:

Increase production of consonant clusters
Increase contrast between liquids and glides

These goals were approached within an overall plan of treatment that also sought to increase this child's abilities to express conceptual relationships using conventional language structures in narratives.

Behavioral Objectives

In contrast to the general goal, behavioral objectives are highly specific in nature. They alert the clinician and patient to exactly what must be done, under what conditions, and with what degree of success. To use such objectives the clinician must be aware of three key terms: behavior, conditions, and criterion.

Behavior. *Behavior* refers to any speech or physical (gestural) activity performed by the patient. The use of an observable behavior as a key part of any behavioral objective is demanded by the scientific need for empiricism. As you will recall, empiricism demands that claims about scientific knowledge must be observable and reliably judged by any interested scientist. They are just as important for the clinician because improvements in a child's organization of syllables, phonemes, and features in the production and perception of speech must be made obvious so that both the patient and clinician can tell if progress is being made.

When writing objectives, clinicians should consider the degree of abstractness of the terms used. A term is more abstract as it is elevated above the level of observable behaviors. Table 5-3 shows two sets of terms. Those in the left column are abstract relative to those on the right. A goal to "develop an awareness of the difference between stops and fricatives" is relatively abstract: It does not tell the reader what a child will be doing to show that he or she has attained "awareness." A number of child behaviors could be used to show that a child is aware of differences between stops and fricatives. The child could "point" to pictures when named with labels that are differentiated only by a difference between stop and fricative manner (e.g., pictures of the letters *c* and *t*, or pictures of a raging sea and a cup of tea. Or the child could "label" these pictures using articulatory gestures resulting in fricative and stop-initial consonants.

Organization of the various levels of the verbal communication model, an obvious abstraction, must be attested to with observations of a child's speech acts. Mager (1962) was describing the observability of behavioral objectives when he wrote the following:

> An instructional objective describes an intended outcome rather than a description or summary of content.
>
> One characteristic of a usefully stated objective is that it is stated in behavioral, or performance, terms that describe what the learner will be DOING when demonstrating his achievement of the objective.
>
> An instructional objective is a statement that describes an intended outcome of instruction.
>
> An objective is meaningful to the extent it communicates an instructional intent to its reader, and does so to the degree that it describes or defines the terminal behavior expected of the learner.
>
> An objective will communicate your intent to the degree you have described what the learner will be DOING when demonstrating his achievement and how you will know when he is doing it.

Table 5-3. TERMS USED IN WRITING BEHAVIORAL OBJECTIVES WITH RELATIVELY HIGH ABSTRACTNESS AND RELATIVELY LOW ABSTRACTNESS

High abstraction	***Low abstraction***
Develop an awareness of	Discriminate
Understand	Point
Know	Label
Communicate	Produce speech
Syllabic complexity	Consonant clusters

Write a separate statement for each objective; the more statements you have, the better chance you have of making clear your intent.

If you give each learner a copy of your objectives, you may not have to do much else.

Similarly, Andrews (1971) stated that

> most unsatisfactory therapy has been performed by students who have not had in mind exactly what they wished to accomplish during the therapy session. While in nearly all instances the student had written one or more goals for the session, these were invariably vague and unmeasurable. One way to overcome this is to write each goal in terms of the behavior or performance desired of the client.

The key terms in the descriptions of objectives given above are *outcome, doing,* and *performance.* All of these relate to the patient, not the clinician. Your generalized goal may be to increase a child's phonemic contrast. But your behavioral objectives must somehow demonstrate that this outcome is shown in something the child is doing that he or she was not doing prior to your clinical intervention. That is, the goal should describe the performance that you expect from the child.

The generalized goals in Table 5-2 can be made less abstract by including statements regarding whether the child will show these "increases" in productive or perceptual behaviors. At the syllabic level, a perceptual goal might be stated as "John will show a knowledge of consonant clusters by pointing to appropriate pictures when the words *sea* and *ski* are spoken by the clinician." A similar productive goal might state "John will label pictures of *sea* and *ski* using appropriate consonant productions." The use of perceptual goals along with productive goals is one of the issues that contrasts some of the major treatment programs developed over the years.

Conditions. As discussed in previous chapters, a child's articulation of a speech sound may be better in some *conditions* and worse in others. The conditions of a child's performance during therapy are primarily determined by the situation that has been constructed by the clinician. The clinician may provide the child with an utterance to be repeated. Articulation of such imitated responses is typically enhanced relative to the child's "spontaneous" responses, which may be prompted by a clinician's request for information during a conversation about some topic, while engaged in some building project, or while telling a story. In general, the more structure the clinician supplies regarding the speech act to be produced by way of sensory inputs to the child, the more organization will be apparent in the child's responses. The clinician's manipulation of these conditions is used to help the child reorganize his or her conceptual system.

When constructing a treatment program, clinicians typically choose to make the conditions of the child's articulatory performance provide greater structure of the verbal responses at the beginning of teaching some aspect of language. The clinician then allows the child to assume more of the organizational task as therapy progresses. In the beginning of treatment, the clinician will provide a variety of cues, models, and instructions to enhance the child's chances of including all of the appropriate features in a speech sound's production. As therapy progresses, the clinician will use fewer cues and prompts so that only natural cues related to speaking situations are necessary for the child to maintain appropriate speech sound production.

The utterances demanded of the child will be made more complex as therapy progresses. The manner in which utterance complexity is manipulated is partially determined by the clinician's view of what is the important determining factor or factors in the cause and maintenance of misarticulation.

A clinician who believes in the primacy of sensory-motor factors will increase syllable length and syllable complexity of utterances produced by the child. He or she may ask the child to introspect about individual gestures used to construct these utterances and make further judgments about the adequacy of the speech sounds produced.

The clinician who believes in the primacy of cognitive-linguistic factors may start by eliciting utterances that are cognitively easier to produce and progressively move to more difficult utterances. The clinician may ask the child questions that require differing levels of language processing on the part of the child as exemplified by Blank and colleagues' (1978) levels I through IV. Example questions at each level are shown in Table 5-4. A level I request requires that the child use language in reference to sensory information that usually captures the child's attention. A level II request maintains its focus on current actions and objects but requires that the child focus attention on particular sensory information. A level III request requires that the child reorganize his or her perceptions of what is immediately present in compliance with the language used by the clinician (e.g., naming objects that are *not* present). In level IV, the child must predict and explain reasons for semantic relationships among objects and actions. The speech used by a child in these conditions will include longer utterances with more complex sentence structure. Both of these are surface characteristics that tend to be related to decreased articulation ability.

Table 5-4. REQUESTS FOR CHILD VERBAL RESPONSES DIFFERING IN LEVEL OF COMPLEXITY ACCORDING TO BLANK AND COLLEAGUES' LEVELS

LEVEL I MATCHING PERCEPTION	
Naming an object seen	"What is this?"
Naming an object heard	"What did you hear?"
Naming an object touched	"What did you touch?"
Imitating a simple sentence	"Say this. . . ."
Remembering a pictured object	"What did you see?"
LEVEL II SELECTIVE ANALYSIS OF PERCEPTION	
Naming an object described by its function	"What do you use to cut paper?"
Recalling items named in a statement	"What did Johnny take to school?"
Recalling other information from a previous statement	"Who? What? Where?"
Naming characteristics of objects	"What color is it?"
Naming functions of objects	"What does it do?"
Identifying differences	"How are these different?"
Citing an example within a category	"Name a bird."
LEVEL III REORDERING PERCEPTION	
Describing subsequent events	"What will happen next?"
Assuming role of another person	"What could he say?"
Generalizing from a series of events	"What happened to all of these?"
Unifying a series of pictures	"Tell a story about these"
Naming an object by exclusion	"Tell me something that is not big or red"
Naming a class of objects by exclusion	"What animals do not have legs?"
Defining words	"What is a . . . ?"
LEVEL IV REASONING ABOUT PERCEPTION	
Predicting change in location	"Where will . . . ?"
Predicting change in structure	"What will happen if . . . ?"
Justifying a prediction	"Why will it . . . ?"
Identifying cause of an event	"Why did that happen?"
Explaining the means to a goal	"Why use a cup?"
Explaining the construction of objects	"Why is this round?"
Explaining the obstacles to an action	"Why can't we . . . ?"

Criteria. The third component of a behavioral objective is a criterion for determining when a particular goal has been achieved. For example, "John will correctly imitate [s] + V syllables in 18 of 20 syllables" contains a 90 percent correct criterion. Criteria are sometimes used to determine when a child is ready to advance from one stage of a treatment program to another. They are also used to determine when a child's treatment program can be terminated.

Unfortunately, we do not currently have much research that would support the use of any particular criterion for either of these purposes. For example, in treatment programs in which a stage of syllable imitations is followed by picture-labeling responses, no one has shown that children who reach a 90 percent criterion in the first stage do better in the second phase than those who reach a 70 percent criterion. The same thing can be said of criteria for terminating therapy. Data from a study of elementary school children who misarticulated /s/ or /r/ suggested that a 75 percent correct criterion in conversational speech may be sufficient for future success (Diedrich & Bangert, 1980). However, we cannot readily generalize such a conclusion to younger children who misarticulate many phonemes.

PROCEDURES

The clinician provides a plan related to what the child is expected to learn in treatment and she must also devise a strategy for causing change in the child's verbal communication processing system. Basic to a clinician's strategy are choices among a variety of clinical factors. In the sections that follow, we present a review of some of these factors. First is the role taken by the clinician. Every clinician should have an underlying notion of the role to execute while interacting with children. Since a chief part of any role assumed by a clinician involves talking to children, the second section is aimed at providing some information useful in learning how to successfully communicate with children. The third section discusses tools the clinician can use to alter a child's verbal communication skills.

Clinician's Role

Treatment programs assume some form of social interaction between clinician and patient. Within this interaction, each person—clinician and patient—assumes a particular role. It is the clinician's responsibility to set this interaction stage in such a manner that a child's progress in development of speech production is enhanced.

Consider the roles you and your physician play. You periodically ask this person to assess your physical condition and make recommendations. The physician runs tests and makes recommendations based on the findings. Sometimes the things you are asked to do are easy and have an immediate payoff (e.g., you are suffering from a throat pain and you basically need to take a prescribed medicine and stay off your feet for a weekend). In this case, the physician's role was largely that of a diagnostician. Sometimes the things you are asked to do involve altering your life-style (e.g., your blood pressure is high and the physician instructs you to lose weight, stop smoking, and exercise for half an hour every day). The physician's job must now expand beyond the role of diagnostician to that of a counselor who must convince you to take a course of action. In most cases the physician will attempt to do this by explaining your condition to you and trying to logically convince you that the course of action is useful and necessary.

Ideally the clinician also plays the role of someone who seeks to understand a person's problem and to bring that person to an understanding of their problem. To be understanding involves a process of acute abstracting or "noticing" on the part of the clinician. The clinician hears more than the patient intends in their utterances. In the case of a person with misarticulations, the clinician notices how speech sounds are articulated at the gestural movement level, what patterns of misarticulation exist, how the misarticulations interact with other levels of communication, and so forth. Speech-language pathologists stand alone in their knowledge of speech disorders, including assessment and treatment. We, more than any other professional, view those with whom we interact as being language users or abusers. From television hucksters who cleverly peddle profit-motivated wares, to the child who stutters or misarticulates, we are simultaneously aware of the simplicity and complexity of human communication. Some of this knowledge must be imparted to the child, either directly or indirectly.

Speech and language are intertwined with the uniqueness of the individual. The speech and language of any human is as individualistic as fingerprints, eye or hair color, gait, or handwriting. The very automaticity of a person's speech production and the manner in which it is closely interrelated with other aspects of cognition and behavior *make it difficult for the client to see the problem as abstractly as we do.* Thus, we must be specialists in broad aspects of human behavior because we manipulate behavioral change embedded in the total cognitive and affective personality of the client. By accepting a child into treatment, the clinician seeks to become an active and positive agent in changing the child's cognitive organization for speech production/perception. The clinician must become highly skilled at directing the client to willingly experiment with doing things differently. The clinician wants to instill in the patient a willingness to experiment with speech sound production. To succeed at this, the clinician must establish the patient's interest in speech and confidence in the clinician. In turn, the clinician must be *interesting, confident,* and *trustworthy.* At the very least the clinician must be *personally* willing to experiment and demonstrate different aspects of speech sound production.

As an initial step, the clinician should cultivate in the patient the sincere belief that he or she is special, not special in a negative or animated way, but special in a *soft-spoken, sensitive, positive* way. Animated speech behaviors of the stereotypical kindergarten or early elementary teacher have no place in the treatment room. As clinicians we are not teaching a lesson or talking down to robots awaiting programming. Rather, we are talking *with* someone who must take an active role in helping themselves.

No clinician can assist the older child in effecting positive behavioral and cognitive change without first achieving his or her permission. In many cases this involves evoking an interest in speech production. The clinician can explain to the child how articulatory gestures are used to produce speech sounds, how speech sounds differ in one context or another, and how the sounds used in words change. While examining these aspects of speech production, the clinician informs the child that this knowledge makes *him or her* special, not because the child talks differently from friends, but because the child knows more about talking than the friends do. Each newly grasped piece of knowledge is put to practical use as rapidly as possible so that it may be used in communication situations, thus altering the child's communication system connection strengths toward the adult norm.

For the child who is too young to view speech as an abstract system whose words, syllables, and speech sounds can be talked about and manipulated like objects, the clinician seeks to help the child communicate in a situation that is meaningful to the child. As the child is using language for some purpose, the clinician provides feedback regarding how well the message was received and what portions of the message were not understood. Having given the child some useful information, the clinician provides an opportunity for the child to reformulate the speech act and try it again. In so doing, the cognitive connections among the child's propositions, concepts, and meaningful units become more closely aligned to those of the clinician.

Our first responsibility is to regard each child or patient as unique and important; our final responsibility is to convince them that we are right. The road to achieving such responsibilities should be regarded as a challenge. As clinicians we learn to be personally objective and positively critical. How do we perceive what *we* do, as we review a videotape, and carefully evaluate *our* performance as related to that of the patient? Do *we*, as clinicians, hold primary or secondary responsibility in the treatment process? Are *we* as willing to accept the responsibility for patient failure as readily as silent commendation for our success?

These are questions we must ask and grow wiser, it is hoped, in seeking the answers. Every clinician who confronts a patient should do so with an understanding that ultimate success is based on knowledge, experience, understanding, and responsibility.

General Procedures

First and foremost, the clinician is involved in a continuing dialogue with the child. Both are using speech acts to accomplish their purposes at any particular moment. Inasmuch as increasing the child's speech production abilities is the clinician's primary purpose, the clinician's speech acts must continually encourage the child to produce speech acts. What are some of the techniques *you* can use to keep children talking or to help them to express themselves? Basically, they involve choosing topics that are of *interest to the child* and *really listening* to what the child says. These two aspects can be built into your treatment goals and in your role.

Consider the characteristics of people you enjoy talking to and those you would rather avoid. The interesting person talks about the same topics you would choose to talk about. The boring person talks about himself, *his* job, *his* hobby, *his* problems. The interesting person pays attention to your comments and considers your position on a topic in formulating his or her own comments. The boring person ignores your point of view and your comments as unimportant or argues against them without really considering their worth.

Perhaps the interesting person truly is enthralled by the same aspects of life that you are, and you have found a kindred soul who likes golf and gin rummy as much as you do. In that case, they will naturally interact with you conversationally in a manner that encourages your conversation. On the other hand, some persons school themselves in being conversationalists. Sales representatives should possess the techniques necessary to make you feel good about your conversations with them. They are probably doing this by structuring the conversation so that you talk mostly about topics of your own choice. The turn in the conversation that takes you to a discussion of your abysmal life insurance situation will probably go largely unnoticed.

One of the first things you can do to show that you are interested in the child is to take notice of something special about him or her that day. Speech is but one factor in the constellation of cognitive/social/behavioral aspects of an individual. From the shining brown eyes of a boy whose speech is unintelligible, to the painted nails of a girl with a postoperative cleft palate, to the strong handshake of an adult dysarthric, the superior clinician is quick to compliment. There must always be numerous positive attributes of a patient to be noticed and commended. To genuinely care about anyone is to acknowledge their weaknesses but to *recognize* their strengths. In your measurements of articulatory abilities and efforts to direct change in their performance, you will have to engage in a large number of comments about the person's failings; you should conscientiously work at balancing the scale by noting the good things as well.

Consider the following greeting of a child entering the therapy room.

Clinician: Good morning, Joe. You look so nice today. Is that a new shirt? Give me a big old handshake.

The clinician comments favorably about the child's appearance and asks for a handshake as a greeting. These are both adult communicative behaviors that are used for the purposes of establishing social contact. The clinician is modeling these for the child and using them to bring the child into a conversation. This greeting is easily modeled and used in a group situation in which the clinician prompts each child to greet others in the group (e.g., "Joe, say good morning to Zack. Zack, look at Joe's new shoes. Tell him how nice you think they look"). Contrast this with the clinician who does not look up when a child enters the room and says "Take your seat. I'll be with you in a minute" while shuffling through papers. Such a "greeting" shows a general lack of interest in the child and does little to foster the onset of communication between the two.

As you talk to a child, you should be aware of your nonverbal communication as well as your outward speech acts. Although we are seriously concerned about a patient's welfare, our facial expressions should not be serious or frowning. Passive or concerned expressions are not the mark of interesting, helpful people. More often than not, they are indicators that someone is wallowing in a cesspool of self-concern. Successful treatment sessions include procedures directed by clinicians who convey enjoyment for what they are doing, including their communicative interaction with the child.

A special case of self-concern occurs for the beginning clinician who experiences great anxiety. For the beginning clinician, anxiety is frequently and generally regarded in a negative manner. For some reason we tend to regard our nervousness or anxiety as being something to overcome. Obviously, our initial clinical experiences done under observation will be less than comfortable and the procedures we employ, poorer than our expectations. Many veteran stage performers are bundles of nerves even after the curtain goes up. Surgeons may pace the floor before performing highly skilled procedures. You get "butterflies" before that very important date. We do not sit quietly when our favorite football team is locked in a tied score with 1 minute to go. In a very real way, anxiety should be regarded as an indicator that we care about what we are doing. It should be regarded as a driving force for improved performance, and not something to fear. You can lessen the negative effects of your anxiety by focusing your attention on the child, rather than your perceptions of self.

The communication between two people will flow naturally when both are judging the intentions of the other and are responding accordingly. The antithesis of this approach involves a common first-year clinician's strategy of "parrotting" what a child says. "How are you today?" "I feel pretty good." "Oh! you feel pretty good." "Do you have a pet?" "Yes, I do." "Oh, you do." "What kind of pet do you have?" "A dog." "A dog." "What's it's name?" "His name is Porky." "Oh, his name is Porky." In essence, repetition causes the conversation to start and stop because the clinician is not adding any new information to the topic. To keep talking, the clinician asks a series of "Wh-" questions. Each new question demands a change in topic. The clinician controls the conversation completely, and the child is left to wonder why he or she should bother to respond. By not adding any new information, the clinician forces the child to try to organize the conversation about each topic. Children with communication disorders often are not skilled at organizing conversations about things and actions that are not present, and they do not have the ability to hold the conversation together. Each time the clinician repeats a child's utterance, the child may choose to simply affirm that the clinician's interpretation of the original utterance was appropriate. Take note of when someone responds to your utterances with a repetition of what you said; typically it will be a case in which the person is intending to find out if he or she interpreted what your intention was.

An additional variable that marks the performance of a skilled clinician is the versatility with which treatment procedures are employed. The need to be versatile is necessitated by the fact that most often we ask patients to experiment with behavioral changes that require effort and skill. As a result, we must be constantly aware of the need to recognize variables such as distraction, inattention, fatigue, tension, or frustration resulting from failure to perform to their, or our, expectations.

Distraction may occur as a result of noise, room temperature, inappropriate lighting, messy or cluttered rooms, or poorly organized treatment procedures. Of these, poorly organized or inappropriate treatment procedures are a direct and controllable responsibility of the clinician. Younger children are frequently expected to perform beyond their ability and, as a result, boredom or misbehavior takes over. Children, in particular, may not know the purpose (or care about the purpose) of what they are doing. Tired, disinterested, or just plain ignorant clinicians may resort to such practices as attempting to have children repeat endless word lists or point to an endless array of pictures as they mutter the alleged stimuli. As such, distraction is not the problem: It is the result of a problem. Inattention, although closely related to distraction, is frequently the result of inappropriate planning. The attention span of young children and even some college students and professors is surprisingly short. As a result, it is important that activities (not games) conform to appropriate interests, age level, relation to the real world of the patient, and most important, the degree of success within which the patient can operate. In doing this, the speech produced by a child should be directly related to the activity and have the purposeful intent of speech acts. The speech produced will thus have an inherent payoff and will be realistic to the purpose of the activity.

Fatigue usually results from sustained, repetitious, and redundant activity. Tennis, golf, and volleyball are usually less fatiguing and much more interesting than calisthenics, jogging, and weight lifting. Though each involves exercise, the former tend to be more fun than the latter (unless, of course, one is a poor loser). Similarly, the treatment session must include, in addition to necessary exercise, those activities in which the clinician and patient have fun. In doing so, the alert clinician recognizes when the patient is beginning to fatigue and moves quickly to a related activity designed to continue, yet relax, performance emphasis.

Tension or frustration typically results from the patient's inability to perform to either his or her own or the clinician's expectations. It is frustrating and demoralizing to constantly fail. Clinicians must recognize that much of what they ask of patients is difficult, and that the patient usually tries very hard to achieve the expected performance criterion level or model of the clinician. When subsequent and continued attempts are inadequate, responses result in tension and frustration. Rather than continue under such conditions, the clinician must recognize the need to divert attention away from the particular task to one in which the patient can experience success. Or, at best, take a moment to just relax, smile, and admit that what we are doing is hard work, and from time to time we need to take a break. In summary, Table 5-5 illustrates negative factors related to consideration of treatment procedures.

These problems can be avoided by treating the interaction with a patient as a conversation. The single most crucial variable facilitating conversation is listening to interpret the child's intent. Too many semi-interested listeners attend to how things are said rather than what and what is not being said. Too frequently, egocentric clinicians and professors prepare personal speeches during the responses of their hopeful listeners rather than listening. To be an effective listener one must be more interested in the what, how, and why of the speaker, than in personal biases, prejudices, insecurities, and judgments. Study the manner in which the clinician in the following examples chose some aspect of the child's utterance to comment on, expand on, or ask for more information about. To do this, the clinician has to be listening to the child. During conversations with friends and others, experiment with listening and response. We think of the world as our laboratory. Scientific methodology (especially experimentation/analysis) is not a technique confined to the classroom or laboratory: it is a life-style. It is fun. Most important, it is personally stimulating and rewarding.

Following the greeting, the clinician's next speech act is intended to establish a conversational topic that is familiar to the child and shows an interest in the child's life.

Clinician: You know, I really don't know a whole lot about your house and today I'd like you to tell me about your bedroom.

Child: It has blue walls . . . a *dresser* . . . a picture . . . a radio.

To choose topics that are of interest to a child, the clinician needs two forms of knowledge: general knowledge of children and specific knowledge about a particular child.

Discovering what is generally interesting to children in a particular age group can be gleaned from activity books aimed at children in different age groups. You can also look into the children's literature section in the school library or the public library. For preschool children, many of the topics revolve around day-to-day experiences of children: getting a new pet, getting along with friends, going on family picnics, and so on. As we saw in Chap. 2, it is from these social interactions that language develops. The child learns

Table 5-5. CLINICIAN PERFORMANCE AND ITS RELATIONSHIP TO NEGATIVE PATIENT RESPONSES

Clinician performance	*Negative patient response*
Anxiety	Distraction
Response parroting	Inattention
Passive facial expressions	Fatigue
Lack of compliment	Tension
Restricted differential feedback	Frustration
Minimal versatility	Failure

appropriate meaningful linguistic units and constructions to deal with these situations. These include syllable structures and phonemic contrasts. Your attempts to alter these aspects of a child's system are more likely to be effective if the types of speech you work with are already partially formed in the child's system. You will be adding a level of refinement to the knowledge the child is already working on.

The older child who is using language to learn can make use of materials that are designed to teach them about experiences beyond their present life circumstances. You can find materials regarding such activities in the textbooks and activities planned by the classroom teachers in your school. If you are not in a school setting, look in the university's education library to see the types of projects that are suggested for children in different age groups. Good places to look are in the science teacher's manuals and books where age-appropriate projects in physical and biological sciences are available. For example, a science text about butterflies could lead a specific child to want to collect pictures of butterflies and discuss their differences in shape, coloring, habitat, and so forth.

You find out what is interesting to your particular child by talking to him or her and listening to what the child says. You can adapt your procedures to any topic, so let the child choose what is important. *Those topics will most likely motivate the child to change speech production skills to make speech more effective.* It is also in these activities and topic realms that the child is going to practice articulation naturally after leaving your office. The changes in connection strengths that you attempt to build in treatment will become stronger and faster if they are used in words and situations similar to the ones you are manipulating. As a stronger phoneme-to-feature connection pattern is made, other nontrained words and higher-order linguistic constructions will also be produced with appropriate articulation.

Having found a topic the child is apparently willing to talk about, the clinician is going to maintain this topic and ask the child to predicate, or add information, about a part of what the child has listed.

Clinician: I have a *dresser* in my bedroom, too. Tell me about yours.

Child: Well, it's made out of wood and has drawers and *junk* all over the top that makes my mom mad.

The clinician will again provide a focus on part of the child's utterance. In this case, the clinician uses a partial repetition of what the child has said, with a rising intonation pattern to signify that she wants the child to elaborate on the "junk." She also notes the similarity between the child's experience and her own. This is a subtle social form of accepting the child as a worthwhile human being and encourages the child to keep talking to this other person.

Clinician: Junk? I have junk and it's really fun stuff. Tell me about yours.

Child: I have this fake snake that looks real and I scare my sister with it ... a bolt that used to be on my brother's bicycle. Then, there's a rock that I found that has a hole in the middle.

The clinician chooses one of these objects to elaborate on and to use as a topic for letter writing. The composition, writing, sending of the letter, and replies will become a topical activity for the child and clinician to talk about as the clinician seeks to model and rehearse changes in the child's articulatory system.

Clinician: I like *rocks*. I have some that you'd like to see and I'd like to see yours. Maybe we could start collecting some. Or we could write to some people and ask them to send us rocks or pictures of rocks. Have you ever written a letter to anyone?

Child: Once I wrote a letter to my grandma after Christmas.

Clinician: That's fantastic! What did you say in your letter?

Child: I thanked my grandma for the present she sent me.

Clinician: You know, when your grandma got your letter you gave her the most wonderful present of all.

Child: How? Why?

Clinician: Because you are very special and wonderful and when you wrote to her to say thank you you made her feel special and wonderful. Let's you and I think of some people to whom we can write letters, for fun, to say thanks, for rocks or whatever. If you'll help me, I'll help you. Who are some people you'd like to write?

Child: My grandmother, my friend who lives far away, and my mother.

Clinician: Let's see! What all do we need, to write letters to all these people? Tell me.

While they are setting about the task of letter writing, the clinician talks to the child about the things that are needed (i.e., stamps, paper, pen, envelopes), where these things come from, which choices they should make in choosing each item, and so forth. The general activities of rock collecting and letter writing can be used as conversational topics as long as the child is interested.

Procedures for Enhancing Articulation

In Chap. 3, the process of using behavioral modification strategies was described as part of the experimental study of children's misarticulations. It was noted that the researcher can control conditions that precede and follow a subject's behavior in an attempt to control the behavior itself. A similar description can be made of the things that a clinician does before and after a child's speech productions in an attempt to enhance the child's articulation. A discussion of some of these procedures follows under the headings of "Antecedent Events" and "Consequent Events."

Antecedent Events. Van Riper (1939) summarized the art of instructing persons to produce speech sounds by listing the following methods of speech sound elicitation: stimulation, phonetic placement, modification of other sounds, and locating words in which the sound is correctly produced. Clinician's were using these techniques when Van Riper wrote that summary and are still using similar techniques today.

Stimulation. Stimulation typically describes a situation in which the clinician models an appropriate production of a speech sound and asks the child to imitate the adult's production with appropriate gestures. This typically takes the form of the adult saying something like "Ok, Zack, you've been saying this word *rabbit* like [wæbɪt]. Now I want you to say it like I do, say [ræbɪt]." In so doing, the clinician will also typically emphasize the speech sound being stimulated, making it louder and longer than typical. The clinician may also cue the child to listen and watch carefully while the target sound is being produced.

In Chap. 3 we noted that many experimental manipulations of children's misarticulations used such "modeling" procedures at various stages of their treatment programs. A child is often asked to imitate syllables or words prior to being asked to produce them alone. In Chap. 4 we saw that the ability to imitate appropriate productions of syllables and words is indicative of a child's ability to produce and combine articulatory gestures and is related to probable success in therapy. Thus, a number of commercially available articulation tests incorporate assessment of children's ability to imitate a speech sound.

Van Riper assumed that the effectiveness of modeling could be enhanced by practice in speech sound discrimination. This refers to a person's ability to perceptually discriminate among accepted and variant forms of sound segments. The rationale underlying exercises designed to improve skill in discrimination prior to production rehearsal of segments has been a topic of long-standing research, inference, and discussion. Generally speaking, the proponents of perceptual or discrimination training exercises assume that subsequent success in effecting articulatory change is related to, or will be enhanced by, the patient's ability to discriminate between the clinician's imitations of error approximations and correct forms. Although continued research is perhaps necessary to determine what relationships exist between practices designed to improve discrimination skill with resultant production improvement, studies thus far do not reveal significantly improved production skills.

Inasmuch as speech is a highly integrated, overlearned, and automatized sensory-motor event, apparently abstract and dichotomized attempts to improve singular elements of the event are highly questionable. We must, however, keep in mind the fact that the patient already possesses a highly organized/integrated system. Humans are uniquely adapted for speech. Regardless of content, structure, and pragmatics, potential for change exists. That is quite a different story than starting from proverbial "scratch." In other words, our attempts to assist patients involve revision and rehearsal within an already relatively well developed and highly complex system.

In a sense, clinicians function in a manner similar to coaches of professional athletes or singers. That is, we work with those who have automatized a highly skilled sensory-motor act. Coaches, professional athletes, and singers realize it would be a waste of time and effort to involve themselves in activities designed to simply discriminate between error behavioral patterns and desired production. In other words, the essence of improving performance, be it athletic, musical, vocal, speech, or articulation, must involve the act undergoing change via active rehearsal. The act of speaking is so inextricably bound to auditory and tactile-kinesthetic feedback and the nature of speech acts as related to expression of propositions for a particular purpose that exercise or rehearsal designed to change or improve any aspect of speaking performance should involve, first and foremost, the act of speaking. This is not to say that inclusion of auditory or perceptual training should be ruled out. On the contrary, exercises in discrimination must be directly related to a patient's speech productions. As patients actively, physically experiment with change, they will be afforded an opportunity to learn to discriminate between variances of their own performance. It is through the latter that efficient and effective change can be realized. In effect, during early treatment procedures involving stimulability, clients learn to compare and contrast their productions to revised internalized standards resulting from ongoing experimentation and experience with personal performance.

Stated simply, one cannot learn how to improve a complex ability that has developed to such a high degree by merely watching or listening to another. This is true of running, singing, playing an instrument, driving a car, painting, swimming, writing, or cabinetmaking. The process of learning to improve any skill must involve active and dynamic rehearsal in performing.

Within the verbal communication model, the provision of a model utterance enhances the child's gestural attempts because the visual and auditory features stimulated impose part of the organization of the utterance. The sensory inputs may stimulate appropriate gestures if the child's organization of word-, syllable-, and phoneme-level connections is not stronger than the input stimulus. Thus, modeling would appear to be an easy approach to organizing a child's system when the child has not established connection strengths that are too strong. In the final section we will suggest that such modeling is an important characteristic of manipulating the younger child's articulatory ability. However, the older child's gestures may be so strongly patterned by his or her current organization at phonemic, syllabic, and word levels that modeling elicits only error productions. Other more direct forms of articulatory instruction are required in such cases.

Phonetic Placement. Phonetic placement techniques involve verbally describing for a child the articulatory positions required for a particular speech sound. This is similar to the articulatory phonetics training you received when you learned that a [p] production was associated with a particular vocal tract configuration (i.e., one in which the vocal tract is closed at the lips and open at the larynx with the nasal cavities shut off). The particular articulator positions required for each error sound would be described, and these positions would be visually demonstrated by the clinician, shown in diagrams, and looked at in a mirror. The differences between the child's sound production and those of the adult's phoneme production would be analyzed and described. Some clinicians sought to develop instruments that could be used to shape the child's vocal tract directly into the necessary configuration.

The clinician is required to analyze the articulatory differences between the child's production and the adult model and provide corrective feedback regarding production. The following paragraphs discuss some of the instructions appropriate for the common error patterns.

Common production errors for stop consonants involve manipulation of place of articulation and voicing. Place of articulation errors occur for the alveolar and velar consonants. Alveolar place of articulation can typically be cued by touch of a sterile tongue blade. The child can be asked to touch the blade, which is then removed, or touch the spot on the roof of the mouth where the blade just touched. Velar productions often cannot be cued in this manner due to the child's gag reflex. Rather, the child may be instructed to move the tongue from front to back in an exaggerated movement from a dental position, or the child may be cued to move the tongue body so that the contact between the teeth and the sides of the tongue moves farther back.

Voicing errors of stops and fricatives involve timing of the onset of voicing and the consonant constriction or constriction release. The typical pattern is to produce voiced rather than voiceless consonants at the beginning of a syllable. This can be counteracted by cueing the child to feel for the onset of laryngeal vibration with the fingers and then exaggerating the delay between consonant release and onset of voicing. In essence, the clinician teaches the child to exaggerate voice onset time. The onset of voicing may coincide with production of fricative constrictions so the child may be cued to feel for voicing and then start and stop voicing while a fricative is produced (e.g., shifting from [s] to [z] while continuing production of the fricative noise).

A similar palpation cue can be used to demonstrate differences between nasal and oral stops. By feeling the vibration of the nose, the child can practice alternating between /m/ and /b/.

When fricatives are produced as stops, the child is producing a complete rather than a partial constriction. The clinician can instruct the child to alter this condition by not touching the articulators together; the child should make a slit between the two articulators instead. This is probably best first attempted at the lips where such manipulations are visible. The child could be shown the difference between a complete bilabial closure [p] and a partial closure [θ]. Similar instructions can be used to cue differences between a dental fricative and a dental stop production. The alveolar and palatal fricatives also involve a central groove in the tongue configuration. This groove can be accentuated by asking the child to press up against the teeth with the sides of the tongue while feeling for the air stream to hit the alveolar ridge. The palatal fricative can be produced by moving the tongue back from this position. Stop productions for affricate sounds can be cued by asking the child to release the stop constriction slowly, holding the fricative slit long enough to produce the required noise.

When liquids are produced as glides, the child is not producing the more complicated tongue shapes required for /l/ and /r/. Instructions to produce these shapes can be given. The tongue position for /l/ requires that the tongue tip be lifted to touch the alveolar ridge. Then the child can be instructed to make sure that he or she does not feel the sides of the tongue touch the teeth so that this sound can be produced as a lateral. Alternately, the child may be instructed to point the tongue tip, then raise it to the alveolar ridge while the mandible is lowered, then raise the mandible. This series of steps should lead to an appropriate central constriction. /r/ can be produced by curling the tongue up and back. This curling can be accomplished while the mandible is lowered and the process is visualized in a mirror. Then the mandible must be raised while holding this position.

These techniques allow the clinician to prompt the child into a static articulatory position that is appropriate for production of a particular speech sound. However, the gestures used to reach those target configurations are often quite unnatural. A speaker does not maximally lower the jaw, curl the tongue up and back, and then produce an [r]. The final target position reached may be appropriate, but the connection strengths to gestures are not readily usable. At best, these techniques should be used to cue the child to the tactile and auditory aspects of a sound's production.

Modification of Other Sounds. The third strategy involves asking a child to produce a speech sound that is appropriately articulated and then shift one or two articulatory gestures to approximate the target production. Van Riper referred to this strategy as *modification of speech sounds.*

From the discussion in Chap. 1, you should realize that sound production results from manipulation of specific articulatory gestures. The turbulent, noiselike airflow of an [s] is created by forcing the breath stream through an apical alveolar constriction. The constriction was created by grooving and raising the tongue tip. If the tongue tip is raised too high, contact is made rather than constriction. The child will either produce a stop consonant or will lower the sides of the tongue, forcing the resultant noisy airflow to be emitted laterally, resulting in what is referred to as a lateral /s/. Similarly, if the tongue tip is pulled too far forward, the constriction will be dental, and the noisy airflow will be of both lower intensity and frequency, resulting in what is referred to as a dental or interdental /s/.

In any case, the problem is not with the resultant sound but with the gestures used to produce the sound. Sound stream lateralization primarily involves apical dental or alveolar contact during production. This is the physiological feature that must be altered. Through the process of development, children have associated inappropriate gestures with the visual and auditory characteristics of particular phonemes. In essence, they most frequently hear our adult standard productions and their own aberrant productions as being equivalent. They have automatized their productions and are frequently only able to hear and feel differences after we have directed change in such a way as to interrupt their habitual production. Asking children to make adjustments in the gestures associated with a sound given only auditory information (i.e., modeling) will fail to the extent that they have habituated their production. As an alternative, directions may be based on moving from segmental productions that share gestures with the target sound (facilitory segments or contexts). Transition to appropriate production may occur with relative ease because the child is starting from an already habituated set of gestures and is asked to modify only one gestural component.

The commonly misarticulated /s/ shares its alveolar constriction with the commonly appropriately produced /t/. The gestural differences involve making a slight, as opposed to a complete, constriction and formation of a central groove in the front of the tongue. An appropriate fricative sound can be cued by asking the child to release a [t] production slowly, then to hold the tongue in the position in which a frication noise is produced. Demonstrate this for yourself by exploding [t] slowly, noting that sustaining aspiration following contact/plosion results in none other than [s]. With regard to lateralized production of /s/, a note of caution is in order. It is possible and frequently the case that those who lateralize /s/ production may also lateralize /t/. Demonstrate this for yourself by maintaining apical alveolar contact during production of /t/ while allowing the release of air pressure to occur laterally around the sides of your tongue. Based on our knowledge of articulatory theory, the latter should come as no surprise. If we consider the number of contexts in which /ts/ occurs (e.g., *cat saw, rats ate; it's nice; Pat's friend*), /st/ (*mistake, stop, best, kiss Tom*), and /tst/ (*let's take, shortstop, flat stick*), it is reasonable to assume that coarticulation, or pre- and postfeature integration, from /s/ to /t/ occurs. Nonetheless, the physiological complexity of /t/ is such that tongue release is visually obvious, easily demonstrated, and readily imitated. Following correct production of [t] and sustaining plosion, we are able to have the patient demonstrate the desired feature replacement. The experienced clinician can readily complete the entire process in a matter of only a few minutes.

Dentalization or interdentalization of /s/ presents only minor change with regard to stimulability toward appropriate production. Here again, production of [t] as a facilitory segment is apropos. Once again, however, a number of considerations are important. Inasmuch as segments [t, d, n, l] each share a common place of production with [s] and occur so frequently in /s/ clusters, they too, are frequently dentalized. For numerous reasons, we tend to overlook (or underhear) dentalized productions of these sounds because dentalization does not noticeably affect the acoustic characteristics of the sound. Again, experiment by producing [t, d, n, l] dentally or interdentally and note that such productions are acoustically acceptable. If, on observation, these sounds are consistently produced dentally or interdentally, initial treatment should include rehearsal designed to automatize production in the elevated apical alveolar region.

An additional variable related to the production of dentalized /s/ warrants particular attention. By the very nature of the fact that apical position is lowered, a recognizable degree of mandibular lowering is also observable. As a result, it is frequently necessary to instruct the patient to elevate or raise the mandible for production of [s]. In doing so, two very important adjustments occur. Elevated mandibular positioning will interfere with apical dental contact and apical alveolar positioning for such sounds as /t, d, n, l/, and /s/ will be facilitated. We can test this ourselves by lowering our mandible, producing /t, d, n, l, s/ dentally or interdentally in the sentence "Tom does not like Sunday school," then elevating the mandible and repeating the sentence correctly. In addition to noting the ease with which you can achieve apical alveolar approximation for the target segments, the relationship of mandibular elevation to the necessity of /s/ approximation should be readily apparent.

A similar shift in articulatory position can be used to alter an appropriately articulated [s] into the palatal [ʃ]. The child is instructed to maintain the [s] and slide the tongue back. This backward tongue gesture can be demonstrated visually by asking the child to observe him- or herself move from an [θ] to an [s].

Without question, the segments [r] and [ɝ] are frequently misarticulated and resistant to stimulation. Our attempts to achieve stimulability are again determined by analysis of how inappropriate approximation is being achieved and directions in which we must move to approach the desired idealized production position. As in production of other continuants, our objective is to achieve desired production in such a way as to provide maximal duration of simultaneous auditory, tactile, and kinesthetic feedback. Typically, imitative attempts to achieve sustained /r/ production result in neutralization toward the vowel /3/. To achieve desired idealized position for production, the tongue must be elevated and retroflexed. Here again, we realize that such an idealized position can be facilitated by mandibular elevation during tongue retraction. For those who find /r/ production difficult, attempts to elevate and retract the tongue with the mandible lowered are accompanied by excessive lingual/mandibular tension and inappropriate production. Demonstrate this for yourself by lowering your mandible and simultaneously elevating and retracting your tongue during sustained phonation. Rather than facilitating production, such practice makes appropriate production extremely unnatural and difficult. On the other hand, appropriate production may be facilitated by experimenting with sustained sound production from [dɝd], [nɝn], [lɝl], [iɝi], or any permutations of potential facilitatory segments that share a raised tongue-tip gesture.

Whenever possible, the clinician should direct desired behavioral change from sound approximations successfully produced by the child or patient in such a way as to minimize physiological complexity or difficulty. *Achieving idealized sound approximations as quickly and easily as possible is crucial to subsequent treatment.* Nothing reinforces our efforts as much as knowing we are succeeding—not just hitting the target, but the bull's-eye.

Target Words. Van Riper noted that many misarticulating children correctly produce their error sound in at least one word. In such cases, the child need not be taught to move the articulators to particular positions: That set of positions is already available. The clinician's task becomes one of isolating the correct production from that word and making it usable in other words.

Consequent Events. As discussed in Chap. 2, children learn to modify their speech and language systems in order to better communicate with the persons in their environment. They naturally alter their productions of words when it becomes apparent that they have been misunderstood, particularly if the misunderstanding leads to their not achieving the intent of their utterance. A relatively natural way for the clinician to respond to a child's misarticulations would be to inform the child how his or her utterance has been misunderstood and to ask for a clarification. For example, if a child were putting blocks together to spell the word *cap* and he asked the clinician for a [ti], the clinician would give the child the *t* block. The child would protest by saying "No, I don't want the [ti], I want the [ti]!" The clinician could then explain, "Oh, you want the [si]. I didn't understand you because you said [ti]. Here, say it with an [s] at the beginning, [si]." When the child improves his production, the clinician complies with the child's request, and the activity continues.

In the name of efficiency, some articulation training programs use artificial reinforcement in an attempt to reinforce correct productions. In a particular activity, the child is instructed that he or she will receive some reward if some number of correct productions of a target sound are produced. These are then tallied in some way, or the child receives some token for each response, which can then be traded in for the reward. Alternatively, clinicians will use "social reinforcement" in which the clinician comments favorably on the child's good articulations.

One problem with this procedure is that it demands a particular interaction between adult and child in which the two are "working on their speech production." Although this is appropriate for the older child, the younger child may not view communicative interaction with the adult in the same light. In such cases, the adult's comments such as "That was a good [s]" are unnatural inasmuch as they do not add information to the conversation. When was the last time someone complimented your articulation in the middle of a project or conversation, or clapped their hands and said "Good trying"?

For the older child who is motivated to work on articulatory abilities, the comments made by the clinician take the form of differential feedback. They inform the child how well he or she is doing. Depending on how the comments are delivered, they may or may not encourage a child to keep trying. One problem arises when the clinician attempting to provide such feedback becomes too predictable. For instance, Wright and Schuckers (1979) reported that clinicians employed the verbal reinforcements *good, O.K.,* and *alright* over 80 percent of the time during treatment procedures. Obviously, constraining ourselves to the application of a restricted repertoire of verbal reinforcement or differential feedback should be avoided. Responses to successful performance should range from *good, tremendous, super, great, fantastic,* and *wonderful,* to a handshake or well-intended and deserved pat on the back.

Wright and Schuckers also indicated that clinicians lacked schedules of administration, novelty, and consistency in the use of differential feedback or reinforcement during treatment procedures. Effective clinicians must attend to the variables included in their own performance as judiciously as they attend to the performance of their patient. The nature of human communication is such that what we do and say and how we do and say it, may have a significant effect on our listener. Much like the conductor of an orchestra, we must maintain an awareness of how our performance both affects and effects individual as well as group performance. In this sense, the treatment session is simultaneously a rehearsal and performance. Although constrained by certain factors of the treatment plan, we each bring unique individuality to performance. Just as we expect orchestra conductors, musicians, actors, and athletes to present unique performances while operating within the rule system of the score, script, or sport, we must recognize that each clinician brings special uniqueness to the treatment session.

Measurement Strategies

In the last chapter, we discussed some of the characteristics of measuring articulatory performance from the perspective that we were evaluating a child to determine if treatment was necessary and what the characteristics of the child's problem were. However, assessment of a child's articulation is a clinical process that continues throughout our contact with a child in treatment. As noted above, behavioral objectives must be measurable in terms of the child's performance. This requires that the child's performance be periodically measured by the clinician. Two basic strategies can be employed in measuring a child's progress through therapy: measurement of success in specific tasks used as treatment procedures and measurement in the child's typical speech.

In the first form of therapy measurement, a clinician lays out a treatment plan, including a set of behavioral objectives. The clinician then measures performance with respect to the objectives. For example, that a child can correctly articulate [s] in 80 percent of a list of words is taken as a measurement of treatment performance.

The primary consideration in use of this form of measurement is that it depends on the validity of the treatment tasks employed. If production practice in nonmeaningful syllables has little to do with improvement in the child's typical speech patterns, then advancement through such program stages can hardly be taken as a measure of success. This is analogous to the use of picture articulation tests to measure a child's articulatory performance. All clinicians know that this task usually overestimates a child's articulatory ability. When the picture-naming task is used as a standardized procedure to compare a child to others, its flaws may not be crucial. However, when we claim that it is a measure of the child's typical articulatory ability, we are standing on shaky ground with these assumptions.

Another problem of using behavioral objectives to measure a child's progress in therapy relates to the mechanics of treatment. No one, least of all children, likes to fail in tasks they are asked to perform. Thus, setting up a program in which a child practices a particular task until it is mastered defines that the child must be failing in a fair percentage of attempts, at least 10 percent if a 90 percent criterion is set. If the child succeeds at greater than 90 percent, he or she is moved to the next step where failure can start again. Learning theorists want the child to succeed to a high degree, often in excess of 95 percent of the child's attempts at a task. However, when a child's program is constructed so that he or she typically succeeds at these rates, then the use of these tasks as a measurement of treatment success becomes meaningless.

An alternative measurement strategy is to use the terminal behavior as the measurement device. If a child's terminal treatment goal is correct production of [s] in conversational speech, then we should periodically measure performance in conversational speech to determine if the goal is being reached. Such measurements should be taken throughout treatment to determine if different stages are useful. If a child's performance in conversational speech is not improving as a result of practicing production of the sound in syllables, then perhaps that practice is not a good treatment component.

Such measurements can be taken relatively easily for the child whose misarticulations involve one or two speech sound errors. The clinician need only record or judge live the child's production of individual phonemes in a conversation. A percentage correct is calculated for each to determine if improvement is taking place. For the child who misarticulates a variety of phonemes, the clinician can measure the overall percentage of consonants correctly produced or individual error patterns such as production of fricatives as stops can be tallied.

Regardless of the measurement procedures employed, we should keep our focus on the behavior we ultimately want to improve and then measure that behavior. If it is not changing, we should question our treatment techniques before we question our measurement techniques.

TREATMENT PROGRAMS

TREATMENT PROGRAM REVIEW

In the following sections, a variety of published treatment programs is described. These are presented in their historical order of appearance. Their makeup reflects the historical development of theories of children's misarticulations as seen in Chap. 3. The first program reviewed is Van Riper's (1939) approach, which is now considered the traditional model of articulation therapy. It emphasized the child's ability to detect auditory characteristics of speech sounds and to use this ability to guide development of production of error speech sounds in words. The second program is McDonald's (1964) sensory-motor approach, which emphasized the importance of the movement patterns underlying articulation and the use of tactile-kinesthetic sensory information in articulation learning as opposed to Van Riper's emphasis on auditory information. The third program is Mowrer, Baker, and Schultz' behavioral modification approach. The fourth program is Winitz' (1974) program which returned to Van Riper's emphasis on auditory information, but focused more on the child's cognitive organization of these inputs than their value as eliciting stimuli for articulatory responses. The final program presented is Hodson and Paden's (1983) approach, which emphasized the cognitive organization of speech sounds by keying on common error patterns.

Van Riper's Traditional Approach

Charles Van Riper was one of the first authors to suggest a coherent treatment plan for children's misarticulations as a chapter in his 1939 book about speech and language disorders. In the discussion that follows, we analyze his approach with regard to goals, clinician roles, and measurement strategies.

Table 5-6 shows the generalized goals of Van Riper's approach to articulation therapy. In this traditional approach to misarticulation therapy, the focus of remediation is a "speech sound." With respect to our model, this focus corresponds to a phoneme unit.

The first goal was to bring the child to an awareness of his or her misarticulations. In this stage of treatment, the child was taught through practice exercises to identify the speech sound error in a small set of five or six words. For example, the clinician might read a passage and misarticulate those words in the same manner that the child does while the child produces some signal that shows that he or she has heard the word error. Or the clinician might read a word list and sometimes misarticulate the target sound and sometimes produce it appropriately, while the child judges the correctness of the production.

The second goal sought to eliminate the influence of possible contributing factors. Physiological factors such as malocclusion would be referred to an orthodontist. Children with obvious motoric problems would be referred to a physical therapist. Emotional problems would be referred to a psychologist. The speech-language pathologist would work to eliminate excessive environmental demands on the child's speech and would work on concomitant speech and language problems.

The third goal involved teaching the child to hear the differences between the error sound and the child's production. Van Riper's view of this process is quite similar to the processing that we suspect occurs in the verbal communication model. For example, he stated the basic relationship between

Table 5-6. GENERALIZED GOALS OF VAN RIPER'S (1939) APPROACH TO TREATMENT OF CHILDREN'S MISARTICULATIONS

Convince the child that he or she has speech errors that must be solved
Eliminate causal factors
Ear training
Elicit correct sound
Strengthen new sound
Make transition to familiar words
Consistently use new sound

the phonemic level and the word level in the following terms: "To the uncorrected lisper, for example, the substitution of *th* for *s* in the word *soup* is entirely natural. The liquid's name just happens to be *thoup*." (p. 224). He also stated the relationship between the word level and the sensory feature level: "Each word is a complex configuration, having within it patterns of muscular movement, patterns of sequences of auditory sensation and a unitary meaning" (p. 225). Van Riper was most concerned with organization of auditory-sensory features of sounds and words, and so this treatment phase sought to teach the child to listen for his or her error sound. The first step involved asking the child to signal when the sound occurred in isolated syllables or in words in connected speech. For example, the clinician would read a sentence with the correctly produced version of the sound, and the child would signal its presence by identifying the word. Next the child would learn to identify and describe the auditory characteristics of the appropriately produced sound and the error approximation. Finally, the child would be taught to contrast and compare the error production with the appropriately produced version. Within the verbal communication model, this stage amounts to calling conscious attention to the auditory and, by virtue of the fact that this training is typically done live, the visual characteristics of the sound the child is attempting to produce and his or her current approximation of that sound.

The fourth goal was to elicit correct production of the target sound. This was done through use of the stimulation techniques, instructions, models, and prompts of the clinician.

The fifth goal was to strengthen the new sound. Van Riper used an analogy between articulatory skills and those skills of musicians and athletes to justify this stage: "Any musician or tennis player will tell us that a new stroke or fingering sequence must be practiced and strengthened a great deal before it is used in competition or composition" (p. 247). To accomplish this strengthening of the articulatory movement patterns involved in production of a speech sound, Van Riper advocated practice in nonmeaningful syllables, even for children who could quickly produce the new sound in words. With respect to the verbal communication model, he sought to strengthen the connections between the feature level and the new phoneme while avoiding the word-level connections that would tend to elicit the use of the old features. In other words, words still have strong connections to the error speech sound, which makes it more difficult for the child to produce the new phoneme in previously learned words. The practice Van Riper used involved prolonging the new sound in syllables, repeating a new sound within a syllable, exaggerating the loudness of the new sound, and describing the tactile and kinesthetic feedback involved in production of the new sound.

In the next phase of training, Van Riper sought to teach the child to use the new sound in words familiar to the child. "In retraining," Van Riper wrote, "we do not merely substitute one sound for another. We build new words, new configurations" (p. 254). In the verbal communication model, this step attempts to rearrange the connection strengths between the word level and the phonemic level. A new phonemic target, or at least a new set of features for an old phonemic target, must be connected to all of the words that were previously learned with inappropriate connections. To bring this process to the child's awareness, exercises would be constructed in which a child would use a substitution of a nonerror sound for another nonerror sound. For example, a child who produced /s/ as [θ] might be asked to read a passage and substitute a [b] for every /f/. Next, Van Riper might have a child substitute the new sound, in this case [s], for a different phoneme target (e.g., /k/). Later, the child would be asked to use the new sound in appropriate words. Then the process of strengthening would be started again, and the child would be asked to prolong the new sound or repeat the new sound until given a signal by the clinician to continue.

In the articulation therapy strategies that preceded Van Riper's, and in some that followed, treatment took the form of a drill routine in which the child reads word lists or sentences to perfect speech production. The stereotypical speech teacher of the time would have students repeatedly practice appropriate sound production in such sentences as "The rain in Spain falls mainly on the plain," apparently seeking to improve articulation of the vowel /e/. However, Van Riper strongly objected to the technique of repeating word lists: "Practice of word lists will have little transfer to real speech situations unless those words are taken out of series and made part of the actual communication function" (p. 264).

The final step in therapy was to foster consistent use of the new sound. The techniques in this stage are designed to make the child his or her own clinician. The child is asked to establish *nuclear situations.* These are speaking occasions in which the child plans ahead of time to pay attention to articulation, noting if errors occur, correcting errors, and attempting to anticipate error productions so the newly learned sound can be used. These situations are agreed on in a treatment session, and it becomes the child's responsibility to report on his or her performance in the next session. Another technique used in this phase is *negative practice,* in which the child purposefully produces the error sound with the old approximation. Van Riper suggested that such voluntary use of the error sound is punishing to the child and makes the child more aware of the word-level cues that precede an error production. These techniques both involve the child's taking conscious control of speech production and a very active part in the planning of his or her own therapy.

Van Riper was clear in the role he assigned to the speech clinician: "The teacher should constantly assume the role of helper or an assistant, placing the entire responsibility on the child" (p. 263). Van Riper suggested that every child, no matter how young, needed to know what he or she was being asked to do and why. In essence, Van Riper was asking that the child be an active, informed learner.

Van Riper did not specifically address the issue of measuring improvement in therapy. Apparently, this approach would be successful if a child could actively control articulation when needed, could design his or her own nuclear situations, and would be willing to continue the therapy process without the clinician's help.

McDonald's Sensory-Motor Approach

As seen in previous chapters, Eugene McDonald (1964a) developed a theory of children's functional misarticulation that focused on the lower levels of the verbal communication model: the syllabic, phonemic, and featural levels. He was quite specific in rejecting the idea that functional misarticulation involved a mislearning of English words: "It is our point of view that a misarticulated sound does not represent something 'wrong' which the child has learned. Rather, a misarticulated sound represents an arrest in the development of specific sensory-motor function" (p. 159). Thus, the goals of McDonald's therapy approach involved sensory-motor aspects of production of individual speech sounds. Inasmuch as he acknowledged the importance of phonetic context in altering the articulation of a particular speech sound, his overall goal was to teach the child to correctly articulate an error sound in all appropriate phonetic contexts. He approached this task with three generalized goals as seen in Table 5-7.

The first goal sought to increase the child's awareness of sensory feedback related to articulation. McDonald sought to teach the child to analyze the auditory aspects of speech sounds as spoken by the clinician and to match these impressions with the tactile and movement patterns felt in the vocal tract. His technique involved teaching the child to verbally describe articulatory contacts and directions of tongue movements for speech sounds that were appropriately articulated. A child who misarticulated /s/ would first be asked to describe movement patterns for speech sounds that contained maximally different features. As therapy progressed, the sounds used would become more like the intended sound.

McDonald sought to teach this ability by asking the child to repeat syllabic strings and then describe their production. Initially, the consonants and vowels contained in these strings would differ from one another maximally with respect to their articulatory features. As the child became more skilled at description, the speech sounds described would become more similar. For example, a child might be asked to repeat the syllable string [kina], chosen because the vowels differ in both height and backness, and the consonants differ in place, manner, and voicing. The child would be taught to

Table 5-7. GENERALIZED GOALS OF McDONALD'S SENSORY-MOTOR APPROACH TO ARTICULATION THERAPY

Heighten auditory, proprioceptive, and tactile sensations associated with articulation
Reinforce child's correct articulation of error sound
Facilitate correct production in phonetic contexts

describe this syllable as first involving a contact between the back of the tongue and the upper molars, [k]. The second contact is between the tip of the tongue and the alveolar ridge, [n]. The tongue movements involved shifting from the back of the tongue to the front of the tongue. The tongue tip moved up to the alveolar ridge and was then lowered. The child would be asked to feel the throat during production to describe when voicing is onset and offset. He or she might be asked to feel the side of the nose to note when vibration of nasal consonant production was felt.

As the child learned to perform such descriptions of maximally distinct speech sounds, the distinctions would be made finer. As the child was able to describe finer distinctions, the particular features that were misarticulated were included, and eventually the child was taught to describe the characteristics of the error approximation and the intended sound (if it was correctly articulated in any phonetic context).

Van Riper concentrated on the auditory characteristics of a speech sound; McDonald concentrated on the child's tactile and proprioceptive feedback during productions. This type of in-depth discussion of the characteristics of speech sounds obviously requires that the child have good language skills and be able to talk about speech as an abstract process.

The second generalized goal was to reinforce the child's correct production of the speech sound. It was hoped that administration of the Deep Test of Articulation would have uncovered at least one two-word context in which the child appropriately articulated the error sound. This two-word context would be practiced with a variety of alterations. The child would be asked to alter the speed and stress pattern of the two word combination. It would be embedded in sentences, and the stress pattern of the sentences would be altered. These stages often involved use of non-English patterns (e.g., the two-word combination "watch sun" is difficult put into a sentence form—"The watch sun is funny"). However, McDonald was convinced that the child's knowledge of English was normal, and this type of practice would provide the needed sensory-motor feedback to develop articulatory control.

The last goal involved spreading the correct production of the appropriate speech sound to the complete range of phonetic contexts. To accomplish this, McDonald altered the correctly produced two-word context. For example, "watch sun" could be changed by altering the word containing the preceding consonant (e.g., "hat sun, pop sun") or the vowel following /s/ could be altered by changing the second word (e.g., "watch sue, watch sea"). The two-word combinations would be altered in stress and rate as practiced before. As the child became accomplished at producing a wide variety of these two-word combinations, the child would be asked to construct sentences in which target words were embedded in a variety of contexts. Reading assignments were also suggested.

McDonald clearly stated his view of the clinician's role: "The use of drill books, games, mimeographed lists and exercises, and similar materials tend to make the therapy program material-and-clinician centered rather than principle-and-client centered" (p. 137). The descriptive ability developed in the first stage of therapy was to be carried on throughout therapy so that the child would become his or her own judge. The child would also be asked to construct practice materials and include these in a notebook. The clinician sought to supply guidance in developing these materials and to help in adequately judging the child's productions.

Mowrer, Baker, and Schutz' Behavioral Modification Approach

Using Van Riper's production goals as a basis, Mowrer, Baker and Schutz (1968) sought to use principles of behavior modification to increase the efficiency of articulation therapy for a particular speech sound. They wrote an instructional program for correction of dentalized [s] that specified in great detail the procedures to be used by the clinician in manipulating the cues that preceded the child's productions and those that would follow. They also specified a set of discrete goals, stating the behaviors that were expected of the child at each stage.

The terminal behavior chosen was correct production of [s] in 100 percent of its uses in all speaking situations. Three subgoals were constructed to reach this goal, each intended to be reached in a single therapy session lasting 15 minutes. Each of the three parts of the program was further divided into subgoals. Part I started with the child's production of the vowel [i], chosen because it is in the child's repertoire of behaviors and involves a high front tongue position. The next step involved production of [is] with the clinician supplying the phonetic instruction to "Close the teeth" during production of the [s]. This instruction was chosen because it is impossible to produce an interdental [s] if the dentition is intact and this instruction is followed. Next, the [i] vowel is dropped because it has served its purpose of helping to evoke the [s], and the child practices producing individual [s] productions. The fourth step involves producing [s] + V syllable productions. The fifth step has the child producing word-initial [s]. This phase of instruction ends with the child producing the [s] + V words in a carrier sentence such as "I see a ______." In the second session, the child produces [s] in (1) polysyllabic words, (2) words containing [s] clusters, (3) simple sentences containing an [s] in the subject noun and in the verb, and (4) [s] in more complex sentence structures. In the final session, the child is prompted to produce [s] while (1) answering questions, (2) filling in a missing word in sentences, (3) retelling a sentence, and (4) recalling.

While the child's speech responses were made longer and more complex through the stages shown above, the clinician was manipulating the types of cues used to prompt the child's speech attempts. These were categorized as echoic, picture-echoic, picture, question, fill-in, and memory. In the *echoic* mode, a child would be asked to repeat an utterance. The model provided in the echoic mode was made either "strong" or "weak" by manipulating the directions used. Strong cues included phonetic placement instructions (e.g., "Close your teeth and say [s]" or "Look in the mirror and make sure your teeth are closed. Now say [s]"). Cues were considered to be weaker if they did not contain this level of instruction (e.g., "Say [s]" or "Try it again"). Pictures were used to gain labeling responses and descriptive responses (e.g., "This is a saw. Say saw"). Note that this was a level I response in Blank and colleagues' (1978) question scheme described in Table 5-4. The type of prompt used was considered weaker as the models were eliminated and the child was prompted with *questions* (e.g., "What is this?"), a level I labeling response. A *fill-in* response involved a longer utterance such as "This is a ______" in which the child filled in the missing item's label. Finally, *memory* prompts were those that would be considered level II by Blank and colleagues (1978) (e.g., "What do we wash our hands with?").

The clinician also manipulated a reinforcement schedule to shape the child's behavior. A correct response was rewarded with a token that could be redeemed for a prize or privilege. Incorrect responses were "punished" by not being rewarded with a token and were followed by the clinician's "No."

An 80 percent correct criterion was established for the final task in each phase. For example, a child at the end of the first phase must be able to correctly produce 8 of 10 words in a posttest. If the child fails this test, he or she either repeats the phase or is dropped from the program.

The clinician's role is relatively automatic. In fact, if it were presently possible to program a computer to judge [s] productions as correct or incorrect, or in this case, whether tongue protrusion has occurred, the program could be executed by a microcomputer.

Winitz' Auditory Conceptualization Approach

McDonald emphasized sensory-motor aspects of children's misarticulation; Winitz (1975) emphasized the child's discrimination of auditory features and categorization of these at the phoneme and syllable levels of analysis. His treatment program has four basic phases as shown in Table 5-8.

In the first stage of therapy, the clinician trains the child to discriminate the clinician's productions of the error sound and the adult form of that sound. This ability is trained in play situations in which the child would have to label or request objects whose names are made homophones by the child's misarticulation. This often requires that the clinician give made-up names to objects (e.g., an object might be labeled as an [θi] so that it could

Table 5-8. WINITZ' (1975) TREATMENT STAGES

Discrimination
Production
Transfer
Retention

be contrasted with a letter *C*, to show the difference between /s/ and /θ/. The clinician might request that the child give him or her the [θi]. If the child gives the clinician the wrong object, the clinician explains the speech sound difference. Similarly, if the child requests the [θi], the clinician responds by giving the child the object with the [θi] label. At times the child will have intended to request the *C*. In those situations, the clinician instructs the child with respect to the reason for the failure to communicate (e.g., "Oh, you wanted the *C*, but you said [θi]. That's why I gave you the wrong thing"). Other procedures used in discrimination training involve the child's pointing to pictures representing the contrast between error sound and child production. At first, the clinician produces the individual words (e.g., *bass bath* and later the contrasts are embedded in sentences—"The bath is cold").

Discrimination training as used by Winitz involves the child's ability to contrast and compare phoneme units or syllable structure units within words and longer utterances. He referred to this as *conceptualization training* when a child's misarticulations involved multiple phoneme errors. For example, a child who produces fricatives as stops would be asked to discriminate a number of stop and fricative phonemes in minimal pairs. A child who deletes final consonants would be asked to discriminate appropriate pairs of words (e.g., *bow -boat*).

Production training took a similar form if a child was able to correctly imitate the error sound in words. The clinician would point out the nature of the child's articulation errors in a conversational setting. If a child told the clinician to write the letter *C* but produced it as [ti], the clinician would respond by writing a *T*. When the child says that the clinician wrote the wrong letter, he or she would explain the phonetic difference between [si] and [ti] and ask the child to try again. Given a good ability to imitate the clinician's model, the child would succeed in the production and would achieve the communicative intent.

If a child is unable to easily imitate the error sound in words, the clinician would construct "nonsense" words for the child to use. These words would contain phonetic contexts in which the child correctly articulated the sound. By using novel words, Winitz hoped to bypass the connections between the error production and the previously learned word, in the same manner suggested by Van Riper. The nonsense words might be associated with novel line drawings or could be used as names of characters that were then manipulated and talked about in a play setting.

When no correctly articulated phonetic contexts were found, Winitz suggested manipulating the individual gestures associated with production of a phoneme until an appropriate production was elicited. These would then be practiced in nonsense syllables within conversations as discussed above.

The next phase of therapy involved transferring the appropriate production of the sound to other words. This amounts to reassociating already known words with new connection strengths at the syllable, phoneme, and feature levels. Winitz would do this through manipulation of nonsense words to form real words. This is one of the procedures used by McDonald to extend the phonetic contexts in which a speech sound was correctly articulated. For example a child who usually dentalizes [s] may produce it appropriately when it is surrounded by velar consonants as in [ɪkski]. The child would construct real words or word combinations from this syllable (e.g., *Dick skis, thick ski*).

Winitz viewed the final stage as one of practicing articulation in other conversational settings. The child and clinician would arrange to practice articulation of the speech sounds in a variety of commonly occurring environments (e.g., with siblings, classmates, parents, and teachers in the classroom). This stage of practice would provide training in articulation of the words, sentence structures, concepts, and propositions most like those in the child's system.

Hodson and Paden's Cyclic Approach

Rather than approaching therapy for articulation as a process in which a single sound or single error pattern is targeted and treated until production is appropriate, Hodson and Paden (1983) organized therapy in *cycles.* Each cycle is of relatively short duration—2 to 4 weeks—and targets a particular speech production error pattern. Each pattern is exemplified by a phoneme that is stimulable in the child's speech. Each session involves a set of steps called review, auditory bombardment, production practice, probing, and a homework assignment.

The activity called *auditory bombardment* involves the clinician reading a list of words containing the speech sound that has been chosen as a target representation of an error pattern. For example, a clinician who has chosen to target final-consonant deletion may chose word-final /p/ as a stimulable target for an individual child. The clinician would then pull together a list of approximately 10 words to represent this pattern (e.g., *mop, rope, map*). These are slowly read to the child as individual words and as parts of sentences through an auditory trainer. The intent is to focus the child's attention on the sound to be produced and its auditory characteristics as seen in both Van Riper and Winitz' approaches.

Next these words are produced in play activities in which the child is asked to name and request pictures or objects that exemplify the target words. The tactile, kinesthetic, auditory, and visual features of the speech sound are discussed as they occur in each of the training words, in much the same manner used by McDonald. Gamelike activities are used to elicit productions of these words as often as possible in the session so that each production can be described. For example, in a session the children might take turns pulling objects out of a bag, naming them, and describing what each can be used for.

The auditory bombardment phase is repeated at the end of a session. Finally, the parents are instructed in the use of that day's words so that the auditory bombardment and production practice may continue at home.

During subsequent sessions, new phoneme exemplars for an error pattern are added, and the old word sets are reviewed. After three to four sessions on one error pattern, a new pattern is introduced.

It is apparent that each of the treatment approaches shares much with the others, partly because all treatment approaches ultimately must deal with a child's perception and production of speech sounds. Whether the clinician believes that he or she is strengthening motor patterns, sensory patterns, or cognitive patterns, the clinician must always have the child listening to speech, talking, and responding to feedback about the performance in each task.

SUGGESTED TREATMENT STRATEGIES

In general, our approach to treatment is a singular process in which the clinician's role is to provide the learner with information regarding phonetic production in the service of language use. As the child incorporates this information into the verbal communication system, his or her speech productions will become more adultlike. The child is helped to associate adultlike sensory features with adultlike categories of phonemes, syllables, words, and propositions. The directness with which the clinician imparts this information will depend on the language level of the child. We draw a line between Nelson's (1985) second and third stages of language acquisition.

As you will recall from Chap. 2, the second stage involves the development of language forms for their use as tools. In the early part of this stage, the child is associating labels with basic concepts of present, ongoing actions such as agent, action, and object. As the child develops more adultlike concepts, he or she will become able to describe featural similarities and differences among objects and actions. Then the child learns to coordinate and express time and space relationships among these basic concepts using tense markers on verbs, temporal terms such as *before* and *after,* and spatial terms such as *up* and *over.* Still later, the child learns to establish causal relationships expressed by complex conjoining of basic agent-action-object sequences with words such as *because, if . . . then,* and *but.* The uses of these linguistic tools will first be social (i.e., they will allow the child to manipulate the behaviors of the persons in the environment). These also become useful as abstract thinking tools, which allow the child to succeed in academic environments and to mentally manipulate agents, objects, actions, and their interrelationships.

The child in the second stage is developing the ability to manipulate these symbols in the absence of the sensory information available in these social interchanges. As the child's language symbols become useful as abstract objects that can be consciously manipulated, the child passes over into the third stage. During this stage, the child learns to view language symbols abstractly. The child will learn to understand that a single word can mean many different things and that many words sometimes mean the same thing. Such knowledge can be seen in the child's developing appreciation of puns and jokes. The child will start to appreciate that stories have definable parts such as characters, settings, and resolutions of plots. Important for our purposes, the child will be learning that words are made up of syllables and speech sounds. This development becomes apparent in the child's ability to rhyme words and to phonetically read novel words.

Van Riper and McDonald's approaches to articulation treatment outlined in the previous section assume that the child is in the third stage. The child is expected to analyze words and syllables for their phonemic content. The child is expected to make abstract judgments about the "correctness" of his or her speech sound productions and is asked to analyze feature similarities and differences among phonemic units. The first of our approaches, entitled "Motoric Automatization of Articulatory Performance," is an extension of these and is intended for such children. In particular, this approach is intended for the older child who misarticulates one or two speech sounds. These children are suspected of having little or no difficulty in the use of language symbols to mark complex relationships among basic concepts including time, space, causality, and so forth. The clinician must keep in mind that children who are treated in this manner must be able to take an abstract view of speech sound production. This is the same abstract view of speech production that some of us may have found difficult to take when we first took courses in phonetics or foreign languages. For those of you who have taken a French course, think of the kinds of manipulations you went through trying to learn to produce the rounded, high, front vowel [y]. Ultimately you may have had to use some cues such as "Start to say the vowel [i]. Now hold your tongue there and round your lips like you are going to say [u]." Such instructions may well be as unintelligible to the younger misarticulating child as his or her speech is to you.

The basic operating procedure in this strategy is to directly teach the child that his or her current phonemic target varies from the adult model in terms of basic gestures of mandibular raising, tongue fronting, and so forth. The child learns to manipulate these independent gestures to produce more appropriate phonemic approximations. The child is asked to actively go about recognizing and reorganizing new phonemic associations for higher-level language units of words and phrases. With the clinician acting as guide, the child learns to practice these productions to make them automatic.

The second approach, entitled "Phonetic Elaboration in Narratives," is intended for the younger child. The basic strategy here is to teach the child to coordinate all levels of language processing simultaneously in the service of supplying information to others. The clinician's role is to provide the child with help in organizing and expressing basic and more advanced meaningful relationships. This is done primarily through storytelling and reading activities in which the clinician adds missing information to the child's system by interpreting the speech acts of others for the child and by providing needed information to the child's utterances. Part of the information that is provided by the clinician will necessarily be related to the organization of syllable shapes, phonemes, and features.

Motoric Automatization of Articulatory Performance

The basis of motoric automatization of articulatory performance is the assumption that revision of overlearned, highly automatic behavior is possible through carefully planned and executed performance rehearsal. Once inappropriate patterns of any behavior are automatized, the process of revising those patterns may differ from development of the original behavior. Perhaps the best examples of automatized error patterns involve the poorly learned athletic gestures resulting in dropped softballs, topped golf balls, and belly flops. Improper learning results in less-than-optimal motor patterns that may result in failure belief systems that compound the difficulty with which appropriate behaviors may be successfully performed or demonstrated—the "I just can't learn this game" syndrome.

Careful coaching and extensive rehearsal of minor adjustments of discrete behaviors must be used to replace previous learning of inadequate or inappropriate behavior. Similarly, ingrained and automatic articulatory patterns resulting in error approximations (disordered articulation) of accepted standards of sound production must be replaced by carefully evaluated/directed and extensively rehearsed behavioral variants. The speech clinician, like the voice, golf, or basketball coach, must realize, accept, and support the fact that rehearsal can and must be viewed as an important and interesting component to improved performance. In so doing, we structure rehearsal to give it meaning, carefully evaluate its results, and enthusiastically reward its improvement.

Stimulability Tasks—Pretraining. Prior to stimulating manipulation of error approximations during early stages of treatment, it may be important to elicit, via imitation, productions of sound segments that the patient produces correctly. This allows the patient to quickly identify with success. You are asking the child to do something that he or she is capable of. Directly and indirectly, you care enough about the child to ensure that he or she succeeds. In so doing, the child will be less likely to confront subsequent tasks with apprehension, pessimism, or negativism. Second, providing a framework within which success is probable, attention can be paid to following your directions and carefully observing your demonstrations. Imitating grossly distorted productions of /m, p, f/ by excessive lip rounding and retraction, for instance, alerts children to their ability to manipulate parameters/components of the articulatory mechanism. In other words, "There are several rather varied ways in which we can produce the same sound, and it's fun to do. Let's see how good we are at doing some fun kinds of things with our speech mechanism, or articulators." Third, the patient is afforded the courtesy of getting to know the direction from which we are coming. The child's awareness of our expectations regarding performance as related to accepted levels of achievement provides an opportunity to learn the so-called rules of the game. Finally, and most important, a model is established within which sound segments are identified, compared, and discriminated. As a result of approaching treatment initiation in such a manner, the patient will be afforded the advantage of knowledge of task requirements before beginning work on articulatory performance, an understandably more difficult and less familiar task. We will have simplified task completion and, most important, prepared our patient for tasks requiring greater effort and attention. On completion of pretraining tasks, the patient and clinician then work together in attempting to achieve desired adjustments of error target positions.

At this point the clinician's knowledge of physiology is of particular importance. Like the golf pro or voice coach, the clinician must be able to first analyze what the patient is doing. We must be able to observe carefully, visually, and auditorily, and then examine conceptually those physiological features underlying error approximations. Every clinician should be able to repeat sentences or converse using error approximations similar to those of the patient. As students, we should practice producing some of the types of speech we will encounter.

Table 5-9 lists several sample sentences in which misarticulations have been embedded. We should be able, with a little practice, to demonstrate our ability to manipulate the parameters of the speech mechanism to interested or convenient listeners including sponsors (parents), alleged friends (fellow students), and others (lovers or spouses). If you find these tasks somewhat difficult, you should be able to better understand the difficulties encountered by our patients as they do their best to achieve our expectations.

It is most appropriate to supply prompts and verbal directions for articulatory gestures according to the *dynamics* of sound production. What we are doing—or trying to do—does not have to be labeled in terms of an orthographic or phonemic description. It is of little value to say "We're going to

Table 5-9. SENTENCES EXEMPLIFIED WITH A VARIETY OF MISARTICULATIONS

I saw a baby boy.
[a tɔ ə beˀɪ bɔɪ]
Larry is so nice.
[wɛwɪ ɪd to naɪ]
Ray was a precious urchin.
[wɛ wʌd ə pwɛdɪd ʊdən]
Studying articulation gives me goose bumps.
[dʌdɪ ʌdɪdʊedʌn dɪb midubʌp]

try to make a better /s/ or /r/ or /k/," or whatever. We first want to get the idea across that what we are going to do will involve some interesting and funny things with our speech mechanisms. It is very much like a musical instrument. And like a musical instrument, there are several ways in which it can be played. In other words, we are going to experiment with different ways in which we can produce sound with our own speech instrument.

Activities designed to provide information concerning anatomy and physiology of the speech and hearing mechanism are important to the future of treatment. Given the opportunity, children are fascinated by graphic information related to the structure and function of their lungs, larynx, oral and nasal cavities, and ears. Other activities incorporated in the treatment process include active participation in learning social functions of speech such as how to introduce themselves and others, giving directions, and telling jokes. Similarly, as the treatment process continues, they should be given the opportunity to act as the speech clinician (or teacher) and direct group members in activities, or pretend that the clinician is their patient. Ultimately, they can work toward a presentation in their classroom concerning what all they are learning about speech. As a final result of learning with highly skilled health professionals they become directly and indirectly aware of the social, academic, scientific, and therapeutic aspects of speech communication.

Production activities should involve manipulation of the various articulatory gestures reviewed in Chap. 1. An [i] can be produced with lip spreading that is gradually shaped to lip rounding. A vowel series such as [i][ɪ][ɛ][eɪ][æ] can be produced to show the movement of the mandible. Tongue-tip movement can be demonstrated and practiced by producing dental stops, alveolar stops, and retroflex stops. Bilabial stops can be contrasted with bilabial fricatives and affricates. Voicing can be manipulated with touch feedback as can nasalization. Non-English sounds have an advantage in such manipulations. Their gestures do not have extensive phonemic connections and can usually be manipulated freely. Children should be encouraged to view what they do in a mirror and listen to the results on audio or audiovideo tape recordings. The structure of their own articulators, for example, and the number, size, and shape of teeth, can be compared with those in textbook pictures and so forth.

Rehearsal. In this section, the process of rehearsing appropriate articulation of a particular consonant is presented in four levels: nonsymbolic, word and word pair, sound-in-context sentences, and narratives. It is crucial to realize that these are not intended to constitute a linear program in which a child is forced to practice production of nonsymbolic units for days or weeks before dealing with words: These are approached as rehearsal units that can be intermingled within a session, within the context of talking about speech production and perhaps constructing an interesting narrative for the children to write out or perform as a skit. For example, a session may be spent in the activity of writing a story about a picnic to be acted out with felt board characters or as a group skit. Such a story will necessarily involve a number of occurrences of each child's error sound production. When these occur, they can be dissected into their constituent sentences, word pairs, and nonsymbolic units for production practice. After these are practiced, they can be comfortably produced by the child as one part of his or her role in the skit or part of the reading of the story. For example, the sentence "Jack surprised Tom" may be part of a story. For a child who misarticulates [s], the two-word combination "Jack surprised" can be pulled out and practiced, as can the nonsymbolic unit [æksɝ]. These levels are discussed below.

Nonsymbolic Units. The gestures manipulated in pretraining will be actively manipulated in rehearsing the target sound's production in nonsymbolic units. A matrix of nonsymbolic sound units is illustrated in Table 5-10. The ability to successfully approximate target segments within VC, CV, and VCV units is the base on which subsequent automatization rests. For the most part, these units are nonsymbolic. They are not, however, "nonsense" syllables. If we consider, for instance, those activities employed by golfers; football, baseball, and basketball players; singers; and instrumentalists, an analogy to the significance of production rehearsal can be better appreciated. Golfers usually take practice swings or actually "shag" balls before a match. Football, basketball, and baseball players spend countless hours rehearsing fundamentals before playing a game. Even immediately before a game they warm up by rehearsing fundamental units of their respective sport. Similarly, musicians rehearse scales, sustain notes, and in general, loosen up before a rehearsal or performance.

Insofar as our work with patients is concerned, careful direction, evaluation, and continuation of rehearsal of nonsymbolic sound units are also important to improved performance. The implication of "nonsymbolic sound unit" is particularly significant. The fact that, for the most part, CV, VCV, and VC units involve only syllabic-, phonemic-, and feature-level processing places minimal linguistic constraint on the speech production mechanism. In other words, in repeating such units as [si, isi, is], the speaker is able to attend to such tasks without being constrained by morphology, syntax, and semantics. This is particularly important to speakers who have learned error approximations to standard sound segments, because the substandard patterns have become embedded in each of the highly interrelated subcomponents of language structure. For this reason, reducing task complexity by elimination of higher-level constraints will result in motoric automatization, which prepares performance generalization of newly learned patterns to more highly constrained acts. In the case of speech production, words, phrases, sentences, and conversation, again the analogy to musicians and athletes is useful in that rehearsal of discrete acts, whether preparatory to playing or singing a composition or scrimmaging or playing a game, prepares the performer for subsequent, more highly constrained events.

The construction of the matrices in Table 5-10 includes primary emphasis of those vowels /i, u, æ, a/ that represent the extremes of the vowel quad-

Table 5-10. NONSYMBOLIC SOUND UNIT REHEARSAL MATRICES

VC	*VCV*	*CV*	*VCCV*
i s	i s i	s i	i t s i
a s	i s a	s a	i t s a
u s	i s u	s u	i t s u
æ s	i s æ	s æ	i t s æ
	a s i		a t s i
	a s a		a t s a
	a s u		a t s u
	a s æ		a t s æ
	u s i		u t s i
	u s a		u t s a
	u s u		u t s u
	u s æ		u t s æ
	æ s i		æ t s i
	æ s a		æ t s a
	æ s u		æ t s u
	æ s a		æ t s a

rilateral. As such, articulator movement to and from target consonant approximations to the vowels /i, u, æ, a/ is greatest. In addition, inasmuch as these vowels are generally longer in duration than other vowels, movements to and from their idealized positions provide maximal auditory, tactile, and kinesthetic feedback. These two factors can be readily demonstrated by rehearsing the segment [s] in the contexts of [isi], [æsæ], [usu], and [asa]. In the context [isi], the apical construction necessary for [i] to [s] and back again to [i] occurs with the mandible fully elevated for the entire unit. To the contrary, the low front vowel [æ] requires mandibular lowering and is, in a sense, antagonistic to production of /s/. When [s] is embedded in an [asa] unit we immediately recognize that tongue and mandibular excursions are far greater than for [isi] and require greater effort and precision. In varying degrees, the same may be said for the units [usu] and [asa]. Note that feedback information resulting from production of such units is maximized, thus enabling the speaker to establish idealized target approximations against which subsequent productions can be matched.

Contrary to several other approaches to articulatory treatment that suggest moving as quickly as possible through "nonsense syllables" to words and phrases, extensive and repeated successful performance of sound units will result in more rapid generalization to words, sentences, and conversational speech. The same may be said regarding treatment approaches that overlook the significance of a hierarchical linguistic system. Therapy systems that initiate treatment at the word or word pair level simply cannot provide "sound" information (pun intended) that is meaningful and pragmatic to the patient.

As we continue our study of motoric automatization of articulatory performance, the significance of successful sound unit rehearsal will become even more apparent. Sound units, whether they are CV, VC, VCV, or VCCV, are the rudiments of speech. Achieving high degrees of success at rudimentary levels facilitates success at more highly complex levels. The same may be said with reference to successful academic/clinical training and professional performance. Preparation and perspiration are infinitely more valuable to successful performance than hope and inspiration.

Word and Word Pairs. Having successfully programmed the articulation of a particular nonsymbolic unit, transition to the word group from which it came should be relatively automatic. The child can then return to the story construction process.

Each child may be made responsible for constructing a notebook containing a variety of nonsymbolic units and their associated word and word pairs. These can be used by the child for continued self-practice in homework assignments or as quiz materials by which each child plays teacher and asks the others in the group to rehearse particular units and to develop their own possible words and word pairs. While guiding the construction of these rehearsal materials, it is advantageous to include those words and word pairs that relate to age/maturational levels and individual interests. Names of family members, pets, characters from favorite stories and TV programs, dolls, and favorite toys are particularly apropos. When given the opportunity, children are sophisticated enough to assist clinicians in developing personalized activities. As opposed to commercially or clinician-prepared "monotonous and mesmerizing" (M & M) word lists that bore patients out of their minds by playing "repeat this," alternative procedures derived from self-generated patient-clinician responsibility lead to sustained cooperative interest and participation. Most important, as a result of cooperative responsibility, the patient more readily understands personal responsibility in recognizing and judging adequacy of personal performance. Ultimately and ideally, the patient learns to become his or her own clinician.

The development of word and word pair lists can also be readily adapted to tasks requiring memory and speed. In addition to accurate sound production, competing with others in a group or bettering one's previous performance leads to improved skill in attending to and recall of words containing target sounds.

Depending on individual skill and progress, patients learn to quickly identify and categorize target sounds according to word-initial, cluster, medial, and final positions. Once production skill has been ingrained during nonsymbolic rehearsal, patients are then frequently able to determine production adequacy within words and word pairs.

Table 5-11 illustrates sample word and word pair lists for the target sound

Table 5-11. WORD AND WORD PAIR LIST FOR [s]

Prevocalic		*Intervocalic*	*Postvocalic*	
Initial	*Cluster*	*Medial*	*Final*	*Word pair*
Sam	scat	passing	pass	Jack sat
seed	ski	receive	niece	jeep seat
soup	scooter	loosen	loose	room soon
saw	scar	bossy	toss	cop saw
sit	skit	kissing	miss	lip sip
sign	sky	nicer	mice	right side

[s]. Note that in addition to relatively common words, high-interest words and word pairs have been included. Notice also that neither words nor word pairs contain more than one occurrence of the target sound.

For patients who are initiating sound change at the word and word pair level, it is important to reduce complexity and difficulty as much as possible. Tongue twisters and sentences loaded with target sounds should be kept on the proverbial shelf until the patient is able to demonstrate high degrees of success. Our responsibilities as clinicians require that we maximize opportunities for success while discretely increasing task complexity. For this reason, initial rehearsals of words and word pair lists should include items with only single occurrences of target sounds. Finally, rapid and accurate production of sound unit, word, and word pair tasks indicates initial progress toward automatization. At this point in the treatment process, patients will be able to assume personal responsibility for repetition of tasks in the classroom and at home. Until patients are able to demonstrate successful performance and degrees of personal direction, parent and teacher involvement in the treatment process should be minimal. This is because parents and teachers do not share our specialized knowledge and clinical skill. As a result, their performance in monitoring or assisting in initial phases of the treatment process might be characterized by uneasiness or perhaps even resentment. (Most teachers do not feel they are employees of speech clinicians.) When their responsibilities are simplified by a patient who understands what is going on, the direction in which he or she is going, as well as what has to be done to get there, parents and teachers will usually become proud and willing partners in the treatment process.

Sound-in-Context Rehearsal Sentences. In addition to isolating sentences from the narrative activity, the clinician can guide a variety of rehearsal situations in which children cue each other for production of their error sounds. Imitative tasks involve repetition of preselected sentences as illustrated in Table 5-12. During these tasks the patient imitates the clinician's repetition of each sentence. Once again, it is important to construct stimulus

Table 5-12. SOUND-IN-CONTEXT REHEARSAL SENTENCES FOR TARGET SEGMENT [s]

Target stimulus	*Sentence*
PREVOCALIC	
Sam	Sam is a good boy.
seed	Plant the seed in the dirt.
soup	The soup is hot.
saw	We saw a big worm.
sit	Don't sit on my foot.
same	We are the same age.
sign	The sign is red.
CLUSTER	
scat	I told the cat to scat.
ski	Don't ski down that big hill.
scooter	Can you ride a scooter.
scar	The cut left a scar.
skip	I can hop, skip, and jump.
skate	Can you roller skate?
sky	The kite was high in the sky.
INTERVOCALIC	
passer	My dad is a good passer.
receive	I will receive good grades.
loosen	Please loosen the jar lid.
bossy	My brother is bossy.
kissing	The monkey was kissing him.
racer	My friend built a new racer.
nicer	Your hair is nicer than mine.
bicycle	I can ride a bicycle.
Icee	Mom bought a root beer Icee.
POSTVOCALIC	
pass	Please pass the pepper.
niece	I am my uncle's niece.
loose	My shoe is too loose.
toss	Toss the ball to me.
miss	Miss Piggy is cute.
face	You have a pretty face.
mice	I like to play with mice.

Table 5-12. (continued).

Target stimulus	*Sentence*
WORD PAIR	
Jack sat	Jack sat in a puddle.
jeep seat	The jeep seat is hard.
room soon	The room soon got cold.
cop saw	That cop saw a cat in the tree.
quit sitting	Please quit sitting on my chair.
cake sale	The cake sale was fun.
right side	The right side of the room is dark.

sentences in conformity with the patient's age, abilities, and interests. Given the fact that, by this time, the patient will have demonstrated abilities to successfully produce target sounds in sound units, words, and word pairs, sentence repetition difficulty will be significantly reduced.

The second phase of sentence rehearsal, word stimulus sentences, is completed by presenting a stimulus word containing the target segment. The patient's task is to repeat the word and embed it in a spontaneously generated sentence frame. As illustrated in Table 5-13, this task, although similar in nature to imitative sentence repetition, requires higher-level performance by the patient. Also included in Table 5-13 are examples of the spontaneous word stimulus sentences. During these tasks, the patient spontaneously produces the stimulus word, followed by a sentence in which it is embedded. Examples of such sound-in-context sentences can be found in Appendix B.

Narratives. Articulation serves the overall process of verbal communication, and its rehearsal should always be related to communicative tasks. A useful format involves the construction of stories that can be written by the children (preferably with the aid of a microcomputer-based word-processing program). These stories can be illustrated, acted out, and read to parents and friends. These stories are particularly useful with elementary-age children and are more effectively presented when using a felt board and felt figures. Table 5-14 illustrates a portion of such a story. Note that this particular sequence has been developed to emphasize and assess the target sounds [s] and [θ]. Each narrative presentation by the clinician is followed by the child's target responses. These responses should be similar or identical to those found in the narrative and should always be in sentence form. Although several other such stories appear in Appendix C, children and clinicians who involve themselves in development of their own stories thoroughly enjoy the challenge and the results.

Although tasks involved in the motoric automatization of articulatory performance have been presented in a quasi-stepwise manner, overlapping of

Table 5-13. WORD STIMULUS SENTENCES AND SPONTANEOUS WORD STIMULUS SENTENCES

Clinician	*Patient*	
Stimulus	***Imitative***	***Spontaneous***
bird	bird	A robin is a bird.
ring	ring	A bathtub ring is gross.
Rita	Rita	Rita wears a curly wig.
friend	friend	You are a good friend.
talker	talker	I am becoming a good talker.
redundant	redundant	I myself personally am redundant.
Spontaneous Stimulus		Response
rat		The rat ate the cheese.
bread		Whole wheat bread is yummy.
rubbers		I wear rubbers in the rain.
rich		Writing books is a hard way to get rich.

Table 5-14. ARTICULATION AUTOMATIZATION STORY: "POKY'S SURPRISE"

Suggested materials: flannelboard, felt figures (turtle, rocking chair, telephone, duck, owl, pond, bushes, ice cream, cake

Target sounds: [s] *and* [θ]

Clinician narrative	*Target response*
1. This is Poky the turtle. Today is his birthday. He is 6-years old. He says, "It's my birthday." What does he say?	It's my birthday.
2. But Poky the turtle is sad. Nobody knows it's his birthday. No one cares. Poky says, "It's sad when no one cares." What does he say?	It's sad when no one cares.
3. Poky says, "I'll just stay home today. No one remembers it's my birthday." Poky sits in his rocking chair. What does he does?	He sits in his rocking chair.
4. All of a sudden, the telephone rings. Poky jumps up and answers the phone. "Hello," he says. "Who's calling?" It was his friend Mitsy, the duck. "Oh, hi Mitsy," says Poky. What does he say?	Oh, hi Mitsy.

Table 5-14. (continued).

5. Mitsy says, "Come on over Poky. Let's swim in my pond." She says, "Let's swim in my pond." What does she say?	Let's swim in my pond.
6. "OK," says Poky. "I'll be right over." Poky hangs up the phone. "I thought someone would know it's my birthday," he says. What does he say?	I thought someone would know it's my birthday.
7. Poky starts walking to Mitsy's house to go for a swim. On the way, he stops at the rabbits' house. "Maybe the rabbits will know it's my birthday," he says. What does he say?	Maybe the rabbits will know it's my birthday.
8. He knocks at their door, but no rabbits are home. Poky walks down the road until he comes to Mr. Owl's nest. "Mr. Owl," he says, "come outside and say hello." What does he say?	Mr. Owl, come outside and say hello.
9. But Mr. Owl is not at home. "Oh, well," says Poky, "it's silly to worry about a dumb birthday." What does he say?	It's silly to worry about a dumb birthday.
10. Poky walks slowly to Mitsy's pond. He says, "I'll just swim in the pond. It's fun to swim on your birthday." What does he say?	It's fun to swim on your birthday.
11. Just then, Poky hears some noise in the bushes. "Who's there?" "It's us," he hears someone say. What does he hear someone say?	It's us.
12. Out from the bushes came Mitsy, the duck, the rabbits, and Mr. Owl. "Surprise!" they say. "Happy birthday, Poky! Eat some cake and ice cream." What do they say?	Happy birthday Poky. Eat some cake and ice cream.
13. "Oh, boy!" says Poky. "You remembered my birthday. That's so nice of you." What does he say?	That's so nice of you.
14. His friends say, "We would never forget your birthday, Poky. Now, let's eat before the ice cream melts." What do they say?	Let's eat before the ice cream melts.

tasks is important to the treatment process. For example a child may take a particular nonsymbolic unit such as [ɪtsi] and derive a number of word units such as *Mitsi* and *fit seems* that can then be put into a number of sentences. The clinician should always keep the child as primary judge of the productions—describing the movement patterns, articulatory contacts, and adequacy of production of each target sound in its context. The child should become teacher as rapidly as possible.

In the same sense, children who misarticulate more than one sound should not complete automatization of one specific target segment before beginning training on another. To the contrary, once training has been initiated through stimulation and sound unit rehearsal, a second target segment can be introduced, while continuing work on the first. Treatment programs should not be viewed as cookbook approaches. Clinicians and clients, unlike sugar, salt, and flour, are highly variable ingredients of the treatment process. Creativity, spontaneity, enthusiasm, adaptability, and sensitivity are variables that cannot be written into a treatment design. Yet, without them, the best treatment designs will be ineffective.

Phonetic Elaboration in Narratives

The techniques employed above made a number of assumptions about a child's abilities. These include that the child is aware of misarticulating a particular sound or sounds, is able to talk about speech production as a topic that is not too abstract, is interested enough in altering articulation to practice nonsymbolic units and make judgments about their adequacy, and finally is able to bind time and space changes in language forms while constructing narratives. The preschool child who misarticulates many phonemes and deletes consonants is not likely to be a sophisticated enough language user to profit from such an approach. For such a child, articulation is one aspect of language ability that is used in communication settings. It is within such settings that the clinician should seek to improve articulation.

Within the approach described here, the clinician establishes communication situations for a group of children. The topic of these situations is a narrative derived originally from a picture depicting commonly occurring childhood experiences such as those in Appendix A and those referred to in Chap. 1. The general goal is for the children to produce more complex stories using appropriate meaningful units of sentences, phrases, words, and their production via more complex syllables, phonemes, and features. Specific goals can be derived for an individual child from the general list cited earlier.

The clinician's primary role is to keep the children involved in constructing and talking about the story. She does this by structuring the social interaction of the children so that each child is taking communicative turns that relate to the story topic. She also supplies the child with information prior to taking a turn that will aid in the child's appropriate communication. Following the child's speech act, the clinician provides feedback about its communicative adequacy, including information about its phonetic production when appropriate. She then ensures that each speech act is consequented by someone's response, either a nonverbal action or another speech act. Each of these aspects of the clinician's actions is discussed in the following sections.

Structuring the Social Interaction. The clinician wants each child to construct speech acts incorporating adequate meaningful linguistic units, syllable shapes, phonemes, and gestures. In order to do this, each child must be given the opportunity to produce speech acts that have an effect on a listener.

The clinician initiates the production of a narrative by asking for a child to start telling a story about a particular picture. Using the first drawing in Appendix A, the clinician might ask for a volunteer ("Who wants to start telling a story about this picture?") or she could direct one of the children to start the story ("Zack, you tell the other children a story about this picture"). If the clinician is working individually with a child she could say, "Tell me a story about this picture." Or, she could set up a situation in which she and the child are going to tell a story to a doll or a puppet.

In any case, the intent is for the child to be speaking with a purpose. The purpose will be to inform the listeners about some aspect of the picture that the child has chosen to include in a story. Contrast this strategy with one in which the child is asked to name pictures for the clinician. Certainly most children will realize that the adult knows the name of the picture and they are not really informing her of anything.

It is important that each speech act be treated as though it were meaningful and had an effect on a listener. The clinician makes sure that someone ackowledges the child's statement and makes a comment related to the child's meaning. For example, if Zack's opening statement was "The lady has ice cream," the clinician could direct another child to ask for more information. ("Joe, ask Zack why she is getting the ice cream.") Joe's speech act, directed at Zack, will consequent Zack's statement (i.e., it will show that it had an effect on a listener). The clinician could also direct one of the other children to add more information about the topic by saying something like "Joe, Zack told you that this woman is getting ice cream. Tell him why she is getting it." The two children's speech acts will compose part of a conversation regarding a single topic with each child intending to supply meaningful information to the other.

The clinician essentially acts to direct the conversational traffic. She wants each child to have a number of opportunities to speak. And she wants to keep each child's speech related to the topic and the other children's speech acts.

Providing Information Prior to a Child's Speech Act. In the examples used above, each child was able to formulate an appropriate utterance that fulfilled the purpose suggested by the clinician. However, the clinician is seek-

Table 5-15. EXAMPLES OF PROMPTS SUPPLYING DIFFERING DEGREES OF INFORMATION

Ask Zack why the lady bought ice cream.
Find out why the lady bought ice cream.
We don't know why she's getting ice cream but I bet Zack knows.
Who can find out why she's doing that?

ing to expand each child's language-processing ability, so she will often be asking children to produce utterances that exceed their present level of functioning. To make it more likely that a child will be successful in these attempts, the clinician supplies the child with needed information while directing him to speak.

The information given will be manipulated by the clinician to suit the child's level of functioning. The examples in Table 5-15 contain a variety of degrees of information. The first prompt, "Ask Zack why the lady bought ice cream," is a direction to ask a particular person a particular question. It contains all of the major constituents of the expected question as seen in the italicized components of "*Why* did *the lady* buy *ice cream*?" The clinician has supplied a purpose for the speech act; now the child needs to organize the given information into a question format by supplying a change in the verb form to "did buy." The second statement contains the constituents of the question to be asked, but the child is not specifically directed to "ask" a particular person: The child must supply this organization. The later examples are missing many of the constituents for the questions that must, therefore, be supplied from the child's own system.

The clinician may provide more of the needed information for a child's speech act by using "cloze" procedures. The clinician provides the scaffolding of an utterance, leaving the child "blanks" to be filled in. For example, the clinician provides more of the constituents for the child by saying

"Ask Zack, 'Why did the mommy buy the . . .'"
or
"Ask Zack, 'Why did the mommy . . . '"
or
"Ask Zack, 'Why did . . .'"

The clinician's expectant pause gives the child the opportunity to fill in the rest of the utterance.

The clinician can use gestures or pointing to denote important linguistic units that need to be used in an expected utterance. For example, "Ask Zack, why the [points to mother] bought [points to ice cream]." Note that the clinician does not really expect the child to produce a mere labeling response; rather she is providing help in producing more complex utterances even when the child is required only to add a label to the overall utterance. As the child is better able to express a particular relationship, this support can be faded.

The clinician also uses the prompts to shape the complexity level of the child's utterance. As suggested in Chap. 1, a variety of levels of abstraction can be found in propositions from labeling to describing to inferencing and finally interpreting. Examples of each level and the prompts a clinician might use to raise the level of a child's utterance are discussed next.

Prompts to Move a Child from Labeling to Describing. At the lowest level of attaching meaningful language to this picture, a child might go through the picture naming the persons and objects. For example, while pointing to each part of the picture a child might construct a story such as

[aɪ ki]	[wedi]	[boi]	[wʌk]	[mæ]
Ice cream . . .	lady . . .	boys . . .	truck . . .	man.

In this story the child has labeled some of the persons and objects in the picture. His syllabic structure is relatively undeveloped inasmuch as he does not produce consonant clusters or all of his final consonants. He has not drawn any basic relationships among these objects. He has not included any of the actions in the picture because they must be inferred from the pictured persons and objects. This child's language is extremely static in nature.

Although many articulation training programs extensively practice single-word labeling responses, this appears to be a dead-end approach with respect to the development of articulation ability. If a child attaches appropriate syllables, phonemes, and features to a picture using only labeling, the "meaning" of the utterances is likely to be associated only with the particular pictured objects. Recall that early vocabulary development occurs within the context of *event representations.* In this case, the child's understanding of *lady* is partially determined as the person who provides goodies to children. We want the child to learn not only to produce the appropriate sounds associated with this word but also to associate it with the concept and label *mother* within a commonly occurring event. We want to use similar event representations and approach articulation and language training in a context of telling stories about commonly occurring events the child has experienced in the past and is likely to experience in the future. When the event does occur again, the child should be that much better prepared to converse and to use language the way it was practiced in therapy. To be included in such a representation, the labels should be included in at least the level of description as portrayed next.

To prompt a child to produce a description instead of a label, the clinician points out a relationship between more than one aspect of the picture and asks the child to relate the two. For example, the clinician could alternately point to the lady and the ice cream and ask the child to "Tell the children about this." Or if she wanted to cue the child to express a relationship between the woman's action and that of the boy who has dropped his glove, she could alternately point to these two persons.

If the child's typical response would be to label an actor, the clinician could encourage the inclusion of an action by starting the utterance for the child while pointing out the action aspect of the utterance to the child. For example, saying "The lady . . . " with a rising intonation indicates that something should follow in the utterance. By pointing from the lady to the ice cream, the child may be cued to start with the clinician's utterance and finish it by adding the indicated aspect of the picture.

The clinician continually encourages the labeling child to expand his utterances to the descriptive level. The basic relationships developed by young children described in Chap. 2 such as agent-action, action-object, and so forth can be prompted in this fashion. While seeking to expand the propositional and conceptual level of a child's speech, the clinician will also be providing a large number of models of their syllabic, phonemic, and featural representations. Consider the following utterances supplied by a clinician prior to a child's speech production:

Clinician: Tell Zack about the *lady. She* is *holding* some *ice cream.* The *lady bought* the *ice cream.* The lady . . . .

The words *lady* and *ice cream* have been modeled twice. The child will use the connections stimulated by these productions during a speech attempt. The child's articulatory organization will be increased by the models provided and the subsequent speech attempts that use these productions in more complex language.

Prompts to Move a Child from Describing to Interpretations and Inferences. A descriptive story is one in which the child draws together a number of simple relationships that describe the actors, actions, and recipients of actions. For example, the following is a descriptive story:

[mami hæ ai kim]	[boi maiʔi]	[boi hæ ba]
Mommy has ice cream.	Boy smiling.	Boy has ball.

Children at this level of development are typically not using all of the syntactic markers that express the relationships between agents and actions and so forth. For example, this child does not produce auxiliary verbs. Basically, he has expressed a simple relationship by saying "Boy smiling," and the auxiliary verb here does not add anything to the meaning.

Such children are also not likely to express time and space relationships among the actions that occurred in the story. For example, when did the boy start to smile, before or after mom got the ice cream? The two choices make differing assumptions about the relationships between the boy's actions and that of the other characters.

To supply such time markers, the child must understand and code the relationships among the basic descriptive sentences. A child who states only the individual sentences is not drawing the proper inferences that tie these various components together into an event representation. Although noting that the boy is smiling, this child does not state the cause of the boy's smile.

Descriptions occur at Blank and colleagues' levels I and II in which the child is able to label objects and actions and can identify the perceptible features of objects and actions. Oftentimes articulation programs seek to practice articulation within the context of producing sentences that describe a picture or scene. However, such practice may become a dead end if the child does not have the opportunity to express relationships across sentence units.

The clinician can encourage use of inferences by posing higher-level questions regarding the picture and by requesting that the child explain relationships between aspects of pictures that cannot be stated with a simple description. For example, pointing to the boy's smile and the ice cream and asking the child to "Explain this" requests a causal statement about the child's smile. Pointing to the dropped glove and the boy who is still playing baseball and saying "What will happen next?" prompts for prediction of a future event and so forth.

The clinician can help scaffold these more complex responses by supplying connective words that express such relationships. Temporal information can be prompted by following a child's utterances with "and then . . ." or "next . . ." (asking for a future event)"; "but first . . ." or "before . . ." (asking for a preceding event); or "while . . ." (asking for a simultaneous event). Spatial information can be prompted with "in . . ." or "next to . . ." or "which was on . . . ." Causal relationships can be prompted by "because . . ."; "so that . . ."; or "in order to . . . ." Adversative relationships are prompted by "but . . ."; "except that . . . ."; or "however . . ." These are useful devices for conversations with friends, a good situation in which to practice. When you talk to your friends, try to elicit specific information without using "Wh- questions." If someone says "John is such a fool" say "Because . . ." rather than "Why?"

Simple one-sentence descriptions of pictures do not allow for complex relationships commonly encountered by children. Such practice does not necessarily mesh the child's articulation practice with linguistic devices such as pronouns, which link different sentences together by reference to a previously named person, or time markers, which express relationships across sentence units by detailing complex time relationships. Consider some fairly simple relationships that involve fairly complex time-space relationships in this picture: "Mom will give the ice cream to Joe so he can share it with Tim. But before he gave it to him, he dropped it." This part of a possible story takes place in the future as noted by the verb *will give*. This makes the verb *can share* future as well, even though it is expressed with a present tense marking. Even the verbs *gave* and *dropped* occur some time in the future, even though their inflections say they are past tense. The person being referred to by the pronoun *he* changes throughout the story and can best be patched together by following the logical flow of the time relationships.

In this level of storytelling, the child expresses time relationships and causality relationships that must be inferred from the basic information shown in the picture. For example, "Two boys were playing catch. One dropped his glove because he saw his mother getting ice cream. He is smiling because she is going to give the ice cream to him." Notice that the first statement expresses a relationship between the two boys that is no longer pictured: The boys are not currently playing catch. The statement that the boy dropped his glove involves the inference that he was wearing the glove before the time segment of this picture. The statement "she is going to" expresses a future event relative to the present state of the picture.

The "because" clause involves an interpretation of the relationship between the game of catch and the woman carrying ice cream. The child must figure out that the woman is one of the boy's mothers and that she is going to give the ice cream to them instead of eating it herself. The use of the pronouns *he* and *she* shows that the child is relating the persons in these statements back to the other statements. Also notice that the child has formed a time line for his story as opposed to the first stories, which involved apparently random naming or describing statements.

The child may even go on to expand this story by changing the perspective from which it is told from that of the child to that of the mother: "Mother called to the boys, 'Come get your ice cream before it melts'." Such changes in perspective commonly occur and alter the expression of time-space relationships. This level of language function is similar to that needed to cope with Blank and colleagues' (1978) levels III and IV. We should take into consideration these levels when we ask children to explain why a particular action occurred and find that their articulation seems to be worse than when we were just asking them to label objects. And we should consider the depth of these relationships when a child fails to advance from being able to articulate simple sentences but fails to offer similar good articulation in the face of formulating a complex relationship.

The language often contained in stories, even children's stories, makes references to the characters' motives and inner feelings. These relationships are constructed by relating the more basic relationships expressed above together. They are not directly observable in the simple actions of the characters but involve an interpretation on the part of the storyteller, listener, or one of the characters of the story. For example, a narrator's role might be added to a story about this picture.

This is a story about a brave little boy. His mommy is giving him a reward because he is the only child on the block who will play with Timmy. Timmy is deaf and the other little children don't like to play with him. They make fun of Timmy and anyone who plays with him.

The narrator's utterance explains the mother's motives and sets the stage that this is a story about an abstraction called "bravery" that cannot be defined without reference to simpler actions, deeds, and characteristics of persons.

Although these types of relationships appear to be quite complex, children normally learn how to express and interpret them within their daily activities. We should use such activities as a knowledge base on which to build better speech and language, rather than trying to teach good articulation of words and phrases that are never encountered by the child.

Providing Feedback. After a child has produced an utterance, the clinician will judge its adequacy with respect to the information being conveyed. The first rule is to make sure that a child's utterance has an effect. The second rule is to make sure that the effect is based on the meaning expressed. If inaccuracies exist, the clinician may provide information to show the child why these inaccuracies cause a communication failure. If the utterance failed to reach the desired level, the clinician may provide more information to help the child reach the desired level.

Inaccuracies in a child's utterance can occur at a variety of levels including concepts, meaningful linguistic units, syllable structures, and phonemes. The clinician reacts to the level of inaccuracy that is most important for a particular child and for a particular utterance. Repairs are made by supplying the child with information regarding the need for the repair and then giving the child a chance to restate the relationship.

The following exchange involves a repair at the conceptual level.

Child: Mommy eat ice cream.

Clinician: The mommy isn't eating the ice cream [points to picture]. See, she isn't lifting it to her mouth, and she doesn't have chocolate on her mouth. She is carrying it to the boys. The mommy bought the ice cream from the man and is taking it to the boys. Now, you explain that.

In his utterance, the child misinterpreted the conceptual relationship regarding what the mother is doing. The clinician pointed out some of the salient features of eating (e.g., lifting to the mouth, ice cream around the mouth) that are not present in the picture. She then provides information about what the mother is doing. Note that the information given is not intended as a model sentence for the child to repeat, such as "She is carrying ice cream." Instead, the clinician provides some options for the child and ties the action of the mother to both the ice cream man and the two children.

Repairs may also be needed at the level of meaningful linguistic units, especially in regard to expressing space-time-causality relationships.

Child: Him playing catch.

Clinician: The boy isn't playing catch right now. See, his glove is on the ground. He dropped his glove to run to his mother. Tell Zack what he is doing.

In this case, the child made numerous errors at the sentence level of meaningful linguistic units. The auxiliary verb *is* is not stated. The pronoun should have been the subjective *he*. The clinician has chosen to pay attention to a higher level of coordination in which the time relationship expressed is not accurate. In explaining this time relationship, the clinician models the other errors (i.e., the subjective *he* and the auxiliary verb). Again, after supplying corrective information, the clinician gives the child a chance to reconstruct the original utterance. In this case, the preferred mode of using this approach is apparent in the presence of a second child to whom the story can be told. When at least two children are present, the clinician can direct the children to communicate with one another so that each speech act has an intended audience and so the clinician can help the speaker formulate and correct utterances without confusing his role with that of the primary listener.

Misarticulations that result in faulty message interpretations can be explained in the same manner. The clinician supplies numerous models of well-articulated utterances for the children to reconstruct in this process. She can also provide feedback about a child's articulation of phonemes and syllables that would confuse the listener, much like Winitz did in his reconfiguration strategies. For example, when the child says [boi hæ ba], the clinician could purposefully question what is meant.

Clinician: The boy has a bow? I don't see any bow.

Child: [nou boi hæ ba] [pointing to ball]

Clinician: Oh he has a ball! You confused me because you said [ba]. You need to lift your tongue up at the end of that word and say [bal].

Again the clinician is fulfilling her role of providing feedback regarding the child's communication attempts. The articulatory instruction that occurs in this meaningful setting should be more effective than drill activities in which the child is not intending to communicate.

The clinician can also use the time following an utterance to increase the level of that utterance. For the child who started out labeling separate persons and objects in the picture, the clinician would seek to have the child expand these labels into descriptions. This may be done by accepting the child's utterance as meaningful, seeking to expand its components by modeling, and giving the child a chance to reformulate the utterance using more of its components.

Child: Ice cream . . . lady . . . boys . . . truck.

Clinician: That's right! This is a lady. She's a mommy. She's buying ice cream for her son. Tell me that part of the story.

In this exchange, the clinician accepts the child's attempt at telling the story as meaningful, much like parents do with their children's first word attempts. She then focuses on one basic relationship—"The lady is buying ice cream." She supplies some information for the child (i.e., that the lady is also a mommy and that she is buying the ice cream for her child who is also in the picture). In order to help the child attach these language symbols to the story, the clinician points to the objects and actions as they are described (i.e., to the lady, to her hand holding, to the ice cream, and to the boy). The clinician always seeks to expand the child's knowledge by expanding the utterances and keeping the utterances on track with a basic story line. The clinician keeps going through the story, pointing out the basic relationships and having the child rehearse them.

For a child who describes what is happening in disconnected sentences, the clinician seeks to provide a story line to organize the child's langauge.

Child: The boy is smiling. The lady has ice cream.

Clinician: He does have a big smile! I think he is happy because he sees his mom with ice cream. He thinks the ice cream is for him. Now you tell that part of the story.

Again, the clinician accepts the child's rendition of the story and seeks to expand on it. She supplies information about the child's reason for smiling. Rather than repeating the child's utterance, the clinician rewords its basic intent. Rather than saying "The boy," she models the use of the pronoun *he*. Rather than repeating "is smiling" she states this relationship as "has a big smile," and so forth. She puts together the relationship between the mother buying ice cream and the child's apparent thought that she will give it to him.

As the child tries to put these relationships together, he will meet with failures, and the clinician seeks to help the child through the rough spots by supplying the missing constituents.

Child: The boy . . . he smiling . . . uh . . .

Clinician: because . . .

Child: cuz mommy ice cream . . .

Clinician: The boy . . .

Child: is smiling because mommy has ice cream.

In these exchanges, the clinician sought first to help the child complete the relationship between the boy's smile and the mother's buying ice cream by supplying the verbal marker for the causal relationship. Then she supplied the start of the utterance to see if the child would complete the whole relationship. However, the relationship stated by the child is not quite accurate, and the clinician will explain the difference between the true relationship and the one that the child has expressed.

Clinician: You said that the boy is happy because his mom has ice cream. Well, that's not quite right. He's not happy because she will eat the ice cream. He's happy because she will give it to him. Explain why the boy is happy.

Child: cause he will eat the ice cream.

When a child can explain a particular aspect of the story, the clinician can tie in another character and new related actions. For example, in this picture the friend can be brought in. This will involve explaining what the two children were doing prior to the picture and perhaps what they will do in the future after they get their ice cream. The truck driver can be discussed, including all of the things that he may have on his truck, how he counts change, how he comes by every day at the same time, and so forth.

Moving to Other Activities. This narrative activity can easily be manipulated to keep younger children entertained. In a small group setting, the "theme" from a particular story such as this one can be turned into a group construction project in which the children cut out and color the characters, the truck, the ice cream, and the toys. While engaged in this project, the clinician keeps everyone talking about the mechanics of the project, directing the children to talk to one another for specific purposes, and keeping Blank and colleagues' (1978) levels in mind. For example, if there are three children and only two sets of scissors and bottles of glue (purposefully contrived by the clinician), someone is always going to be requesting tools from someone else. The clinician guides this process: "Joe, what do you need to do next?" [level III]... "I dunno" ... "Well, you drew your ice cream cone on the paper and now you want to cut it. What do you need to cut?" [level II] ... "scissors" ... "Who has some scissors?" ... "Zack and Sue" ... "Does Zack have the big ones or the little ones?" [level II] ... "big ones" ... "Tell him you need the big scissors" ... "Zack, I need big scissors . . . ."

We would approach Blank and colleagues' earlier levels within the process of constructing the materials needed to act out the story. The children in a group would be prompted to ask one another for the things they need, (i.e., construction paper of particular colors, scissors of particular sizes, and so forth). As they are doing this, the clinician would model the higher-order levels (e.g., "Oh, you need scissors so that you can cut the paper" or "You need the big scissors because you are cutting a big piece of paper").

When the group has constructed the objects used in the story, they can act it out. Now the clinician helps each child construct appropriate dialogue to go along with the story line. For example, one child would play the mother and would be prompted to interact with the ice cream man and then the two boys who are playing. The clinician would help everyone in the story construct an appropriate dialogue that follows the story line.

In this manner, the children are learning to associate appropriate syllable shapes, phonemes, and features with conceptual classes and higher levels of utterance organization while acting out typical everyday scenarios. They are learning the language code that will allow them to efficiently recall and retell such happenings. And they are learning appropriate articulation for all of these language activities.

CLASSROOM ACTIVITIES

1. Write appropriate articulation goals for the misarticulating children whose speech you analyzed in Chap. 4.
2. Each student should take a consonant phoneme and devise a set of rehearsal matrices for that sound. List as many cues to appropriate articulation as possible for that sound.
3. Record a storytelling session with a misarticulating child in which you systematically seek to raise the level of responding from labeling to describing, or from describing to interpreting/inferencing. Target 10 misarticulations during this story and provide appropriate feedback.
4. Describe the types of objects you would have preschool children construct to enact the story from the first picture in Appendix A. Make a list of questions you would be able to ask the children during this construction project at Blank and colleagues' (1978) four levels.

References

Abbs, J., Gracco, V., & Cole, K. (1984). Control of multidimensional coordination: Sensorimotor mechanisms in speech motor programming. *Journal of Motor Behaviors, 16*, 195–231.

Andrews, J. R. (1971). Operationally written therapy goals in supervised clinical practicum. *ASHA 13*, 385–387.

Andrews, N., & Fey, M. E. (1986). Analysis of the speech of phonologically impaired children in two sampling conditions. *Language, Speech & Hearing Services in Schools, 17*, 187–198.

Angle, E. H. (1899). Classification of malocclusion. *Dental Cosmos 41*, 248–264, 350–357.

Aslin, R. N., & Pisoni, D. B. (1980). Some developmental processes in speech perception. In G. H. Yeni-Komshian, J. F. Kavanaugh, & C. A. Ferguson (Eds.), *Child phonology: Vol. 2 Perception*. New York: Academic.

Bangs, J. (1942). A clinical analysis of the articulatory defects of the feebleminded. *Journal of Speech and Hearing Disorders, 7*, 343–356.

Bankson, N. W., & Bernthal, J. E. (1982). A comparison of phonological processes identified through word and sentence imitation tasks. *Language Speech & Hearing Services in Schools, 13*, 96–99.

Barton, D. (1980). Phonemic perception in children. In G. H. Yeni-Komshian, J. F. Kavanaugh, & C. A. Ferguson (Eds.), *Child Phonology: Vol. 2 Perception*. New York: Academic.

Best, C., Hoffman, H., & Robson, R. (1981). Perceptual equivalence of acoustic cues in speech and nonspeech perception. *Perception and Psychophysics, 29*, 191–211.

Blank, M., Rose, S., & Berlin, L. (1978). *The language of learning: The preschool years*. New York: Harcourt, Brace, Jovanovich.

Broen, P., Strange, W., Doyle, S., & Heller, J. (1983). Perception and production of approximant consonants by normal and articulation-delayed preschool children. *Journal of Speech and Hearing Research, 26*, 601–608.

Brown, R. (1973). *A first language*. Cambridge, MA: Harvard University Press.

Bruner, J. (1983). *Child's talk*. New York: Norton.

Camarata, S., & Gandour, J. (1984). On describing idiosyncratic phonological systems. *Journal of Speech and Hearing Disorders, 49*, 262–266.

Camarata, S. M., & Schwartz, R. G. (1985). Production of object words and action words: Evidence for a relationship between phonology and semantics. *Journal of Speech and Hearing Research, 26*, 50–53.

Campbell, T. F., & Shriberg, L. D. (1982). Associations among pragmatic functions, linguistic stress, and natural phonological processes in speech-delayed children. *Journal of Speech and Hearing Research, 25*, 547–553.

Carrier, J. K. (1970). A program of articulation therapy administered by mothers. *Journal of Speech and Hearing Disorders, 35*, 344–353.

Carter, E. T., & Buck, M. W. (1958). Prognostic testing for functional articulation disorders among children in the first grade. *Journal of Speech and Hearing Disorders, 23*, 124–133.

Catts, H. W., & Kamhi, A. G. (1984). Simplification of /s/ stop consonant clusters: A developmental perspective. *Journal of Speech Hearing Research, 27*, 556–561.

Chomsky, N., & Halle, M. (1968). *The sound pattern of English*. New York: Harper & Row.

Compton, A. (1970). Generative studies of children's phonological disorders. *Journal of Speech and Hearing Disorders, 35*, 315–339.

Compton, A., & Hutton, S. (1978). *Compton-Hutton Phonological Assessment*. San Francisco: Carousel.

Costello, J., & Ferrer, J. (1976). Punishment contingencies for the reduction of incorrect responses during articulation instruction. *Journal of Communication Disorders 9*, 43–61.

Costello, J., & Onstine, J. (1976). The modification of multiple articulation errors based on distinctive feature theory. *Journal of Speech and Hearing Disorders, 41*, 199–215.

Daniloff, R. G., Wilcox, K., & Stephens, M. I. (1980). An acoustic-articulatory description of children's defective /s/ production. *Journal of Communication Disorders, 15*, 347–363.

Darley, F., Aronson, A., & Brown, J. (1975). *Motor speech disorders*. Philadelphia: Saunders.

DeCasper, A. J., & Fifer, W. P. (1980). Of human bonding: Newborns prefer their mother's voices. *Science, 208*, 1174–1176.

Diedrich, W. M., & Bangert, J. (1980). *Articulation learning*. Houston: College-Hill Press.

Dinnsen, D. A., & Elbert, M. (1984). On the relationship between phonology and learning. In M. Elbert, D. A. Dinnsen, & G. Weismer (Eds.), *Phonological theory and the misarticulating child* (ASHA Monograph No. 22). Rockville, MD: ASHA.

Dodd, B. J. (1976a). A comparison of the phonological systems of mental age matched, normal, severely subnormal and Down's syndrome children. *British Journal of Disorders of Communication, 11*, 27–42.

Dodd, B. J. (1976b). The phonological systems of deaf children. *Journal of Speech and Hearing Disorders, 41*, 185–197.

Dubois, E. M., & Bernthal, J. E. (1978). A comparison of three methods for obtaining articulatory responses. *Journal of Speech and Hearing Disorders, 43* 295–305.

Dworkin, J. P., & Culatta, R. A. (1985). Oral structural and neuromuscular characteristics in children with normal and disordered articulation. *Journal of Speech and Hearing Disorders, 50* 150–156.

Eimas, P. (1975). Auditory and phonetic coding of the cues for speech: discrimination of the r-l distinction by young infants. *Perception and Psychophysics, 18*, 341–347.

Eilers, R. E., Wilson, W. R., & Moore, J. M. (1977). Development changes in speech discrimination in infants. *Journal of Speech and Hearing Research, 20*, 766–780.

Elbert, M., & Geirut, J. A. (1986). *Handbook of clinical phonology: Approaches to assessment and treatment*. London: Taylor & Francis.

Elbert, M., & McReynolds, L. V. (1978). An experimental analysis of misarticulating children's generalization. *Journal of Speech and Hearing Disorders, 21*, 136–150.

Elbert, M., Shelton, R. L., & Arndt, W. B. (1967). A task for evaluation articulation change: 1. Development of methodology. *Journal of Speech and Hearing Research, 10*, 281–288.

Everleigh, K. F., & Warr-Leeper, G. A. (1983). Improving efficiency in articulation screening. *Language, Speech & Hearing in Schools, 14*, 223–232.

Faircloth, M. A., & Faircloth, S. R. (1970). An analysis of the articulatory behavior of a speech-defective child in connected speech and in isolated-word responses. *Journal of Speech and Hearing Disorders, 35*, 51–61.

Ferguson, C. A., & Farwell, C. B. (1975). Words and sounds in early language acquisition: English initial consonants in the first fifty words. *Language, 51*, 419–439.

Fodor, J. (1986). *The modularity of mind*. Cambridge, MA: MIT Press.

Folkins, J., & Abbs, J. (1975). Lip and jaw motor control during speech: Responses to resistive loading of the jaw. *Journal of Speech and Hearing Research, 18*, 207–220.

Fowler, C. A. (1985). Current perspectives on language and speech production: A critical review. In R. G. Daniloff (Ed.), *Speech science*. San Diego: College-Hill.

Fudala, J. (1974) *Arizona Articulation Proficiency Scale: Revised*. Los Angeles: Western Psychological Services.

Fujimura, O. (1986). Relative invariance of articulatory movements: an ice berg model. In J. Perkell & D. Klatt (Eds.), *Invariance and variability in speech processes* (pp. 226–243). Hillside, N.J.: Erlbaum.

Goldman, R., & Fristoe, M. (1969). *Test of Articulation*. Circle Pines, MN: American Guidance Service.

Greenlee, M. (1973). Some observations on initial English consonant clusters in a child two to three years old. *Papers and Reports on Child Language Development, 6,* 97–106.

Grillner, S. (1982). Possible analogies in the control of innate motor acts and the production of sounds in speech. In S. Grillner, B. Lindblom, J. Lubker, & A. Persson (Eds.), *Speech motor control* (pp. 217–229). London: Pergamon.

Halliday, M. A. K. (1975). *Learning how to mean: Explorations in the development of language.* London: Arnold.

Hawkins, S. (1984). On the development of motor control in speech: Evidence from studies of temporal coordination. In N. Lass (Ed.), *Speech and language: Vol. II. Advances in basic research and practice.* New York: Academic.

Haynes, W. O., & Steed, S. F. (1987). Multiphonemic scoring of articulation in imitative sentences: some preliminary data. *Language, Speech & Hearing in Schools, 18,* 4–14.

Hillenbrand, J. (1983). Perceptual organization of speech sounds by infants. *Journal of Speech and Hearing Research, 26,* 268–282.

Himmelwright Gross, G., St. Louis, K. O., Ruscello, D. M., & Hull, F. M. (1985). Language abilities of articulatory-disordered school children with multiple or residual errors. *Language, Speech & Hearing in Schools, 16,* 171–186.

Hodson, B. W. (1980). *The assessment of phonological processes.* Danville, IL: Interstate.

Hodson, B. W., & Paden E. P. (1981). Phonological processes which characterize unintelligible and intelligible speech in early childhood. *Journal of Speech and Hearing Disorders, 46,* 369–373.

Hodson, B. W., & Paden, E. P. (1983). *Targeting intelligible speech.* San Digeo: College-Hill Press.

Hodson, B. W., Chin, L., Redmond, B., & Simpson, R. (1983). Phonological evaluation and remedication of speech deviations of a child with a repaired cleft palate: A case study. *Journal of Speech and Hearing Disorders, 48,* 93–98.

Hoffman, P. R. (1983). Interallophonic generalization of /r/ training. *Journal of Speech and Hearing Disorders, 48,* 215–221.

Hoffman P. R., and Damico, S. K. (1988). Cluster-reducing children's identification and production of /sk/ clusters. *Journal of Clinical Linguistics and Phonetics, 2,* 17–27.

Hoffman, P. R., Daniloff, R. G., Bengoa, D., & and Schuckers, G. H. (1984). Misarticulating and normally articulating children's identification and discrimination of [r] and [w]. *Journal of Speech and Hearing Disorders, 50,* 46–53.

Hoffman, P. R., Schuckers, G. H., & Daniloff, R. G. (1980). Developmental trends in correct /r/ articulation as a function of allophone type. *Journal of Speech and Hearing Research, 23,* 746–756.

Hoffman, P. R., Schuckers, G. H., & Ratusnik, D. L. (1977). Contextual-coarticulatory inconsistency of /r/ misarticulation. *Journal of Speech and Hearing Research, 20,* 631–643.

Hudgins, C. V., & Numbers, F. C. (1942). An investigation of the intelligibility of the speech of the deaf. *Genetic Psychology Monograph, 25,* 289–392.

Ingram, D. (1976). *Phonological disability in children* (pp. 29–44). New York: Elsevier.

Ingram, D. (1981). *Procedures for the phonological analysis of children's language.* Baltimore: University Park.

Irwin, O. C. (1947a). Infant speech: consonant sounds according to place of articulation. *Journal of Speech Disorders, 12,* 397–401.

Irwin, O. C. (1947b). Infant speech: consonant sounds according to manner of articulation. *Journal of Speech Disorders, 12,* 402–404.

Jakobson, R. (1968). *Child language, aphasia, and phonological universals.* A. R. Keiler (Tr.). The Hague: Mouton.

Kelso, S., Saltzman, E., & Tuller, B. (1986). The dynamical perspective on speech production data and theory. *Journal of Phonetics, 14,* 29–39.

Kenney, K. W., & Prather, E. M. (1984). *Coarticulation Assessment in Meaningful Language.* Tucson: Communication Skill Builders.

Kent, R. D. (1976). Anatomical and neuromuscular maturation of the speech mechanism: Evidence from acoustic studies. *Journal of Speech and Hearing Research, 19,* 421–447.

Kent, R. D. (1982). Sensorimotor aspects of speech development. In R. N. Aslin & M. R. Peterson (Eds.), *Development of perception: Psychological factors.* New York: Academic.

King, R. R., & Berger, K. W. (1974). *Diagnostic assessment and counseling techniques for speech pathologists and audiologists.* Pittsburgh: Stanwix.

Klein, H. (1984). Procedure for maximizing phonological information from single word responses. *Language Speech & Hearing Services in Schools, 15,* 267–274.

Kuhl, P. K. (1980). Perceptual constancy for speech-sound categories in early infancy. In G. H. Yeni-Komshian, J. F. Kavanaugh, & C. A. Ferguson, (Eds.), *Child phonology: Vol. 2 Perception.* New York: Academic.

Kuhl, P. K. (1981). Discrimination of speech by nonhuman animals: Basic auditory sensitivities conducive to the perception of speech-sound categories. *Journal of the Acoustical Society of America, 70(2),* 340–349.

Kuhl, P. K., & Meltzoff, A. (1982). The bimodal perception of speech in infancy. *Science, 218* 1138–1144.

Leonard, L. B., Newhoff, M., & Mesalam, L. (1980). Individual differences in early child phonology. *Applied Psycholinguistics, 1,* 7–30.

Leonard, L. B., Schwartz, R. G., Folger, M., & Wilcox, M. (1978). Some aspects of child phonology in imitative and spontaneous speech. *Journal of Child Language, 5,* 403–417.

Leonard, L. B., Schwartz, R. G., Chapman, K;, Rowan, L. E., Prelock, P. A., Terrell, B., Weiss, A. L., & Messick, C. (1982). Early lexical acquisition in children with specific language impairment. *Journal of Speech and Hearing Research, 25,* 554–564.

Leopold, W. (1947). Speech development of a bilingual child: a linguists record: 2. Sound learning in the first two years. Evanston, IL: Northwestern University Press.

Lieberman, A. & Mattingly, I. (1985). The motor theory of speech perception revised. *Status Report on Speech Research* SR-82/83. Haskins Laboratory: New Haven, CT.

Locke, J. L. (1980). The inference of speech perception in the phonologically disordered child: 2. Some clinically novel procedures, their use, some findings. *Journal of Speech and Hearing Disorders, 45,* 444–468.

Locke, J. L. (1983). *Phonological acquisition and change.* New York: Academic.

Lowe, R. J. (1986). Phonological process analysis using three position test. *Language Speech & Hearing Services in Schools, 17,* 72–79.

Mager, R. (1962). *Preparing instructional objectives.* Palo Alto: Fearon.

Mason, R., & Proffit, W. (1974). The tongue-thrust controversy: Background and recommendations. *Journal of Speech and Hearing Disorders, 39,* 115–132.

Mazza, P., Schuckers, G. H., & Daniloff, R. G. (1979). Contextual-coarticulatory inconsistency of /s/ misarticulation. *Journal of Phonetics, 7,* 57–69.

McClelland, J. L., & Elman, J. L. (1986). Interactive processes in speech perception: The TRACE model. In J. L. McClelland, D. E. Rumelhart, & PDP Research Group (Eds.), *Parallel distributed processing: Explorations in the microstructure of cognition: vol. 2. Psychological and biological models.* Cambridge, MA: MIT Press.

McDonald, E. T. (1964a). *Articulation testing and treatment: A sensory motor approach* (pp. 103, 137, 159). Pittsburgh: Stanwix House.

McDonald, E. T. (1964b). *A deep test of articulation: picture form.* Pittsburgh: Stanwix House.

McDonald, E. T. (1964c). *A deep test of articulation: sentence form.* Pittsburgh: Stanwix House.

McGurk, H., & McDonald, J. (1976). Hearing lips and seeing voices. *Nature, 264,* 746–748.

McMahon, K., Hodson, B., & Allen, E. (1983). Phonological analysis of cerebral palsied children's utterances. *Journal of Childhood Communication Disorders, 7,* 23–35.

McNutt, J. C., (1977). Oral sensory and motor behaviors of children with /s/ or /r/ misarticulations. *Journal of Speech and Hearing Research, 20,* 694–703.

McNutt, J. C., & Hamayan, E. (1984). Subgroups of older children with articulation disorders. In R. G. Daniloff (Ed.), *Articulation assessment and treatment issues.* San Diego: College-Hill.

McReynolds, L. V., & Elbert, M. (1981a). Criteria for phonological process analysis. *Journal of Speech and Hearing Disorders, 46,* 197–204.

McReynolds, L. V., & Elbert, M. (1981b). Generalization of correct articulation in clusters. *Applied Psycholinguistics, 2,* 119–132.

McReynolds, L. V., & Engmann, D. (1975). *Distinctive feature analysis of misarticulations.* Baltimore: University Park.

McReynolds, L. V., & Huston, K. (1971). A distinctive feature analysis of children's misarticulations. *Journal of Speech and Hearing Disorders, 36,* 155–166.

Mecham, M., Berko, M., & Berko, F. (1960). *Speech therapy in cerebral palsy.* Springfield, IL: Thomas.

Miller, G. (1951). Speech perception. In S. S. Stevens (Ed.), *Handbook of experimental psychology.* New York: Wiley.

Miller, G., & Nicely, P. (1955). An analysis of perceptual confusions among some English consonants. *Journal of the Acoustical Society of America, 27,* 338–352.

Miyawaka, K., Strange, W., Verbrugge, R., Liberman, A. M., Jenkins, J. J., & Fujimura, O. (1975). An effect of linguistic experience: the discrimination of [r] and [l] by native speakers of Japanese and English. *Perception and Psychophysics, 18,* 331–340.

Monnin, L., & Huntington, D. A. (1974). Relationship of articulatory defects to speech-sound identification. *Journal of Speech and Hearing Research, 17,* 352–366.

Moskowitz, B. A. (1971). *The acquisition of phonology.* Unpublished doctoral dissertation, University of California, Berkley.

Mowrer, D. E., Baker, R. L., & Schutz, R. E. (1968). Operant procedures in the control of speech articulation. In H. Sloane & B. MacAulay (Eds.), *Operant procedures in remedial speech and language training.* Boston: Houghton Mifflin.

Nelson, K. (1985). *Making sense: The acquisition of shared meaning.* New York: Academic.

Nober, E. (1967). Articulation of the deaf. *Exceptional Children, 33,* 611–621.

Ojeman, G. (1983). Stimulation mapping of language. *The behavioral and brain sciences,* 2, 189–230.

Oller, D. K. (1980). The emergence of the sounds of speech in infancy. In G. H. Yeni-Komshian, J. F. Kavanagh, & C. A. Ferguson (Eds.), *Child phonology: Vol. 1 Production.* New York: Academic.

Oller, D., & Eilers, R. (1983). Speech identification in Spanish- and English-learning 2-year-olds. *Journal of Speech and Hearing Research, 26,* 50–53.

Oller, D. K., Weiman, L., Doyle, J., & Ross, C. (1975). Infant babbling and speech. *Journal of Child Language, 3,* 1–11.

Panagos, J. (1974). Persistence of the open syllable reinterpreted as a symptom of language disorder. *Journal of Speech and Hearing Disorders, 39,* 23–31.

Panagos, J. M., & Prelock, P. A. (1982). Phonological constraints on the sentence productions of language-disordered children. *Journal of Speech and Hearing Research, 26,* 171–177.

Panagos, J., Quine, H., & Klich, P. (1978). Syntactic and phonological influences in children's articulations. *Journal of Speech and Hearing Research, 22,* 841–848.

Papandropoulow, I. & Sinclair, H. (1974). What is a word?: Experimental study of children's ideas on grammar. *Human Development, 17,* 241–258.

Paul, R., & Shriberg, L. D. (1982). Associations between phonology and syntax in speech-delayed children. *Journal of Speech and Hearing Research, 25,* 536–546.

Perkell, J. S. (1980). Phonetic features and the physiology of speech production. In B. Butterworth (Ed.), *Language production.* New York: Academic.

Powell, J., & McReynolds, L. V. (1969). A procedure for testing position generalization from articulation training. *Journal of Speech and Hearing Research, 12,* 629–645.

Powell, T. W., & Elbert, M. (1984). Generalization following the remediation of early- and later-developing consonant clusters. *Journal of Speech and Hearing Disorders, 49,* 211–218.

Prather, E. M., Hedrick, D. L., & Kern, C. A. (1975). Articulation development in children aged two to four years. *Journal of Speech and Hearing Disorders, 20,* 179–191.

Read, C. (1971). Preschool children's knowledge of English phonology. *Harvard Educational Review, 41,* 1–34.

Rosenbek, J., & Wertz, R. (1972). Review of fifty cases of deveolopmental apraxia of speech. *Language, Speech and Hearing Services in the Schools 1,* 23–33.

Rumelhart, D. E., McClelland, J. L., & PDP Research Group (1986). *Parallel distributed processing: Explorations in the microstructure of cognition: Vol. 1 Foundations.* Cambridge, MA: MIT Press.

Sander, K. (1972). When are speech sounds learned? *Journal of Speech and Hearing Disorders, 37,* 55–63.

Schwartz, R. G., & Leonard, L. B. (1982). Do children pick and choose? An examination of phonological selection and avoidance in early lexical acquisition. *Journal of Child Language, 9,* 319–336.

Scollon, R. (1979). A real early stage: An unzippered condensation of a dissertation of child language. In E. Ochs & B. Schiefflin (Eds.), *Developmental pragmatics.* New York: Academic.

Searle, J. (1969). *Speech acts.* Cambridge: Cambridge University Press.

Shattuck-Hufnagel, S. (1979). Speech errors as evidence for a serial ordering mechanism in speech production. In W. E. Cooper & E. Walker (Eds.), *Sentence processing: Psycholinguistic studies presented to merrill garrett.* Hillsdale, NJ: Erlbaum.

Sherman, D., & Geith, A. (1967). Speech sound discrimination and articulation skill. *Journal of Speech and Hearing Disorders, 10,* 277–280.

Shriberg, L., & Kwiatkowski, J. (1980). *Natural process analysis.* New York: Wiley.

Shriberg, L., & Kwiatkowski, J. (1982). Phonological disorders: 3. A procedure for assessing severity of involvement. *Journal of Speech and Hearing Disisorders, 47,* 256–270.

Shriner, T. H., Holloway, M. S., & Daniloff, R. G. (1969). The relationship between articulatory deficits and syntax in speech defective children. *Journal of Speech and Hearing Research, 12,* 319–325.

Silverman, F. H. (1977). *Research design in speech pathology and audiology: asking and answering questions.* Englewood Cliffs, N.J.: Prentice-Hall.

Slis, I. H., & Cohen, A. (1969). On the complex regulating of the voiced-voiceless distinction. *Language and Speech, 12,* 80–102.

Smit, A. B., & Bernthal, J. E. (1983). Performance of articulation disordered children on language and perception measures. *Journal of Speech and Hearing Research, 26,* 124–136.

Snow, K. (1961). Articulation proficiency in relation to certain dental abnormalities. *Journal of Speech and Hearing Disorders, 26,* 209–212.

Snow, K., & Milisen, R. (1954). The influence of oral vs. pictorial representation upon articulation testing results. *Journal of Speech and Hearing Disorders, Monograph Suppl. 4,* 29–36.

Spriestersbach, D., & Curtis, J. (1951). Misarticulation and discrimination of speech sounds. *Quarterly Journal of Speech, 37,* 483–491.

Stark, R., & Tallal, P. (1978). Analysis of stop consonant production errors in developmentally dysphasic children. *Journal of the Acoustical Society of America, 66,* 1706–1712.

Stephens, M. I., Hoffman, P. R., & Daniloff, R. G. (1986). Phonetic characteristics of delayed /s/ development. *Journal of Phonetics, 14,* 247–256.

Strange, W., & Broen, P. A. (1980). Perception and production of approximant consonants by 3-year-olds: A first study. In G. H. Yeni-Komshian, J. F. Kavanagh, & C. A. Ferguson (Eds.), *Child phonology: Vol. 2 Perception.* New York: Academic.

Tallal, P., & Stark, R. (1981). Speech acoustic cue discrimination abilities of normally developing and language-impaired children. *Journal of the Acoustical Society of America,* 568–574.

Templin, M. C. (1947). Spontaneous vs. imitated verbalization in testing pre-school children. *Journal of Speech and Hearing Disorders, 12,* 293–300.
Templin, M. C., (1957). *Certain language skills in children.*(Institute of Child Welfare Monograph No. 26). Minneapolis: University of Minnesota Press.
Templin, M. C., & Darley, F.L. (1960). *The Templin-Darley Test of Articulation.* Iowa City: State University of Iowa, Bureau of Educational Research and Service, Extension Division.
Travis, L. E., & Rasmus, B. (1931). The speech sound discrimination ability of cases with functional disorders of articulation. *Quarterly Journal of Speech, 17,* 217–226.
Van Riper, C. (1939). *Speech correction: Principles and methods* (pp. 224, 225, 247, 254, 263, 264). Englewood Cliffs, NJ: Prentice-Hall.
Van Riper, C., & Erickson, R. (1969). *Predictive Screening Test of Articulation.* Kalamazoo: Western Michigan University, Continuing Education Office.
Warren, R. (1970). Perceptual restoration of missing speech sounds. *Science, 167,* 392–393.
Waterson, N. (1971). Child phonology: a prosodic view. *Journal of Linguistics, 7,* 170–221.
Weiner, F. F. (1979). *Phonological process analysis.* Baltimore: University Park.
Weiner, F. F. (1981). Treatment of phonological disability using the method of meaningful minimal contrast: Two case studies. *Journal of Speech and Hearing Disorders, 46,* 97–103.
Weismer, G., & Elbert, M. (1982). Temporal characteristics of "functionally" misarticulated /s/ in 4- to 6-year old children. *Journal of Speech and Hearing Research, 25,* 275–287.
Weismer, G., Dinnsen, D. A., & Elbert, M. (1981). A study of the voicing distinction associated with omitted, word-final stops. *Journal of Speech and Hearing Disorders, 46,* 97–103.
Weiss, C. (1980). *Weiss Comprehensive Articulation Test.* New York: Teaching Resources.
Werker, J. F., & Tees, R. C. (1984). Cross-language speech perception: Evidence for perceptual reorganization during the first year of life. *Infant Behavior and Development, 7,* 49–64.
Williams, D., & McReynolds, L. V. (1975). The relationship between discrimination and articulation training in children with misarticulations. *Journal of Speech and Hearing Research, 18,* 401–412.
Williams, H., & Nottebohm, R. (1986). Auditory responses in avian vocal motor neurons: amotor theory for song perception in birds. *Science, 211,* 279–282.
Winitz, H. (1969). *Articulatory acquisition and behavior.* Englewood Cliffs, NJ: Prentice-Hall.
Winitz, H. (1975). *From syllable to conversation.* Baltimore: University Park Press.
Wright, S. I., & Schuckers, G. H. (1980). Differential feedback used by speech and language clinicians. *Journal of Communication Disorders, 13,* 1–8.
Zemlin, W. R. (1981). *Speech and hearing science: Anatomy and physiology* (pp. 314–316, 378–387). Englewood Cliffs, NJ: Prentice-Hall.

Appendix A

*Speech Elicitation Illustrations**

*All figures in Appendix A except that on p. 280 are reproduced by permission from G. Schuckers and C. Wilcox. *Let's Share*. © 1983 by Word Making Productions, Salt Lake City, Utah.

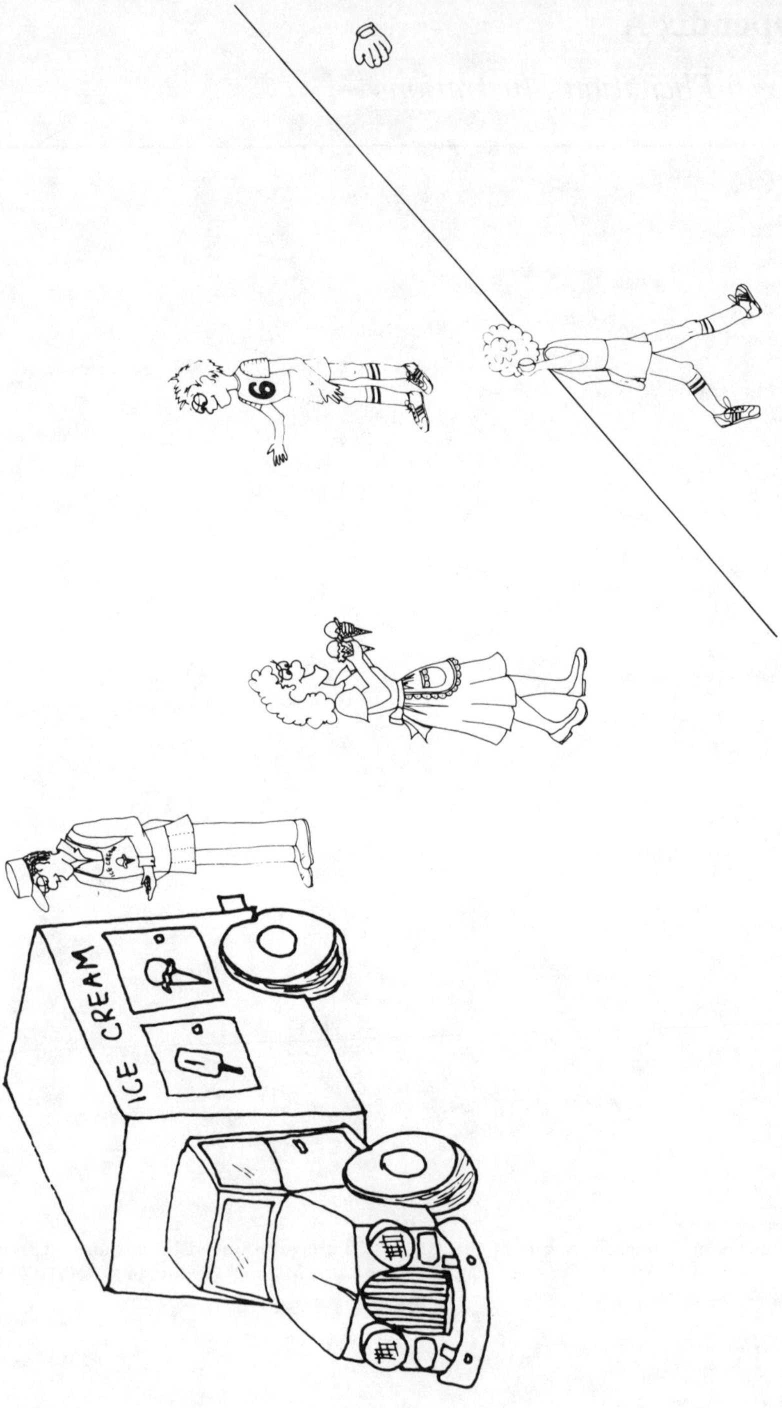
ICE CREAM
6

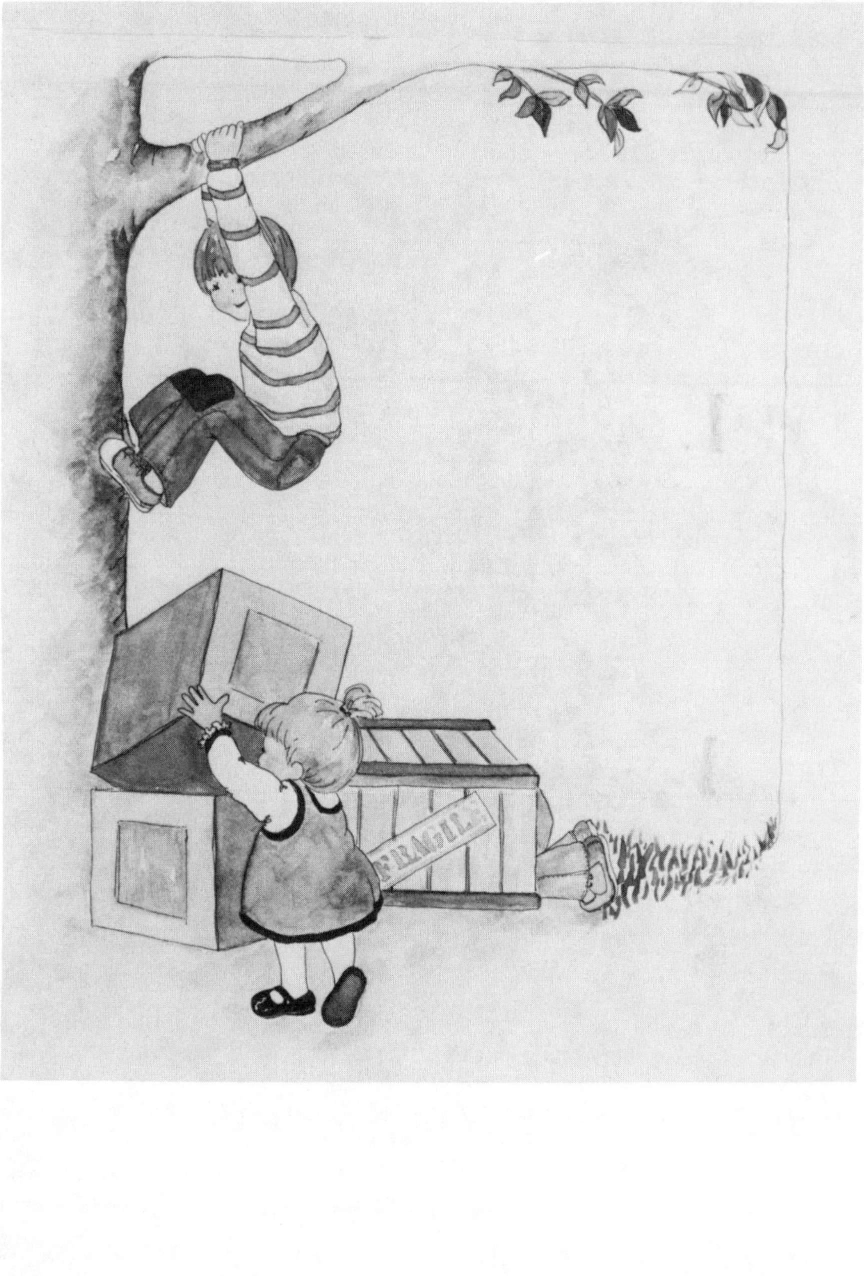
FRAGILE

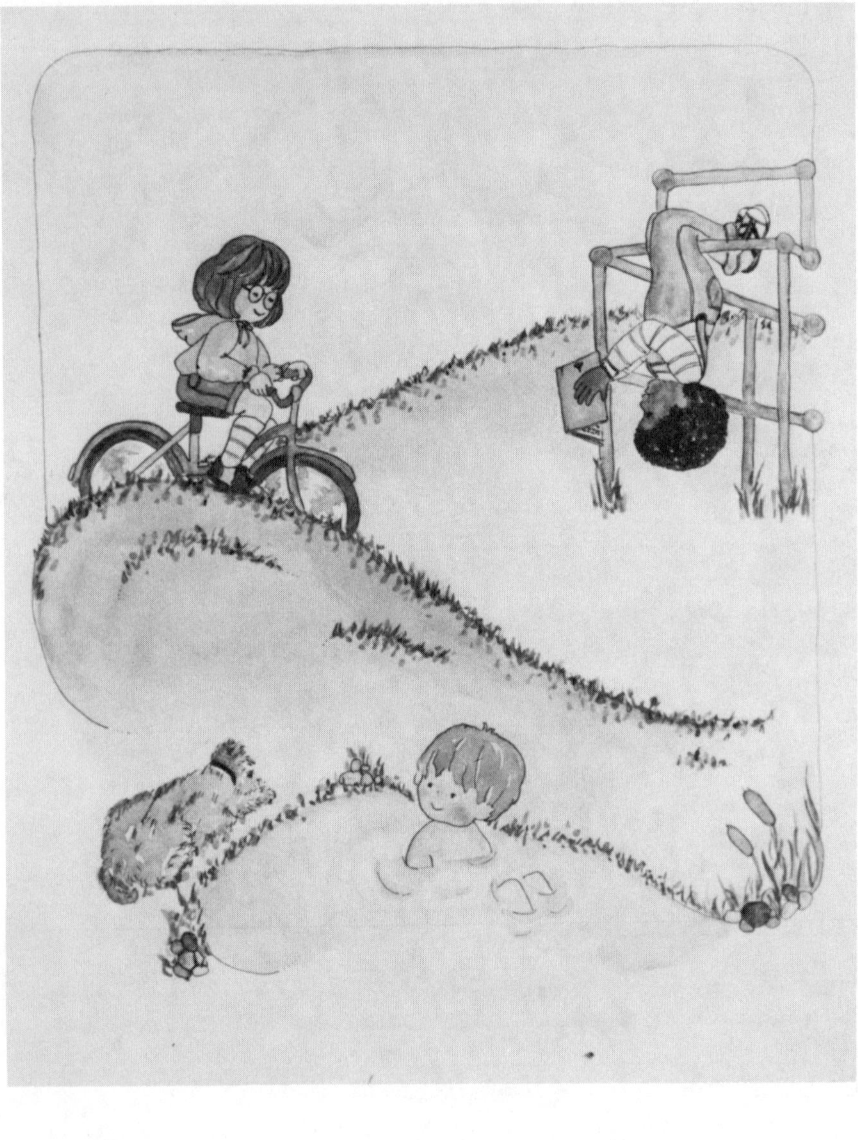

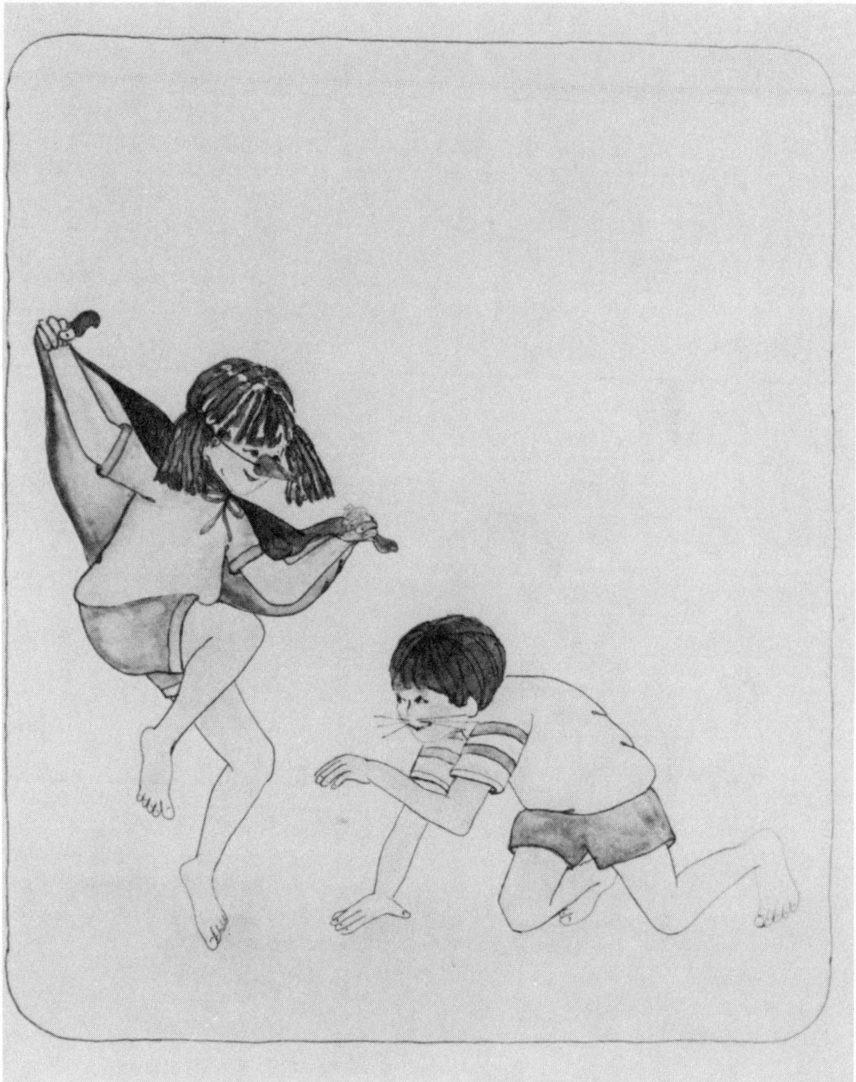

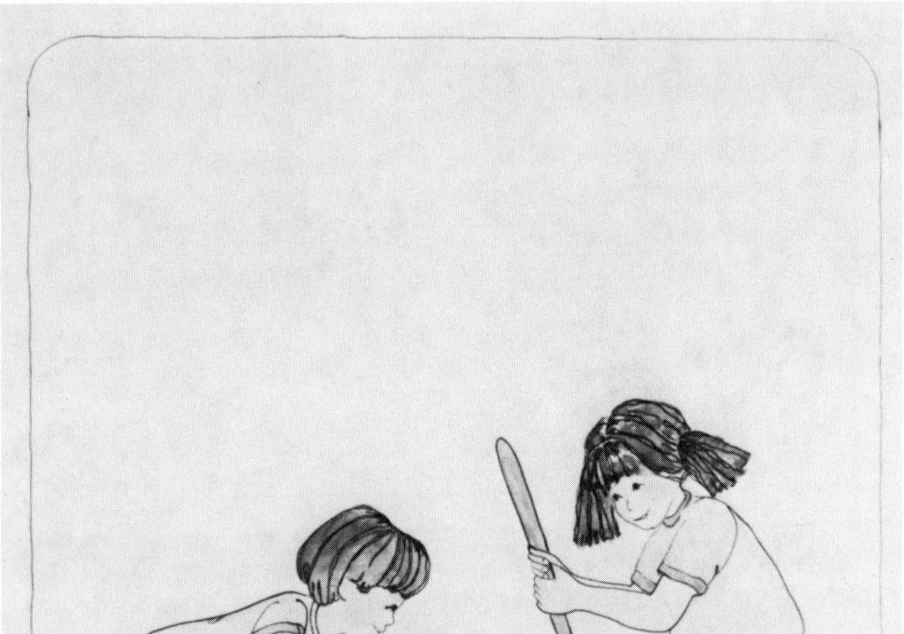

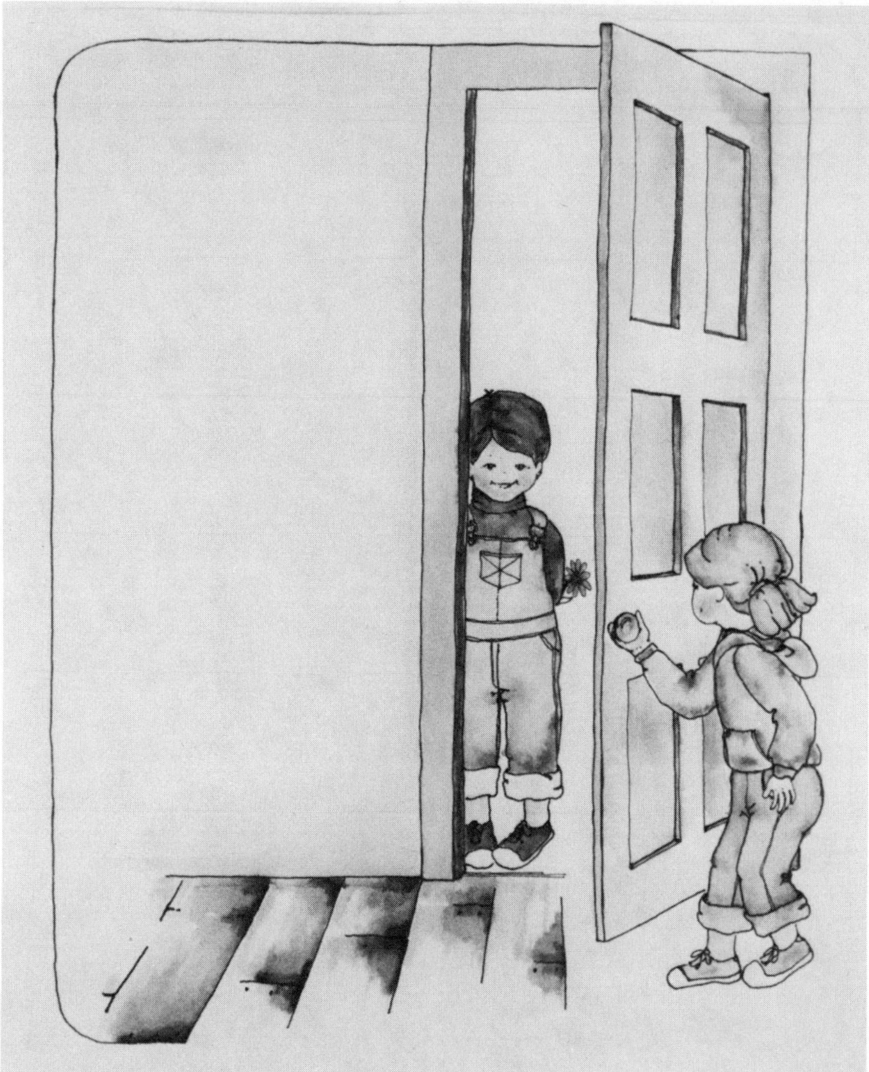

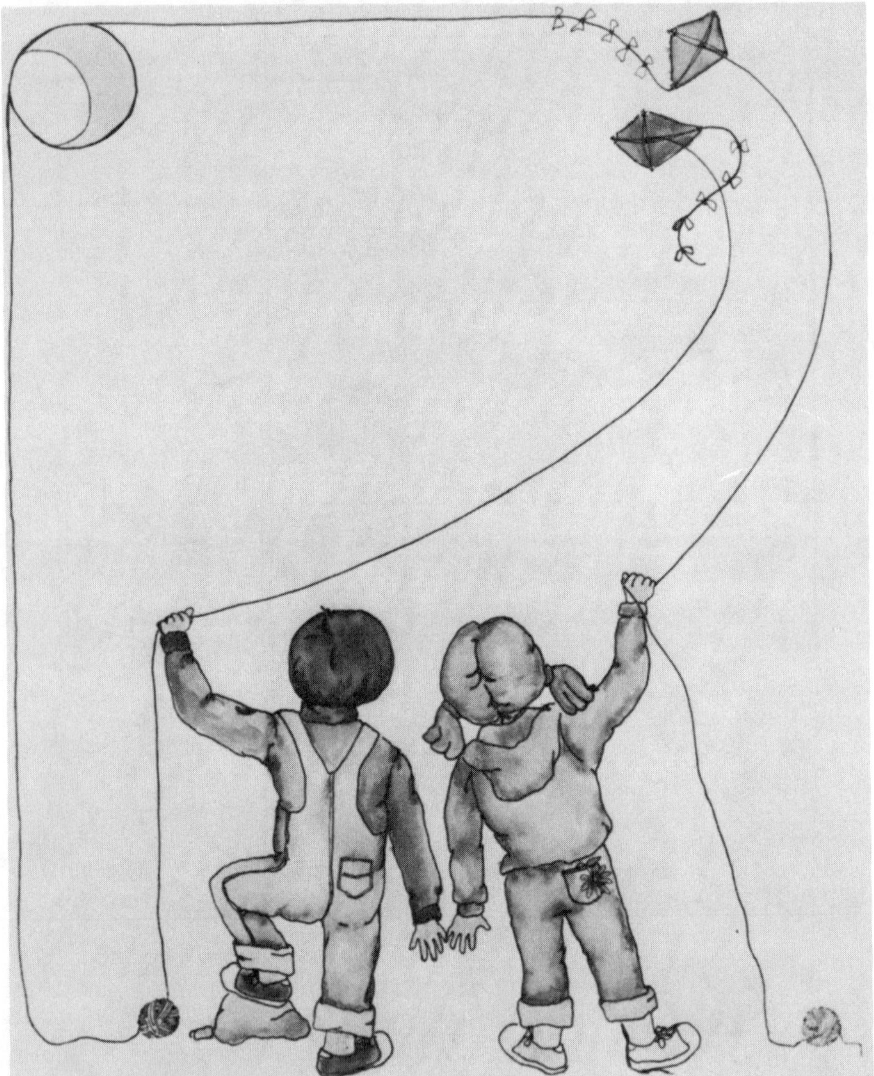

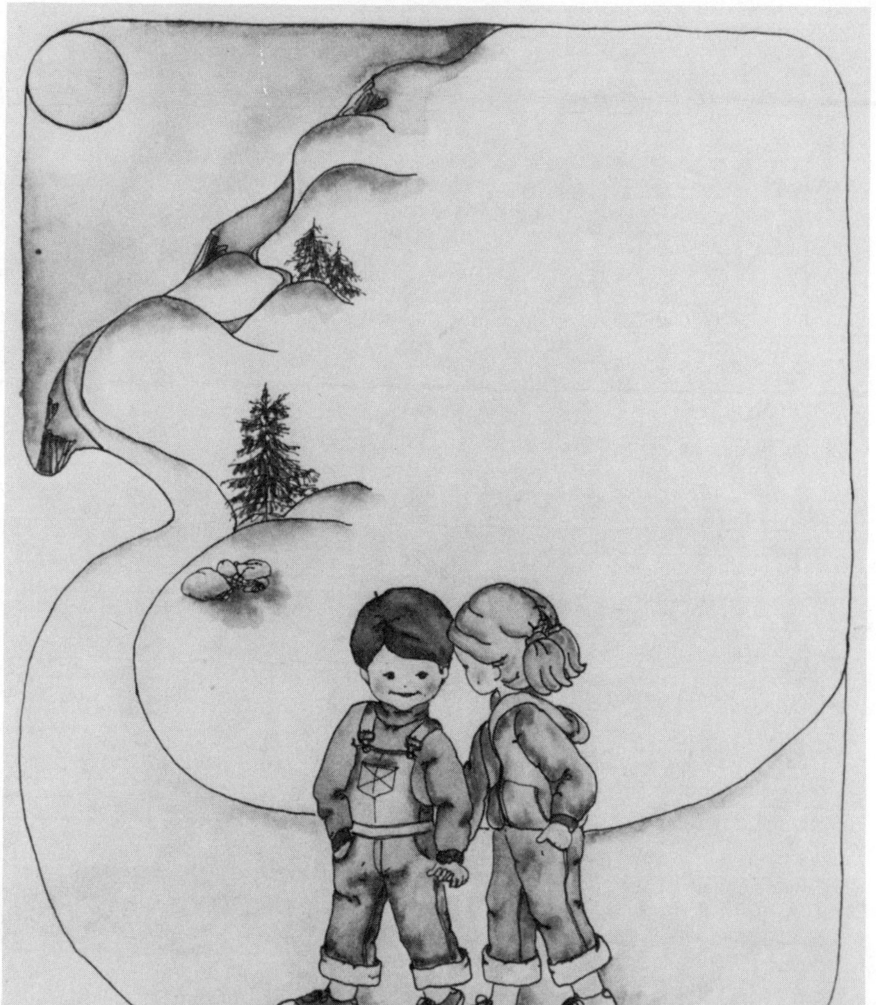

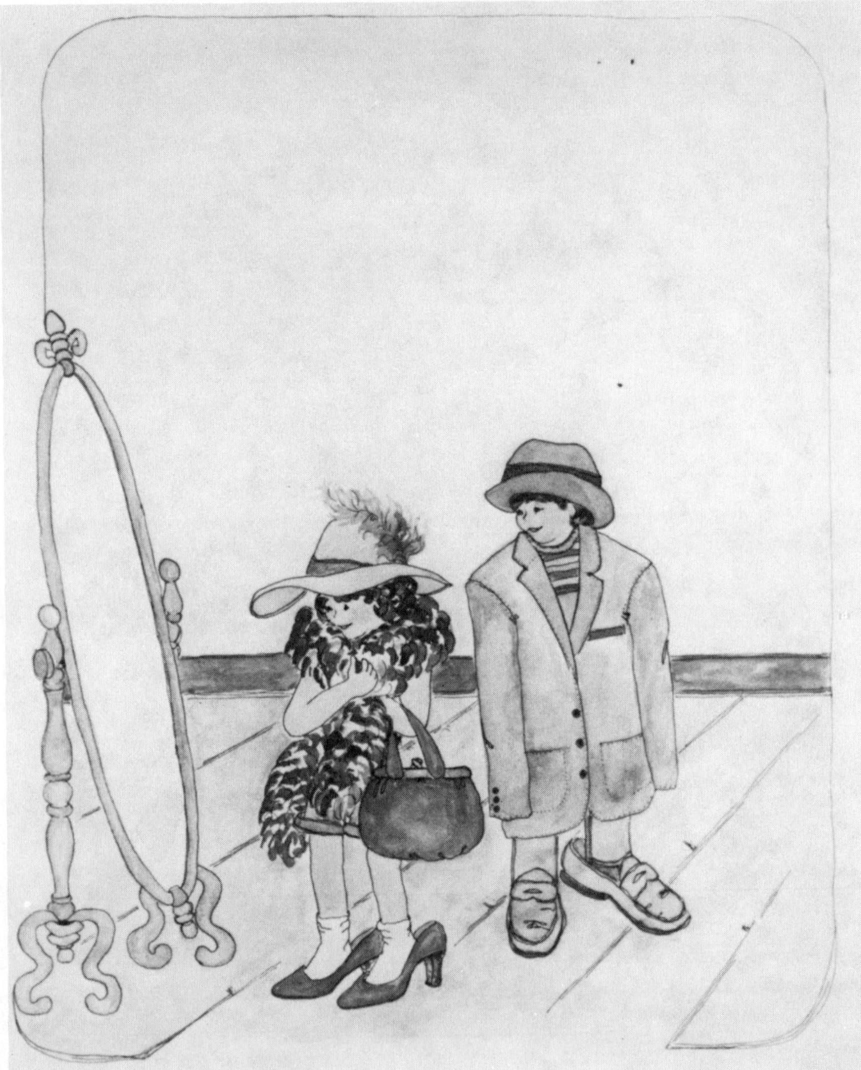

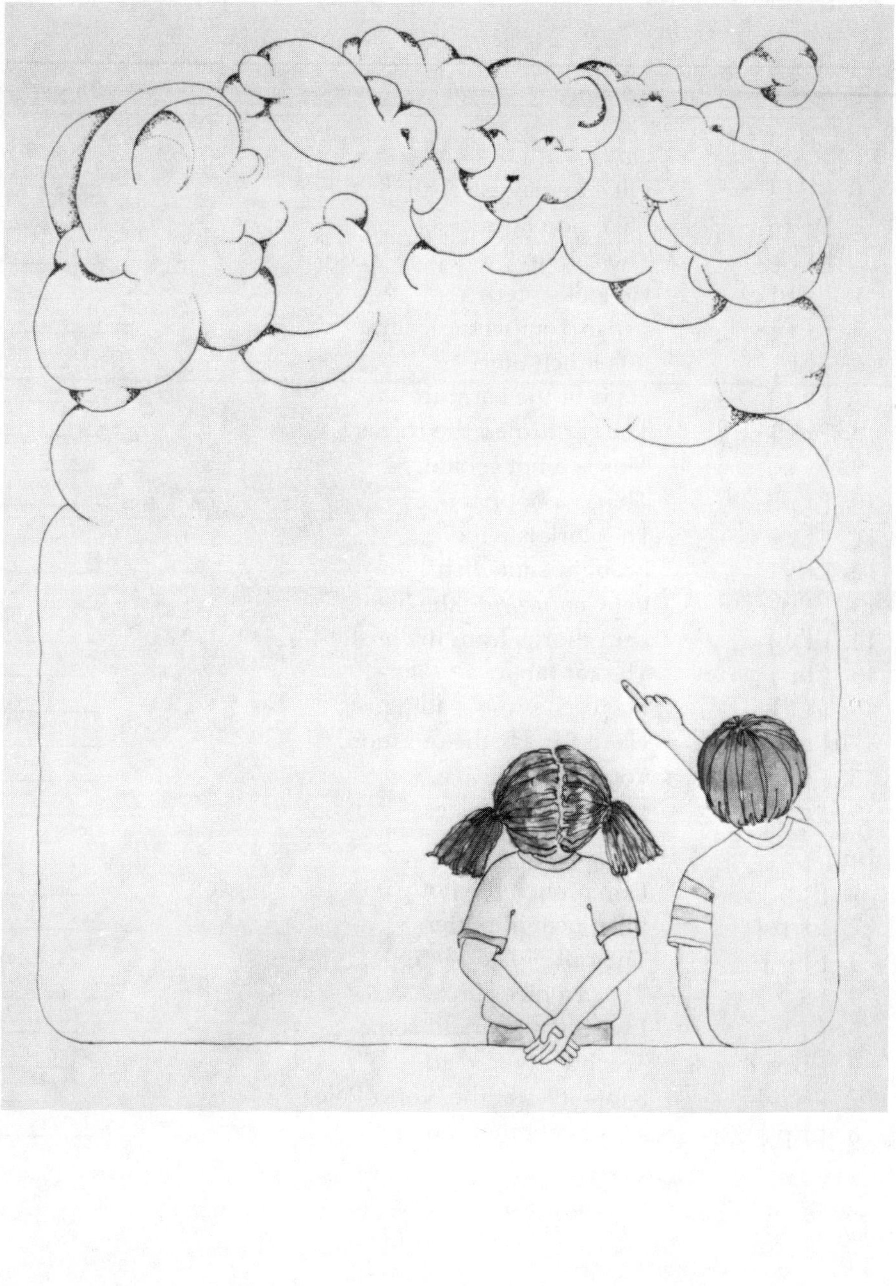

Appendix B

Sound-in-Context Survey

Context	*Sentence*	*Target*
[t]		
1. [k t]	I like to play baseball.	______
2. [p t]	I like pop tarts.	______
3. [f t]	The calf took a nap.	______
4. [s t]	He looks tired.	______
5. [ʃ t]	I wish Tom would come.	______
6. [t t]	It is lunch time.	______
7. [θ t]	He is in the bathtub.	______
8. [r t]	The car turned the corner.	______
9. [t k]	This is a hot cookie.	______
10. [t p]	This is a hot pan.	______
11. [t f]	That fork is mine.	______
12. [t s]	I caught some fish.	______
13. [t tʃ]	Let Charles ride the bike.	______
14. [t θ]	I cut thorns from the bushes.	______
15. [t r]	The cat ran away.	______
16. [i t]	He teaches me reading.	______
17. [æ t æ]	Have Pat ask the question.	______
18. [u t u]	You two can leave.	______
19. [a t a]	I got all the cookies.	______
[p]		
1. [t p]	Don't touch the hot pan.	______
2. [k p]	I like peanut butter.	______
3. [f p]	The calf pulled the rope.	______
4. [s p]	That's a nice pen.	______
5. [ʃ p]	I wish Patty would come.	______
6. [tʃ p]	Teach Patty to read.	______
7. [θ p]	Santa lives at the North Pole.	______
8. [r p]	This is not their pony.	______

9. [p t]	Don't jump too high.	________
10. [p k]	We made chocolate-chip cookies.	
11. [p f]	Tom will chop firewood.	________
12. [p s]	The ship sailed away.	________
13. [p ʃ]	Please stop shouting.	
14. [p t]	The ripe cherries are good.	________
15. [p θ]	I can jump three feet.	________
16. [p r]	Sit on the top row.	________
17. [i p i]	Keep eating your food.	________
18. [œ p œ]	Clap after the show.	________
19. [u p u]	My new poodle is black.	________
20. [a p a]	Don't stop on the road.	________

[k]

1. [t k]	He ate candy before supper.	________
2. [p k]	My cap came off.	________
3. [f k]	This is a safe car.	________
4. [s k]	Mother has the house key.	________
5. [ʃ k]	The push cart was full.	________
6. [tʃ k]	The latch can't be opened.	________
7. [θ k]	His tooth came out.	________
8. [r k]	My car can go fast.	________
9. [k t]	Let's take turns jumping rope.	________
10. [k p]	Bring me the black pen.	________
11. [k f]	Bring the book for the teacher.	________
12. [k s]	I will cook supper.	________
13. [kʃ]	Rick shot a deer.	________
14. [k tʃ]	I drank cherry pop.	________
15. [k θ]	Jack thought the game was fun.	________
16. [k r]	Thank Robert for the gift.	________
17. [i k i]	He keeps money in the safe.	________
18. [æ k æ]	I saw a black ant.	________
19. [u k u]	Are you cool by the window?	________
20. [a k a]	Put the rock on the table.	________

[s]

1. [t s]	I like hot soup.	________
2. [k s]	Dick saw a bird.	________
3. [p s]	The cop sat in the car.	________
4. [f s]	The calf saw a cow.	________

5. [ʃ s]	Push some boxes in here.	______
6. [tʃ s]	Butch sat in the big chair.	______
7. [θ s]	Give me my bath soap.	______
8. [r s]	You are so big.	______
9. [s t]	He looks tired.	______
10. [s k]	The baby likes candy.	______
11. [s p]	Mother bakes pies.	______
12. [s f]	Tom likes fish.	______
13. [s ʃ]	He likes sugar cookies.	______
14. [s tʃ]	Tom likes chocolate cake.	______
15. [s θ]	Let's think of a new game.	______
16. [s r]	She makes ribbons.	______
17. [i s i]	He sees a dog.	______
18. [æ s æ]	Pass Andy the paper.	______
19. [u s u]	I have a new suit.	______
20. [a s a]	Put the sauce on the meat.	______

[ʃ]

1. [t ʃ]	I took a hot shower.	______
2. [k ʃ]	You look short.	______
3. [p ʃ]	Put it on the top shelf.	______
4. [f ʃ]	Ralph shouted at me.	______
5. [s ʃ]	He likes short-cake.	______
6. [tʃ ʃ]	This watch should work.	______
7. [θ ʃ]	The bath shop is closed.	______
8. [r ʃ]	There are sheep in the pasture.	______
9. [ʃ t]	The fish tugged the line.	______
10. [ʃ k]	I wash cars on Saturday.	______
11. [ʃ p]	The fish pulled on the worm.	______
12. [ʃ f]	Mom cooked fish for supper.	______
13. [ʃ s]	Push Sam in the wagon.	______
14. [ʃ t ʃ]	We ate fresh cherries.	______
15. [ʃ θ]	I will wash three towels.	______
16. [ʃ r]	He will finish reading.	______
17. [i ʃ i]	This is the key she lost.	______
18. [æ ʃ æ]	Mr. Nash asked the question.	______
19. [u ʃ u]	This is a new shoe.	______
20. [a ʃ a]	I will wash all my clothes.	______

Context	Sentence	Target
[f]		
1. [t f]	The cat found her dish.	______
2. [k f]	We will look for you.	______
3. [p f]	The cap fell on the ground.	______
4. [s f]	Everyone likes fun.	______
5. [ʃ f]	Make a wish for me.	______
6. [tʃ f]	Watch for the cars.	______
7. [θ f]	I saw the tooth fairy.	______
8. [r f]	We are fine.	______
9. [f t]	The leaf turned brown.	______
10. [f k]	See the safe car.	______
11. [f p]	The chief put his pipe away.	______
12. [f s]	I have enough soap.	______
13. [f ʃ]	The beef should be cooked.	______
14. [f tʃ]	I ate enough chocolate.	______
15. [f θ]	He chopped off three limbs.	______
16. [f r]	The calf ran away.	______
17. [i f i]	He feeds the birds.	______
18. [æ f æ]	Don't laugh at me.	______
19. [u f u]	This is a new food.	______
20. [a f a]	I took off on a plane.	______
[r]		
1. [p r]	Keep reading the book.	______
2. [p r]	The cop ran fast.	______
3. [b r]	Bob reads books.	______
4. [b r]	The cab ran fast.	______
5. [f r]	Jeff reads the comics.	______
6. [f r]	The thief ran away.	______
7. [v r]	Save Rita's place.	______
8. [v r]	I love rabbits.	______
9. [t r]	Pete reached second base.	______
10. [t r]	The fat rat was eating.	______
11. [d r]	My dad reads books.	______
12. [d r]	My dad ran home.	______
13. [s r]	My class reads books.	______

14. [s r]	The mouse ran away.	______
15. [z r]	John was reading.	______
16. [z r]	The cows ran away.	______
17. [ʃr]	I wish Rick would play.	______
18. [ʃr]	Let's wash Randy's bike.	______
19. [ʃr]	Let's wash Rita's bike.	______
20. [ʃr]	The dish rack is blue.	______
21. [k r]	Dick reads books.	______
22. [k r]	The sick rat died.	______
23. [g r]	Peg reads a lot.	______
24. [g r]	The pig ran away.	______
25. [p ɝ]	The pearl was big.	______
26. [p ɝ]	The cop earned a medal.	______
27. [b ɝ]	The bird flew away.	______
28. [b ɝ]	Bob earned a toy.	______
29. [f ɝ]	The furnace was hot.	______
30. [f ɝ]	Jeff earned fifty cents.	______
31. [v ɝ]	We will leave early.	______
32. [v ɝ]	Let's leave early.	______
33. [t ɝ]	Pete earns his money.	______
34. [t ɝ]	My turtle likes flies.	______
35. [d ɝ]	The dirt was black.	______
36. [d ɝ]	My dad earns money.	______
37. [s ɝ]	Mom served lunch.	______
38. [s ɝ]	Pete's early today.	______
39. [z ɝ]	John was early.	______
40. [z ɝ]	My dessert was good.	______
41. [k ɝ]	Jack earned a medal.	______
42. [k ɝ]	The curb is yellow.	______
43. [g ɝ]	That girl is nice.	______
44. [g ɝ]	Peg earned some money.	______
45. [ʃ ɝ]	The shirt was blue.	______
46. [ʃ ɝ]	I met Shirley.	______
47. [ʒ ɝ]	I measured the table.	______
48. [ʒ ɝ]	The pleasure is mine.	______
49. [p ɚ]	The skipper eats fish.	______
50. [p ɚ]	Pass the pepper and salt.	______
51. [bɚ]	My neighbor eats fish.	______

52. [bɚ]	The fibber asked a question.	________
53. [fɚ]	A gopher eats plants.	________
54. [fɚ]	It's safer at home.	________
55. [vɚ]	Never eat too much cake.	________
56. [vɚ]	Never act like a fool.	________
57. [tɚ]	Peter eats pickles.	________
58. [tɚ]	Peter added two and two.	________
59. [dɚ]	The ladder and paint fell.	________
60. [dɚ]	A spider eats flies.	________
61. [sɚ]	It's nicer each day.	________
62. [sɚ]	Use a saucer and cup.	________
63. [zɚ]	A miser eats anything.	________
64. [zɚ]	The loser added a point.	________
65. [kɚ]	The baker eats pies.	________
66. [kɚ]	The baker added salt.	________
67. [gɚ]	A tiger eats meat.	________
68. [gɚ]	The bigger apple is mine.	________
69. [ʃɚ]	The usher acted funny.	________
70. [ʃɚ]	The usher eats candy.	________
71. [ʃɚ]	The window washer eats outside.	________
72. [ʃɚ]	The mop pusher acted funny.	________
73. [b r]	John brags too much.	________
74. [p r]	The priest was fat.	________
75. [p r]	The pony pranced home.	________
76. [b r]	The breeze is nice.	________
77. [f r]	The balloon was free.	________
78. [f r]	The cat freed the mouse.	________
79. [f r]	Frank wasn't home.	________
80. [f r]	I saw Francis.	________
81. [t r]	He climbed the tree.	________
82. [t r]	The mouse was trapped.	________
83. [d r]	I had a funny dream.	________
84. [d r]	This is a drab day.	________
85. [k r]	I like ice cream.	________
86. [k r]	I caught a crab.	________
87. [g r]	He is greedy.	________
88. [g r]	I like my grandma.	________

Context	Sentence	Target
[s]		
1. [k s k]	The old man makes keys.	______
2. [t s k]	He was a great skier.	______
3. [n s k]	The mean skier fell down.	______
4. [p s k]	He keeps keys in his pocket.	______
5. [k s t]	It takes teamwork to win.	______
6. [t s t]	The hot steam burned his hand.	______
7. [n s t]	He climbed ten steep hills.	______
8. [p s t]	Drop Steve off at the gym.	______
9. [k s n]	John never looks neat.	______
10. [t s n]	The cats need milk.	______
11. [n s n]	Cover your mouth when sneezing.	______
12. [p s n]	The dog will keep sneezing.	______
13. [k s p]	He likes peanut butter cookies.	______
14. [t s p]	Paul eats peanut butter every Friday.	______
15. [n s p]	He rode a ten-speed bike.	______
16. [p s p]	Pam keeps peeking through the window.	______
17. [k s k]	He rode a black scooter.	______
18. [t s k]	Pat scooped up the mud.	______
19. [n s k]	I live near the green school.	______
20. [p s k]	May keeps Kool-Aid in the refrigerator.	______
21. [k s t]	She talks too much.	______
22. [t s t]	The foot stool is broken.	______
23. [n s t]	The tall man stooped over.	______
24. [p s t]	The cops tooted their horn.	______
25. [k s n]	My mother bakes noodles.	______
26. [t s n]	The man took a short snooze.	______
27. [n s n]	He had fun snooping around.	______
28. [p s n]	The pup snooped around the garage.	______
29. [k s p]	Jack's poodle won third prize.	______
30. [t s p]	Tony ran from the white spook.	______
31. [n s p]	I need a clean spoon.	______
32. [p s p]	I keep spoons in a bag.	______
33. [k s k]	My teacher drinks coffee.	______
34. [t s k]	Pat's cough was better.	______
35. [n s k]	The cut left a thin scar.	______

36.	[p s k]	Mother keeps calling for me.	______
37.	[k s t]	The boy looks tall.	______
38.	[t s t]	The cat stopped running.	______
39.	[n s t]	The barn stall was empty.	______
40.	[p s t]	The teacher helps Tom.	______
41.	[k s n]	Nick's naughty dog chewed the rug.	______
42.	[t s n]	The cats knocked over the dish.	______
43.	[n s n]	The lion snarled at the hunter.	______
44.	[p s n]	He keeps nodding his head.	______
45.	[k s p]	We waded in Jack's pond.	______
46.	[t s p]	The boy held the cat's paw.	______
47.	[n s p]	The paint left a green spot.	______
48.	[p s p]	The cop spotted the robber.	______

Appendix C

Articulation Automatization Stories

PLANTING A GARDEN

Suggested materials: Flannelboard, felt figures (boy, birl, watering can, lettuce seeds)

Target sounds: /r/ and /l/

Narrative	***Target response***
1. Today our story is about planting a garden. Do you know who is going to plant the garden? Two children named Robbie and Lisa. This is a girl. Her name is Lisa. Lisa is a girl. Is Lisa a boy?	No, Lisa is a girl.
2. Here is a boy. His name is Robbie. What is his name?	His name is Robbie.
3. One day Robbie said to Lisa, "Lisa, let's plant a garden." Listen to what Robbie says: "Let's plant a garden." What did Robbie say?	Let's plant a garden.
4. Lisa says, "Oh, Robbie, I like your idea." What does Lisa say?	I like your idea.
5. So they went down into the cellar. Where did they go?	Into the cellar.
6. Lisa looked around. She said, "Robbie, do you see a watering can?" What did she ask Robbie?	Do you see a watering can?
7. Soon, they found a spade, a hoe, and some other tools. Then they went outside. Robbie said, "Let's plant it here." What did he say?	Let's plant it here.
8. What kind of seeds do you think they will plant?	(elicit response)
9. Now, listen to what Robbie says: "Here are the lettuce seeds." What does he say?	Here are the lettuce seeds.

10. Then they dug the dirt. Robbie and Lisa dug up the dirt. What did they do?	They dug up the dirt.
11. They put in the seeds and covered them up. What did they do?	They covered up the seeds.
12. Then Lisa said, "Here's a little water." What did she say?	Here's a little water.
13. Then they watered the lettuce. Lisa said, "I hope it grows." Robbie said, "I hope it grows." What did they say?	I hope it grows.
14. And it did. Did you ever plant any seeds?	(elicit response)

THE FOOTBALL GAME

Suggested materials: Flannelboard, felt figures (two boys, one man, tickets, car, hot dog, Coke, corn dog, Cracker Jack, goal posts, football)

Target sounds: /k/ and /g/

Narrative	***Target response***
1. This is Kenny. He is in our story. Who is this?	This is Kenny.
2. This is Kenny's dad. He is in our story. Who is this?	This is Kenny's dad.
3. This is Gary. He is Kenny's friend. He is in our story. Who is this?	This is Gary.
4. One night, Kenny's dad comes home from work. He says to Kenny, "I have a surprise for you. I have some tickets to the football game this weekend." What does dad have? What are the tickets for?	He has tickets. For the football game.
5. Kenny says, "Yay! I like football. Can Gary come with us?" "Yes, he can," says dad. "I have three tickets." "Oh, good," says Kenny, "Gary can come." What does Kenny say?	Gary can come.
6. On Saturday morning, Kenny is out of bed early. He tells dad, "I want to get to the game early." "Don't worry," says dad. "The game doesn't start until one o'clock." What time does the game start?	One o'clock.

7. At noon, dad says, "It's time to get Gary and go to the game." Kenny, Gary, and dad drive to the stadium. They park the car and walk to the gate. What do they do?	They park the car and walk to the gate.
8. The ticket taker tears their tickets as they enter. Who tears the tickets?	The ticket taker.
9. "Would you like to get something to eat?" asks dad. "Yes, we would," say Kenny and Gary. "What would you like?" Dad asks. 'I would like a hot dog and a Coke," says Kenny. What does Kenny want?	A hot dog and Coke.
10. Gary says, "I would like some Cracker Jack and a corn dog." What does Gary want?	Some Cracker Jack and a corn dog.
11. Dad says, "I would like some coffee with cream and sugar." What does dad say?	Some coffee with cream and sugar.
12. "Let's go find our seats," says dad. "It's time for the kickoff." What does dad say?	It's time for the kickoff.
13. The first half of the game is very exciting. Both teams score touchdowns. Both teams kick field goals. What do the teams do?	Score touchdowns and kick field goals.
14. At halftime, the score is tied. Kenny says, "I'm worried. I hope the Tigers win." What does Kenny say?	I hope the Tigers win.
15. Gary says, "This is a close game." What does Gary say?	This is a close game.
16. "I hope the second half is as good as the first," says dad. The second half is exciting. With six seconds left, the score is still tied. The kicker comes in to kick a field goal. What is the kicker going to do?	Kick a field goal.
17. Kenny, Gary, and dad are on the edge of their seats. The kick is up—it's good! "The kick is good!" says Gary. What does Gary say?	The kick is good.
18. Kenny says, "The Tigers win." What does Kenny say?	The Tigers win.

19. Kenny, Gary, and dad leave the stadium. "That was a good game," says dad. What does dad say?	That was a good game.
20. Dad asks Kenny, "What position would you like to play if you were a football player?" Kenny says, "I would like to be a quarterback." What does Kenny say?	I would like to be a quarterback.
21. Dad asks Gary, "What position would you like to play?" Gary says, "I would like to be a kicker." What does Gary say?	I would like to be a kicker.
22. Kenny, Gary, and dad drive home. They had a good time at the football game. What did they have?	A good time at the game.

KEN AND ROBERT GO TO THE ZOO

Suggested materials: Flannelboard, felt figures (two boys, bicycle(s), cage, bear, camel, tiger, raccoon, rattlesnake)

Target sounds: /k/ and /r/

Narrative	***Target response***
1. Ken called his friend Robert one Saturday morning. "Robert," Ken said, "Do you want to go to the zoo with me?" Robert said, "That's a great idea. Let's go to the zoo Ken." What did Robert say?	Robert said, Let's go to the zoo Ken.
2. The boys rode their bikes to the zoo. The zoo was not far from Robert's house. Robert and Ken rode their bikes to the zoo. What did Robert and Ken do?	Robert and Ken rode their bikes to the zoo.
3. When they got to the zoo, the boys began to walk around and look at the animals. First, Ken and Robert saw a bear in a big cage. What did Ken and Robert see?	Ken and Robert saw a bear in a big cage.
4. "I hope he doesn't get out," Ken said. "Me too," said Robert. "Let's see what is in the next cage." There was a	

camel in the next cage. What was in the next cage?

There was a camel in the next cage.

5. "He's pretty big," Robert said. "I've seen a lot of pictures of camels before, but this is the first real one I've ever seen. I've seen pictures of camels before." What did he say?

   I've seen pictures of camels before.

6. "I've seen camels in pictures, too," Ken said. "And also on TV. I didn't think camels were so big, though." What did he say?

   I didn't think camels were so big.

7. "I wonder what other animals we can see here," Robert said. "Oh, a lot of different animals," Ken said. "We can see tigers and raccoons." What can they see?

   They can see tigers and raccoons.

8. "Great!" Robert said. "I like this zoo. Let's look at all of the animals." They looked at all the animals. They even found rattlesnakes in a cage. Ken and Robert found rattlesnakes in a cage. What did Ken and Robert find?

   Ken and Robert found rattlesnakes in a cage.

9. Soon it was time for them to leave. "I liked the tiger and the camel best of all," Ken said. "What did you like best, Robert? I liked the tiger and the camel." What did Ken say?

   I liked the tiger and the camel.

10. "I liked the raccoons and the rattlesnakes," Robert said. "The raccoons looked so funny and the rattlesnakes were scary. I liked the raccoons and the rattlesnakes." What did he say?

    I liked the raccoons and the rattlesnakes.

11. "We have to go now, but maybe we can come back soon," Robert said. "I like this zoo." "Me, too," said Ken. Robert and Ken rode their bikes home. What did Robert and Ken do?

    Robert and Ken rode their bikes home.

WHERE IS TIPPY?

Suggested materials: Flannelboard, felt figures (kitten, boy, sofa, tree, fireman, ladder)

Target sounds: /s/ and /t/

Narrative	***Target response***
1. Tippy is a little kitty. Tippy is a little kitty. What is Tippy?	Tippy is a little kitty.
2. Tippy is Bobby's pet. Tippy is Bobby's pet. Whose pet is Tippy?	Tippy is Bobby's pet.
3. Bobby goes to school every day. He goes to school every day. Where does Bobby go?	He goes to school every day.
4. After school Bobby plays. After school Bobby plays. What does Bobby do?	After school Bobby plays.
5. Bobby plays with Tippy. He plays with Tippy. What does Bobby play with?	He plays with Tippy.
6. One day, Bobby runs home from school and says, "I am home, Tippy. I am home, Tippy." What does Bobby say?	I am home, Tippy.
7. "Come here, Tippy," says Bobby. "Come here, Tippy." What does Bobby say?	Come here, Tippy.
8. Bobby looks for Tippy. He looks for Tippy. What does Bobby do?	He looks for Tippy.
9. "Mommy, I can't find Tippy," says Bobby. "I can't find Tippy." What does Bobby say?	I can't find Tippy.
10. "I want Tippy," says Bobby. "I want Tippy." What does Bobby say?	I want Tippy.
11. "Please don't cry, Bobby," says Mommy. "Please don't cry." What does Mommy say?	Please don't cry.
12. "We will find Tippy," says Mommy. "We will find Tippy." What does Mommy say?	We will find Tippy.
13. "Let's look under your bed," says Mommy. "Let's look under your bed." What does Mommy say?	Let's look under your bed.
14. "Tippy is not under my bed," says Bobby. "Tippy is not under my bed." What does Bobby say?	Tippy is not under my bed.

15. "Look behind the sofa," says Mommy. "Look behind the sofa." What does Mommy say?	Look behind the sofa.
16. "Tippy is not behind the sofa," says Bobby. "Tippy is not behind the sofa." What does Bobby say?	Tippy is not behind the sofa.
17. Bobby runs outside. He runs outside. What does Bobby do?	He runs outside.
18. Bobby looks everywhere. He looks everywhere. What does Bobby do?	He looks everywhere.
19. "Little Tippy," yells Bobby. "Little Tippy." What does Bobby yell?	Little Tippy.
20. "Little Tippy is lost," says Bobby. "Little Tippy is lost." What does Bobby say?	Little Tippy is lost.
21. Bobby looks up the tree. He looks up the tree. What does Bobby do?	He looks up the tree.
22. Bobby sees Tippy. He sees Tippy. What does Bobby see?	He sees Tippy.
23. "I found Tippy," says Bobby. "I found Tippy." What does Bobby say?	I found Tippy.
24. "Mommy, Tippy can't get down. Tippy can't get down." What does Bobby say?	Tippy can't get down.
25. "We will telephone the fireman," says Mommy. "We will telephone the fireman." What does Mommy say?	We will telephone the fireman.
26. Mommy telephones the fireman. Mommy telephones the fireman. What does Mommy do?	Mommy telephones the fireman.
27. Bobby hears the siren. He hears the siren. What does Bobby hear?	He hears the siren.
28. The fireman puts up the ladder. The fireman puts up the ladder. What does the fireman do?	The fireman puts up the ladder.
29. The ladder is by the tree. The ladder is by the tree. Where is the ladder?	The ladder is by the tree.
30. The fireman climbs the ladder. The fireman climbs the ladder. What does the fireman do?	The fireman climbs the ladder.
31. The fireman saves Tippy. He saves Tippy. What does the fireman do?	He saves Tippy.
32. Bobby hugs Tippy. He hugs Tippy. What does Bobby do?	He hugs Tippy.

33. "Don't you hide again, Tippy," says Bobby. "Don't you hide again." What does Bobby say?	Don't you hide again.

A TRIP TO THE TOY STORE

Suggested materials: Flannelboard, felt figures (girl, boy, gray station wagon, woman, red frog, golden goose, gold wagon, green wagon)

Target sounds: /d/ *and* /g/

Narrative	***Target response***
1. Our story is about a girl named Debbie and her brother, Gary. What are their names?	Their names are Debbie and Gary.
2. They like to play games and draw pictures. What do they like to do?	They like to play games and draw pictures.
3. On Monday, their mother asked them, "Do you want to go downtown and buy a wagon?" What did their mother ask?	Do you want to go downtown and buy a wagon.
4. Both Debbie and Gary were delighted about their mother's idea. How did they feel?	They were delighted.
5. They quickly decided that they would get a green wagon. What did they decide?	They decided they would get a green wagon.
6. Debbie ran to get her coat and Gary hurried to get his, too. What did they do?	Debbie and Gary ran to get their coats.
7. They went outside and got in mother's gray station wagon. Where did they go?	They went outside and got in mother's gray station wagon.
8. Mother said to them, "Debbie, you are a good girl, and Gary, you are a good boy, so you may get two wagons if you would like." What did mother say?	Debbie, you are a good girl, and Gary, you are a good boy, so you may get two wagons.
9. "That is wonderful!" said Debbie. "That is great," said Gary. What did they say?	Debbie said, "That is wonderful. "Gary said, "That is great."
10. Debbie said, "I am going to get a gold wagon." What did Debbie say?	I am going to get a gold wagon.
11. "My wagon is going to be green," said Gary. How will Gary's wagon look?	Gary's wagon is going to be green.

12. Just then mother turned onto Davis street. Where did mother turn?	She turned on Davis street.
13. Debbie looked ahead and she saw Gibbons department store. What did Debbie do?	She looked ahead and saw Gibbons department store.
14. Mother parked the car and said, "Children, be very good inside the store." What did mother say?	She said, "Children, be very good inside the store."
15. Once they were inside the store they saw a stuffed red frog and a big golden goose. What did they see?	They saw a stuffed red frog and a big golden goose.
16. Gary said, "Debbie, look. Down there are the dolls." What did Gary say?	Debbie, look. Down there are the dolls.
17. Debbie told Gary, "Let's look around and find the wagons." What did Debbie want to do?	Debbie wanted to look around and find the wagons.
18. About that time, they turned the corner and they saw wagons of every description. What did they do?	They turned the corner and they saw wagons of every description.
19. Gary searched for a green wagon and Debbie looked for a gold one. What did they look for?	Gary searched for a green wagon and Debbie looked for a gold one.
20. Debbie looked up and grinned. She saw a gold wagon at the end of the row. What did Debbie do?	Debbie looked up and grinned. She saw a gold wagon at the end of the row.
21. About that time Gary yelled, "Debbie, here is a green wagon!" What did Gary do?	Gary yelled, "Debbie, here is a green wagon."
22. Mother said, "Debbie and Gary, have you decided which wagons you are going to get?" What did Mother say?	Debbie and Gary, have you decided which wagons you are going to get?
23. Together they said, "Yes, we have found the wagons we want to get." What did they say?	Yes, we have found the wagons we want to get.
24. Mother paid for the wagons and the children loaded them in the car. What happened?	Mother paid for the wagons and the children loaded them in the car.

THE BIG JUMP

Suggested materials: *Flannelboard, felt figures (king, dogs, boy, stick, boxes, castle)*

Target sounds: /d/ and /dj/

Narrative	***Target response***
1. Once upon a time, in a land far away, there lived a king. In those days nobody could have a dog for a pet—except the king. The king kept all the dogs himself. What did the king do?	He kept all the dogs himself.
2. The king had many, many kinds of dogs. He had big ones and little ones, thin ones and fat ones. When the king took his dogs out to play, all the children would come to look. They looked at the king's dogs because they didn't have any dogs themselves. Did the children have any dogs?	No, the children didn't have any dogs.
3. One day, a little dog ran away from the king. It ran to a little boy named Jerry. Jerry bent down to pet the little dog. What did Jerry do?	Jerry bent down to pet the dog.
4. Jerry said, "Go back. I'm not the king. You have to go back to the king because only kings can have dogs." But the puppy would not leave. He wagged his tail and barked. Then the little dog just jumped up and down. What did the little dog do?	The little dog just jumped up and down.
5. "Look at that!" said the king. "My dog likes you. If you were a king, you could keep this dog." Jerry was very sad. He wanted to be a king so he could keep the dog. Jerry wanted to keep the dog. What did Jerry want?	Jerry wanted to keep the dog.
6. "Could I be a king?" asked Jerry. "What do I have to do to become a king?" The king laughed. He said, "A king has to do many things." What did he say?	A king has to do many things.

7. "Well," said the king, "for one thing, a king has to know how to do the Big Jump." "What is the Big Jump?" asked Jerry. In a flash, the king was gone. Jerry saw the king way up on top of his castle. "How did you do that?" asked Jerry. "Did you jump up there all by yourself?" What did Jerry ask?	Did you jump up there all by yourself?
8. "Yes," said the king, "that was the Big Jump. All kings can jump like that." Then the king said, "You can keep the dog if you can jump up there." What did the king say?	You can keep the dog if you can jump up there.
9. Jerry said, "Can I keep the dog for just one day?" The king nodded. He said, "You can keep the dog for just one day." What did the king say?	You can keep the dog for just one day.
10. Jerry said, "All right. I will try to jump up there. I will go right home and practice." So Jerry went home to practice jumping. Where did Jerry go?	Jerry went home to practice jumping.
11. When Jerry got home, he practiced jumping over some different boxes. He could jump to the top of one box, and even two boxes. But he could not jump to the top of three boxes. He tried but he tumbled down to the ground. What happened to Jerry?	Jerry tumbled down to the ground.
12. So Jerry got a stick to help him jump. "This stick will help me jump over these different boxes." What did he say?	The stick will help me jump over these different boxes.
13. So Jerry piled up the boxes—one, two, three, four boxes. He wanted to get a running start. He was getting ready to jump. Jerry jerked back his stick and tightened his jaw. What did Jerry do?	Jerry jerked back his stick and tightened his jaw.
14. It was a good trick. Now Jerry could jump over four boxes when he used his stick. But he could not go over five boxes. He tried and tried but he	

Narrative	Target response
didn't go any higher. Did Jerry jump any higher?	No. He didn't jump any higher.
15. Then the little dog did something funny. He began to jump on one box. Then he jumped up to the next box. He began to jump all the boxes. What did the little dog do?	The little dog began to jump all the boxes.
16. That gave Jerry an idea. He said, "Good dog. Now I know how to do it because you showed me how. C'mon, let's show the king that I can jump to the top of his castle." So Jerry and the dog ran down to the castle. What did they do?	Jerry and the dog ran down to the castle.
17. When Jerry got to the castle all the children were there. He began to jump the steps one at a time. All the children watched Jerry jump. What did they do?	All the children watched Jerry jump.
18. All the children laughed at Jerry. They said, "We can all do that way ourselves." "Yes," said the king, "Jerry showed you how. Now Jerry deserves to keep the dog." What did the king say?	Now Jerry deserves to keep the dog.
19. "Oh, thank you," said Jerry, "and thank you, too, little dog." Jerry dropped to his knees to shake the dog's paw. What did Jerry do?	Jerry dropped to his knees to shake the dog's paw.
20. Jerry said, "You are my very own dog now and we are both happy. I will name you Jolly." So Jerry named his dog Jolly because they were both happy. What did Jerry name his dog?	Jerry named his dog Jolly.

THUMPER THE FROG

Suggested materials: Flannelboard, felt figures (frog, lilypad, turtle, elf)

Target sounds: /f/ and /θ

Narrative	***Target response***
1. This is a story about Thumper. Thumper is a frog. What is Thumper?	Thumper is a frog.

2. Thumper likes to sit on his lilypad. He likes to daydream. Thumper wishes he could be another animal (sigh). He closes his eyes. He starts dreaming. Thumper begins flapping his front legs. What does Thumper do?	Thumper begins flapping his front legs.
3. Thumper thinks he is a moth. What does Thumper think he is?	Thumper thinks he is a moth.
4. He is a beautiful green moth. Thumper flaps his legs fast. What does Thumper do?	Thumper flaps his legs fast.
5. He starts going up and down. Splash! Thumper falls off the lilypad! What happens to Thumper?	Thumper falls off the lilypad.
6. Down, down, down goes Thumper. Thud! Thumper falls on a rock. What sound does Thumper make when he falls on the rock? What happens to Thumper?	Thud! Thumper falls on a rock.
7. The rock starts moving. Thumper knows he is not dreaming. Now, he is out of the water. Thumper is on a turtle. Thumper meets Fred, the turtle. Who does Thumper meet?	Thumper meets Fred the turtle.
8. "I want to go home," says Thumper. "I'll take you there," says Fred. "Go north fifty feet," says Thumper. What does Thumper say?	"Go north fifty feet," says Thumper.
9. Fred follows Thumper's directions. What does Fred do?	Fred follows Thumper's directions.
10. "There is my lilypad," says Thumper. It is underneath his favorite tree. Where is Thumper's lilypad?	It's underneath his favorite tree.
11. "Thank you, Fred," says Thumper. What does Thumper say?	"Thank you, Fred," says Thumper.
12. Thumper is sitting on his lilypad. Oops! Thumper's foot slips off the pad. What happens to Thumper?	Thumper's foot slips off the pad.
13. Thumper falls into the water again. He closes his eyes. He is dreaming again. Thumper's tail moves back and forth. What does Thumper's tail do?	Thumper's tail moves back and forth.

14. Thumper thinks he is a fish. What does Thumper think he is?
    Thumper thinks he is a fish.
15. Thumper cannot swim like a fish. Down, down, down goes Thumper! A thousand fish come to help Thumper. Who comes to help Thumper?
    A thousand fish come to help Thumper.
16. The fish takes Thumper back to his lilypad. Thumper says, "Thank you, fish." What does Thumper say?
    Thumper says, "Thank you, fish."
17. Thumper hops from one lilypad to another. He hops onto the ground. Once again, Thumper closes his eyes. He is dreaming again. Thumper stretches his neck. Thumper thinks he is a giraffe. What does Thumper think he is?
    Thumper thinks he is a giraffe.
18. Thumper is hungry. He looks for a leaf. What does he look for?
    Thumper looks for a leaf.
19. Ouch! Thumper bumps into some thorns. What happens to Thumper?
    Thumper bumps into some thorns.
20. Thumper opens his eyes quickly. He does not want to be a giraffe either. Now, Thumper is walking through a forest. What is Thumper doing?
    Thumper is walking through a forest.
21. He closes his eyes again. He starts dreaming again. He walks very slowly. Thumper acts tough and fearless. How does Thumper act?
    Thumper acts tough and fearless.
22. Thumper thinks he is a wolf. What does Thumper think he is?
    Thumper thinks he is a wolf.
23. He is not afraid. Thumper hunts for food. What does Thumper hunt for?
    Thumper hunts for food.
24. Thumper smells something burning. The forest is in fire! What is on fire?
    The forest is on fire.
25. Thumper dashes out of the woods. He runs for fifteen minutes. How long does he run?
    He runs for fifteen minutes.
26. He opens his eyes again (sigh). Thumper does not want to be a wolf either. Thumper looks around. "I am

in a field," says Thumper. What does Thumper say?	"I am in a field," says Thumper.
27. The field is near a farm. What is near a farm?	The field is near a farm.
28. Thumper hops toward the farm. Thumper sees a calf. What does Thumper see?	Thumper sees a calf.
29. He looks all round him. Thumper also sees thirty cows. What else does Thumper see?	Thumper sees thirty cows.
30. The cows start mooing at Thumper. Thumper laughs at the cows. What does Thumper do?	Thumper laughs at the cows.
31. He closes his eyes again. He starts dreaming again. Thumper opens his mouth. What does Thumper do?	Thumper opens his mouth.
32. "Moo," says Thumper. Thumper thinks he is a cow. What does Thumper think he is?	Thumper thinks he is a cow.
33. The cows start running after Thumper. What do the cows do?	The cows start running after Thumper.
34. Thumper opens his eyes quickly. Thumper hops down a rough path. What does Thumper do?	Thumper hops down a rough path.
35. The cows stop chasing Thumper. Thumper stops hopping. He is tired. Thumper huffs and puffs. What does Thumper do?	Thumper huffs and puffs.
36. The cows are far away now. Thumper rests for five minutes. How long does Thumper rest?	Thumper rests for five minutes.
37. Thumper falls asleep. What does Thumper do?	Thumper falls asleep.
38. An elf finds Thumper sleeping. Who finds Thumper sleeping?	An elf finds Thumper sleeping.
39. "Don't be afraid," says the elf. What does the elf say?	"Don't be afraid," says the elf.
40. "I will help you find your pad," says the elf. Thumper follows the elf. What does Thumper do?	Thumper follows the elf.
41. Both go down the rough path. Who goes down the rough path?	Both go down the rough path.

42. Finally Thumper sees his lilypad. Thumper says, "Thank you, Mister Elf." What does Thumper say?	Thumper says, "Thank you, Mister Elf."
43. Thumper hops onto his lilypad. "I feel safe on my lilypad," says Thumper. What does Thumper say?	"I feel safe on my lilypad," says Thumper.
44. It's not worth being another animal. Thumper says, "I am a fine frog." What does Thumper say?	"i am a fine frog," says Thumper.
45. "I just want to be me," says Thumper. Thumper puts a smile on his face. What does Thumper do?	Thumper puts a smile on his face.
46. "I'm Thumper, a fine frog," says Thumper. What does Thumper say?	"I'm Thumper, a fine frog."

TEETH FOR FATHER FISH

Suggested materials: Flannelboard, felt figures (five fish, false teeth, store, birthday cake)

Target sounds: /f/ and /θ/

Narrative	***Target response***
1. This is a story about a family of fish. There are five fish in the family. How many fish are there in the family?	There are five fish in the family.
2. These two are brother fish. Who are these two?	These two are brother fish.
3. This big one is sister fish. Sister fish is rather fat. Which fish is rather fat?	Sister fish is rather fat.
4. The fish wearing the bathrobe is mother fish. She is wearing a bathrobe. What is mother fish wearing?	Mother fish is wearing a bathrobe.
5. The last fish doesn't have any teeth. This is old father fish. Old father fish doesn't have any teeth. Who doesn't have any teeth?	Old father fish doesn't have any teeth.
6. One day, mother fish, fat sister fish, and the fish brothers got to thinking. Who got to thinking?	Mother fish, fat sister fish, and the fish brothers got to thinking.
7. Fat sister fish says, "Do you remember what day Thursday the fifth is?" What does she say?	Do you remember what day Thursday the fifth is?

8. The fish brothers laughed. Who laughed?	The fish brothers laughed.
9. They said, "We know it's not Friday the fifth." What did they say?	We know it's not Friday the fifth.
10. All of a sudden, mother fish said, "I think Thursday the fifth is old father fish's birthday. Thursday the fifth is his birthday." What day is his birthday?	Thursday the fifth is his birthday.
11. Sister fish says, "That's right. It's old father fish's birthday." Whose birthday is it?	It's old father fish's birthday.
12. Everyone said at once, "What can we give him for his birthday?" What did everyone say?	What can we give him for his birthday?
13. They thought and thought for a long time. They thought for a long time. What did they do for a long time?	They thought for a long time.
14. Finally, mother fish flapped her fins and said, "I know what he wants. The best thing for father is a set of false teeth. False teeth is the best present for him!" What is the best present for him?	False teeth is the best present for him.
15. Everyone said, "False teeth? That's a fine thought." What did they say?	False teeth? That's a fine thought.
16. Mother fish said, "I think he'll like them. They'll be good for lots of things." What will they be good for?	They'll be good for lots of things.
17. So, they all went downtown to the fish tooth store and bought a set of false teeth. They bought the teeth at the fish tooth store. Where did they buy the teeth?	They bought the teeth at the fish tooth store.
18. Then they swam home. When they got there, old father fish was floating, taking his nap. Father fish was just floating. What was father fish doing?	Father fish was just floating.
19. They swam to father fish. Then, all together, they yelled, "Happy Birthday, father fish!" What did they yell?	Happy Birthday, father fish.
20. Old father fish jumped with a splash!	

He said, "I thought that everyone had forgotten." What did he say?	I thought everyone had forgotten.
21. Fat sister fish said, "Here's your present. This gift is for you." What did fat sister fish say?	This gift is for you.
22. Old father fish opened the package. "False teeth! What a surprise!" he said. The false teeth really surprised him. What surprised him?	The false teeth surprised him.
23. Old father fish said, "They'll be good for a lot of things." What did he say?	They'll be good for a lot of things.
24. He said, "Thank you, family." What did he say?	Thank you, family.
25. "Let me try them on for size," he said. "I'll try them on for size. What did he do?	He tried them on for size.
26. "They're a perfect fit," said old father fish. "They fit perfectly." How did they fit?	They fit perfectly.
27. And so, old father fish was happy on his birthday. He smiled a fish smile and then swam away to eat his birthday fish cake. He can eat his birthday fish cake now. What can he eat now?	He can eat his birthday fish cake now.

BAKING SOME COOKIES

Suggested materials: Flannelboard, felt figures (woman, two girls, bowl, flour, milk, mixer, fork, spatula, cookie cutters—cat, kangaroo, seal, squirrel—chocolate cookies)

Target sounds: /s/ and /k/

Narrative	***Target response***
1. This is Kim. Who is this?	This is Kim.
2. This is Sue. Who is this?	This is Sue.
3. This is Mom. Who is this?	This is Mom.
4. Mom says, "Let's bake some cookies." What does she say?	Let's bake some cookies.
5. Kim and Sue want to help. They say, "Can we help bake some cookies?" What do Kim and Sue say?	Can we help bake some cookies?

6. Mom says, "O.K. Yes, you can help me." What does she say?	Yes, you can help me.
7. Mom gets out a big bowl. What does she get out?	Mom gets out a big bowl.
8. Next, Mom gets out a mixer, fork, spatula, and the cookie cutters. Mom says, "We will need all these things to make the cookies." What do they need to make the cookies?	They need a mixer, fork, spatula, and cookie cutters.
9. Can you think of anything else they need?	(elicit response)
10. First, Mom sifts flour. She pours and sifts flour. What does Mom do first?	She pours and sifts flour.
11. Next, Mom pours milk. She pours milk in the bowl. What does Mom do next?	She pours milk in the bowl.
12. They use milk and flour to make the cookies. What do they use?	They use milk and flour.
13. What else do they need to bake cookies? Can you guess?	They need eggs, sugar, and chocolate.
14. Mom says, "Now we can mix." Kim and Sue say, "We want to help mix." They say, "We want to help mix the cookies." What do they say?	We want to help mix the cookies.
15. Kim and Sue help mix the cookies. Who helps mix the cookies?	Kim and Sue help mix the cookies.
16. Mom says, "It's time to cut out the cookies. Let's cut out the cookies." What does Mom say?	It's time to cut out the cookies.
17. Kim says, "Let's use the animal cookie cutters. Let's use the cat, kangaroo, seal, and squirrel." What cookie cutters do they use?	They use the cat, kangaroo, seal, and squirrel.
18. It's time to bake the cookies. Sue puts the cookies in the stove. Where does Sue put the cookies?	Sue puts the cookies in the stove.
19. The stove is hot. Mom says, "Be careful, the stove is hot." What does Mom say?	Be careful, the stove is hot.
20. Kim and Sue have to wait for the cookies. They go outside to color a picture. Where do Kim and Sue go?	They go outside to color a picture.

21. It's later now. The cookies are finished baking. Mom takes the cookies out of the stove. She calls Kim and Sue from outside. What does Mom do?	She takes the cookies out of the stove. She calls Kim and Sue from outside.
22. Mom says, "First, the cookies must cool." What does Mom say?	First, the cookies must cool.
23. Mom says, "When the cookies are cool, we will spread the icing on." What does Mom say?	When the cookies are cool, we will spread the icing on.
24. Sue and Kim stay inside while the cookies cool. They cut out pictures and color. What do they do?	They cut out pictures and color.
25. When the cookies are cool, Mom calls Kim and Sue back to the kitchen. What does Mom do?	She calls Kim and Sue back to the kitchen.
26. "The cookies are cool now." Mom says, "It's time to make the icing. Let's make chocolate icing." What does Mom say?	The cookies are cool now. Let's make chocolate icing.
27. Sue and Kim help ice the cookies. They help ice the cookies. What do they do?	They help ice the cookies.
28. Now the cookies are all made. They are all made. Are the cookies made?	Yes, they are made.
29. Sue and Kim have made many cookies. The count the cookies they have made. They count sixty-six cookies. How many cookies do they count?	They count sixty-six cookies.
30. Sue and Kim are very happy. They are happy because they have so many cookies. Why are they happy?	They are happy because they have so many cookies.
31. Sue says, "We can take some cookies to school tomorrow. Let's take some cookies to school." What does she say?	Let's take some cookies to school.
32. Mom says, "O.K. You can take some cookies to school." She says, "You can take some to school." What does she say?	Yes, you can take some cookies to school.
33. Sue says, "Thank you, Mom." Kim says, "Thank you, Mom." What do they say?	They say, "Thank you, Mom."

THE CANOE TRIP

Suggested materials: Flannelboard, felt figures (boy, girl, canoe, lake, paddle, canteen, cave, bat)

Target sounds: /t/ and /k/

Narrative	***Target response***
1. Today's story is about some boys and girls at camp. Here is a boy and a girl. Their names are Tommy and Kathy. What are their names?	Their names are Tommy and Kathy.
2. They have been at camp for one week. They ride horses, go swimming in the pool, and make lots of pretty things in the craft shop. They make lots of pretty things in the craft shop. What do they make in the craft shop?	They make lots of pretty things in the craft shop.
3. Today they are doing something special. They are taking a canoe trip today. What are they doing today?	They are taking a canoe trip today.
4. Tommy says, "Come on Kathy. The other kids have already left. It's time to go. I put the canoe in the lake." What does Tommy say?	I put the canoe in the lake.
5. Kathy runs to the lake. She is ready to go now. Tommy says, "I don't have a map. Did you take the map from the picnic table?" What does Tommy ask?	Did you take the map from the picnic table?
6. Kathy says, "No, I didn't take it. But we won't need it. We won't get lost." What does Kathy say?	We won't get lost.
7. Tommy says, "O.K. Hop in. We're ready to go. Please sit down. Take the paddle and put it in the water." Where does Tommy say to put the paddle?	Take the paddle and put it in the water.
8. Tommy and Kathy are paddling as fast as they can. They want to catch up with the others. Tommy says, "I am thirsty. I want a drink. Please get the canteen from the cooler." What does Tommy say?	Please get the canteen from the cooler.
9. Kathy says, "I am thirsty, too. I would like a drink. What is in the canteen?	

Is it water or Kool Aid?" What does Kathy ask?	Is it water or Kool Aid?
10. Tommy says, "Here, taste it. It is Tiki Punch." What is it?	It is Tiki Punch.
11. Tommy and Kathy have been in the canoe for a long time. They are getting tired. Kathy says, "It is very pretty here. There are lots of trees on shore. Let's stop to take a hike." What does Kathy say?	Let's stop to take a hike.
12. Tommy says, "That's a good idea. We can put the canoe up on those rocks." What does Tommy say?	We can put the canoe up on those rocks.
13. Tommy and Kathy get out of the canoe. Kathy says, "It's so quiet here." Is it quiet here?	Yes, it's so quiet here.
14. Tommy and Kathy are walking down a tiny path. Suddenly, they stop. Up ahead they see a dark cave. What do they see ahead?	Up ahead they see a dark cave.
15. Tommy says, "Should we go inside? There might be a lot of pretty rocks." What might be inside?	There might be a lot of pretty rocks.
16. Tommy and Kathy go inside the cave. Kathy says, "It's so dark and scary. I want to go back." What does Kathy say?	It's so dark and scary. I want to go back.
17. Tommy says, "In a minute. I want to see a bit more." They creep into the cave a little bit more. What do they do?	They creep into the cave a little bit more.
18. All of a sudden, SWOOSH! What do you think it is?	(elicit response)
19. It is a big black bat! Tommy screams, "Yikes! A bat! Let's get back to the canoe!" What does Tommy say?	Let's get back to the canoe.
20. Tommy and Kathy saw a big black bat in the cave. What did they see in the cave?	They saw a big black bat in the cave.
21. Tommy and Kathy run to the canoe. Kathy says, "Let's get back to camp and tell the other kids!" What does Kathy say?	Let's get back to camp and tell the other kids.

22. Tommy says, "Wow! That was something! A big black bat! I hope the kids don't think we're pretending." What does Tommy say?	I hope the kids don't think we're pretending!
23. Do you think Tommy and Kathy are pretending?	(elicit response)

STEVE AND VICKY VISIT A CAVE

Suggested material: Flannelboard, felt figures (boy, girl, TV, cave, large stone, treasure box, frog)

Target sounds: /v/ and /s/

Narrative	***Target response***
1. Today we have a story about a boy named Steve. Here he is. This is Steve. Who is this?	This is Steve.
2. Steve has a friend who lives next door. Her name is Vicky. What is her name?	Her name is Vicky.
3. Steve wants to go see Vicky, so he knocks on the door. Steve says, "I have something to tell you." What does Steve say?	I have something to tell you.
4. Vicky is watching TV; she always watches TV. Yes, Vicky loves to watch TV. What does Vicky love?	Vicky loves to watch TV.
5. She opens the door and says, "Come on in and watch TV with me. This show is very funny." What does she say?	This show is very funny.
6. "No," says Steve. "We're going on a walk. I found something today and I want to show it to you." So, Steve and Vicky leave the house. What do Steve and Vicky do?	Steve and Vicky leave the house.
7. Vicky and Steve walk down the street. They walk farther and farther away from the house until they come to a scary, dark forest. Vicky is sort of scared. How does Vicky feel?	Vicky is sort of scared.
8. Steve finally stops walking and says, "Okay, Vicky, look over there." What does he say?	Look over there.

9. "Oh, my gosh! What a surprise!" Vicky can see a big cave. What can Vicky see?
   Vicky can see a big cave.
10. "All right," says Steve. "I hope you aren't afraid of going in. Let's go into the cave." What does Steve say?
   Let's go into the cave.
11. "I'm not afraid much," says Vicky. So they climb down the stones. Vicky and Steve climb down the stones. What do Vicky and Steve do?
   Vicky and Steve climb down the stones.
12. It got darker and darker in the cave. It got very hard to see where they were going. Vicky says, "I have to leave soon." What does Vicky say?
   I have to leave soon.
13. "Oh, come on," says Steve. "Don't be scared. Look! The surprise is under this stone." What does Steve say?
   The surprise is under this stone.
14. They soon get to a large stone. Vicky wonders what could be under it. Steve lifts up the stone. What does Steve do?
   Steve lifts up the stone.
15. "Here it is!" says Steve. Sure enough. There is something under the stone. Steve says, "I have a secret treasure box." What does Steve say?
   I have a secret treasure box.
16. "Wow," says Vicky. "What's in it?" Vicky wants to see it. What does Vicky want?
   Vicky wants to see it.
17. Steve slowly opens the box. Out comes a big frog. Vicky screams and starts to leave. What does she do?
   Vicky screams and starts to leave.
18. Vicky calls out, "What a mean trick to play on me! I'll never visit the cave again." What does she say?
   I'll never visit the cave again.
19. Steve just laughs and laughs. He knows Vicky isn't really mad. What does Steve do?
   Steve just laughs and laughs.
20. He hurries out of the cave and what do you think happens? Sure enough, Vicky is hiding by the entrance of the cave. Vicky yells "BOO" and frightens Steve. Vicky scares Steve. What does Vicky do?
   Vicky scares Steve.

21. They look at each other angrily, but then both of them start smiling. They went home together. They were smiling and very happy. What were they doing?	They were smiling and very happy.

Index